SMALL ANIMAL SURGERY SECRETS

taper — Monocryl 3-0,4-0

cuttingedge- Ethilon 3-0,4-0

SMALL ANIMAL SURGERY SECRETS

JOSEPH HARARI, DVM, MS, DACVS

Visiting Associate Professor
Department of Veterinary Clinical Medicine and Surgery
University of Illinois
College of Veterinary Medicine
Urbana, Illinois

HANLEY & BELFUS, INC./ Philadelphia

Publisher: HANLEY & BELFUS, INC.
              Medical Publishers
              210 South 13th Street
              Philadelphia, PA 19107
              (215) 546-7293; 800-962-1892
              FAX (215) 790-9330
              Web site: http://www.hanleyandbelfus.com

Note to the reader: Although the information in this book has been carefully reviewed for correctness of dosage and indications, neither the authors not the editor nor the publisher can accept any legal responsibility for any errors or omissions that may be made. Neither the publisher nor the editor makes any warranty, expressed or implied, with respect to the material contained herein. Before prescribing any drug, the reader must review the manufacturer's current product information (package inserts) for accepted indications, absolute dosage recommendations, and other information pertinent to the safe and effective use of the product described. This is especially important when drugs are given in combination or as an adjunct to other forms of therapy.

Library of Congress Cataloging-in-Publication Data

Small animal surgery secrets / edited by Joseph Harari.
      p. cm. — (The Secrets Series®)
   ISBN 1-56053-355-2 (alk. paper)
   1. Dogs—Surgery. 2. Cats—Surgery. 3. Veterinary surgery. I. Harari, Joseph.
II. Series.

   SF991.S5953 2000
   636′.0897—dc21

                                                  00-023119

SMALL ANIMAL SURGERY SECRETS   ISBN 1-56053-355-2

Last digit is the print number: 9 8 7 6 5 4 3 2 1

CONTENTS

Contents

CONTRIBUTORS

Kenneth E. Bartels, DVM, MS
McCasland Professor of Laser Surgery, Cohn Chair for Animal Care, Department of Veterinary Clinical Sciences, Oklahoma State University, College of Veterinary Medicine, Stillwater, Oklahoma

Trevor Bebchuk, DVM
Assistant Professor, Department of Veterinary Anesthesiology, Radiology, and Surgery, University of Saskatchewan, Western College of Veterinary Medicine, Saskatoon, Saskatchewan, Canada

Randy Boudrieau, DVM, DAVC
Professor of Surgery, Department of Clinical Sciences, Tufts University, School of Veterinary Medicine, North Grafton, Massachusetts

Elaine Caplan, DVM, DAVCS, DABVP
Assistant Professor of Surgery, Surgery Oncology Fellow, University of Illinois, College of Veterinary Medicine, Urbana, Illinois

Bradley R. Coolman, DVM, MS
Veterinary Surgical Services, Fort Wayne, Indiana

Curtis W. Dewey, DVM, MS, DACVIM (Neurology), DAVCS
Assistant Professor of Neurology and Neurosurgery, Department of Small Animal Medicine and Surgery, Texas A&M University, College of Veterinary Medicine, College Station, Texas

Dianne Dunning, DVM, MS, DACVS
Assistant Professor, Department of Companion Animal Surgery, Louisiana State University, School of Veterinary Medicine, Baton Rouge, Louisiana

Nicole Ehrhart, VMD, MS, DAVCS
Assistant Professor, Department of Veterinary Clinical Medicine, University of Illinois, College of Veterinary Medicine, Urbana, Illinois

Randall B. Fitch, DVM, MS, DACVS
Assistant Professor, Veterinary Teaching Hospital, Colorado State University, College of Veterinary Medicine, Fort Collins, Colorado

J. David Fowler, DVM, MVSc, DACVS
Professor, Department of Veterinary Anesthesiology, Radiology, and Surgery, University of Saskatchewan, Western College of Veterinary Medicine, Saskatoon, Saskatchewan, Canada

Lynetta Freeman, DVM, DACVS
Research Fellow, Department of Surgical Research and Development, Ethicon Endo-Surgery, Inc., Cincinnati, Ohio

Thomas Fry, DVM, MS, DACVS
Cascade Veterinary Specialists, Issaguah, Washington

Cathy Greenfield, DVM, MS, DACVS
Associate Professor, Soft Tissue and Oncologic Surgery, Department of Veterinary Clinical
Medicine, University of Illinois, College of Veterinary Medicine, Urbana, Illinois

Joseph Harari, DVM, MS, DACVS
Visiting Associate Professor, Department of Veterinary Clinical Medicine, University of Illinois College of Medicine, Urbana, Illinois

Robin H. Holtsinger, DVM
South Florida Veterinary Surgical Services, Inc., Fort Lauderdale, Florida

Giselle Hosgood, BVSc, MS, FACVSc, DACVS
Professor, Small Animal Surgery, Department of Veterinary Clinical Sciences, Louisiana State
University, School of Veterinary Medicine, Baton Rouge, Louisiana

Ann L. Johnson, DVM, MS, DACVS
Professor, Department of Veterinary Clinical Medicine, University of Illinois, College of Veterinary Medicine, Urbana, Illinois

Spencer A. Johnston, VMD, DACVS
Associate Professor, Department of Small Animal Clinical Sciences, Virginia Tech and University
of Maryland, Virginia-Maryland Regional College of Veterinary Medicine, Blacksburg, Virginia

Lisa Klopp, DVM, DACVIM (Neurology)
Surgical Referral Service, Fort Atkinson, Wisconsin

Elizabeth J. Laing, DVM, MS, DACVS
Surgical Referral Service, Fort Atkinson, Wisconsin

Leigh A. Lamont, DVM
Resident in Anesthesiology, Department of Veterinary Clinical Medicine, University of Illinois,
College of Veterinary Medicine, Urbana, Illinois

Otto I. Lanz, DVM, DACVS
Assistant Professor, Department of Small Animal Clinical Sciences, Virginia Tech and University
of Maryland, Virginia-Maryland Regional College of Veterinary Medicine, Blacksburg, Virginia

Andrea L. Looney, DVM
Staff Anesthesiologist, Intensive Care Unit, MSPCA/Western New England Animal Center,
Rowley Memorial Hospital, Springfield, Massachusetts

Douglas M. MacCoy, BS, DVM, DACVS
Veterinary Surgical Associates Inc., Coral Springs, Florida

Sandra Manfra Marretta, DVM, DACVS, DAVDC
Associate Professor, Small Animal Surgery and Dentistry, Department of Veterinary Clinical
Medicine, University of Illinois, College of Veterinary Medicine, Urbana, Illinois

Steven L. Marks, BVSc, MS, MRCVS, DACVIM
Assistant Professor of Internal Medicine, Department of Veterinary Clinical Sciences,
Louisiana State University, School of Veterinary Medicine, Baton Rouge, Louisiana

Timothy McCarthy, DVM, PhD, DACVS
Surgical Specialty Clinic for Animals, Beaverton, Oregon

Sheila McCullough, DVM, MS, DACVIM
Clinical Assistant Professor, Small Animal Medicine and Intensive Care Service, University of Illinois, College of Veterinary Medicine, Urbana, Illinois

Lin McGonagle, MSPT, BS, LVT
Physical Therapist and Veterinary Technician, Genoa, New York

Ronald M. McLauglin, Jr., DVM, DVSc, DACVS
Associate Professor, Department of Small Animal Surgery, Animal Health Center, Mississippi State University, College of Veterinary Medicine, Mississippi State, Mississippi

Holly Sumner Mullen, DVM, DACVS
Chief of Surgery, Emergency Animal Hospital and Referral Center, California Veterinary Surgical Practice, San Diego, California

Marie-Eve Nadeau, DVM, MS
Teaching Associate, Department of Veterinary Clinical Medicine, University of Illinois, College of Veterinary Medicine, Urbana, Illinois

Dennis Olsen, DVM, MS, DACVS
Assistant Professor, Small Animal Surgery, Department of Clinical Sciences, Kansas State University, College of Veterinary Medicine, Manhattan, Kansas

Sheldon Padgett, DVM, MS, DACVS
Metropolitan Veterinary Hospital, Akron, Ohio

Mary K. Quinn, DVM
Resident, Small Animal Surgery, University of Illinois, College of Veterinary Medicine, Urbana, Illinois

Robert M. Radasch, DVM, MS, DAVCS
Senior Surgeon, Dallas Veterinary Surgical Center, Dallas, Texas

MaryAnn Radlinsky, DVM, MS, DACVS
Assistant Professor, Department of Clinical Sciences, Kansas State University, College of Veterinary Medicine, Manhattan, Kansas

Kristi M. Sandman, DVM
Resident/Teaching Associate, Department of Veterinary Clinical Medicine and Surgery, University of Illinois, College of Veterinary Medicine, Urbana, Illinois

Bernard Seguin, DVM, MS, DACVS
Fellow, Surgical Oncology, The Comparative Oncology Unit, Colorado State University, College of Veterinary Medicine, Fort Collins, Colorado

John T. Silbernagel, DVM
Teaching Associate, Department of Veterinary Clinical Medicine, University of Illinois, College of Veterinary Medicine, Urbana, Illinois

Charles William Smith, DVM, MS, DACVS
Professor and Head, Small Animal Surgery, Department of Veterinary Clinical Medicine, University of Illinois, College of Veterinary Medicine, Urbana, Illinois

Steven F. Swaim, DVM, MS
Professor, Scott-Ritchey Research Center and Department of Small Animal Surgery and Medicine, Auburn University, College of Veterinary Medicine, Auburn University, Alabama

D. Michael Tillson, DVM, MS, DACVS
Assistant Professor, Department of Small Animal Surgery and Medicine, Auburn University, College of Veterinary Medicine, Auburn University, Alabama

PREFACE

Small Animal Surgery Secrets follows the paradigm of the immensely popular human text, *Abernathy's Surgical Secrets,* in providing students, house officers, practitioners (and yes, even specialists) with pertinent perioperative information in a highly readable form. Practical surgical topics were selected to enhance the reader's knowledge base as an aid for clinical rounds, examinations, and case management. The text begins with general concepts of surgery, followed by sections devoted to soft tissue, orthopedic, neurologic, oncologic, and dental operations. The final chapters contain information on the field of veterinary surgery as a specialty. The format of relevant (and sometimes irreverent) questions and answers, plus recommended readings, will hopefully stimulate novice and experienced surgeons and provoke discussions on the clinic floor.

A broad group of contributors from around the country in academic, private, and industrial practice were asked to prepare salient features of surgery-related conditions based on their experience and expertise. The author' breadth in backgrounds provides a healthy, diverse approach to a traditional clinical sciences discipline. I'm sure readers will appreciate that many of the described "pearls of wisdom" are based on clinical successes as well as failures.

I am indebted to Bill Lamsback of Hanley & Belfus, who saved this book for me as I bounced between the East and West Coasts and then landed in the Midwest. My colleagues and the administration at the University of Illinois are gratefully acknowledged for permitting me the time to complete this project; our Word Processing Center deserves credit for transforming reams of handwritten pages into an organized text. Lastly, I thank the numerous contributors who were willing to share professional secrets with their colleagues.

Joseph Harari, DVM, MS, DACVS

I. General Concepts

1. WOUND HEALING

Joseph Harari, M.S., D.V.M., Dip. A.C.V.S.

1. Why should surgeons need an understanding of wound healing?
The cornerstone of surgery is the restoration of function. Recovery of organ or limb function is based on cells and tissues regaining biologic integrity by healing from wounds created naturally or iatrogenically.

2. What is a wound?
Disruption of normal anatomic continuity and metabolic functions of body structures, including organs, tissues, and cells.

3. List common causes of wounds.
- Surgery
- Trauma (vehicular, firearm, fights)
- Neoplasia
- Topical medications
- Infection
- Chemicals
- Excessive temperatures
- Irradiation

4. What is wound healing?
The physiologic restoration of organ structure and function. It is characterized by cellular and biochemical processes occurring in an organized and sequential pattern lasting from days to months to years.

5. How do wounds heal?
1. After **wounding, inflammation** occurs within minutes and lasts for 1–3 days. This is also called the **lag** or **substrate** phase and is characterized by vasoconstriction followed by vasodilation and vascular fluid leakage secondary to release of chemical mediators (histamine, serotonin, prostaglandins) by mast cells and platelets. Neutrophils and monocytes migrate into the wound for phagocytosis and enzymatic destruction of foreign and host cellular debris. *In situ* macrophages release chemotactic substances to stimulate fibroplasia, angiogenesis, and collagen synthesis.
2. Between days 3 and 21, the **repair** or **proliferative** phase occurs. It is characterized by fibroblastic proliferation, capillary infiltration, and reepithelialization. Fibroblasts produce an amorphous ground substance and collagen, which is responsible for wound tensile strength. Vascular invasion supplies oxygenation and nutrition, whereas epithelial proliferation provides surface coverage of the wound.
3. After the repair phase, and lasting months to years, is the **maturation** or **remodeling** phase. It is characterized by increased cross-linking of collagen fibers, development of a basketweave arrangement of the fibers, and deposition of the fibers along lines of stress.
4. The final phase of healing is **contraction,** which is characterized by a concentric decrease of tissue area as a result of myofibroblasts. These cells contain actin, a contractile protein found in muscle cells. They undergo cellular contraction, which results in a rearrangement and reduction of the surrounding tissue matrix.

6. What is the basis for wound strength?
Collagen is the major structural protein of connective tissue. In wounds, the initial type III is replaced by type I in the maturation phase. The strength of wound tissue approximates (80%) but

never equals that of normal tissue and is related to cross-linking of collagen fibers, not continued deposition.

7. What marker is used to assess wound strength?
Hydroxyproline is assayed as an indicator of collagen content in the wound. The maximum rate of increasing wound strength occurs between days 5 and 12 postwounding.

8. Describe the categories of wound healing.
- **First intention** or **primary wound closure** is apposition of tissues by sutures, staples, tapes, or adhesives.
- **Second intention** or **secondary wound** closure occurs when large cutaneous wounds are allowed to close by granulation, epithelialization, and contraction without the use of sutures, staples, and so forth.
- **Third intention** wound healing is surgical closure of a granulating (second intention) wound after excision of granulation tissue or freshening of epithelial margins. These wounds heal more rapidly than primary wound closures because the inflammatory and proliferative phases of healing have already occurred.

9. What is granulation tissue?
A mixture of capillaries, lymph vessels, fibroblasts, macrophages, amorphous matrix, collagen, and elastin fibers developing within 1 week after injury. Its gross appearance (red and granular) is based on reforming capillary buds and loops. It provides a barrier to infection, a bed for epithelialization, and a cellular source for wound contraction and support.

10. Which cells are most important in influencing neovascularization, granulation tissue formation, and epithelial migration in healing wounds?
Macrophages—by their secretion of various growth factors, chemoattractants, and proteolytic enzymes.

11. Which growth factors are important in wound healing?
- Platelet-derived growth factors (initiate cellular division)
- Transforming growth factors (increase collagen synthesis)
- Epidermal growth factor
- Fibroblast and insulin-like growth factors—secreted by platelets, macrophages, and fibroblasts

12. Which factors affect wound healing?
Local
- **Vascularity** provides oxygenation and delivery of nutrients to cells and tissues.
- **Foreign material** can delay healing by exacerbating inflammation and promoting infection.
- **Dead space and fluid accumulation** inhibit cellular migration and increase risk of infection.
- **Irradiation** within 2 weeks of surgery decreases fibroblast formation, collagen synthesis, and capillary regeneration.
- **Bacterial infection** impedes healing because of persistent inflammation, tissue necrosis, and accumulation of fluids.
- **Lavage solutions** (lactated Ringer's, saline, 0.05% chlorhexidine, 0.1% povidone-iodine) can promote healing by reducing contamination.
- **Nonadherent dressings** promote epithelialization, whereas **adherent gauze dressings** mechanically débride contaminated wounds.
- **Surgical technique** promotes healing if Halsted's principles are followed.

Systemic

- **Hypoproteinemia** may delay fibroplasia, decrease wound strength, and produce edema.
- **Uremia** depresses granulation, epithelialization, and wound strength.
- Long-term, high doses of **corticosteroids** inhibit the inflammatory phase and decrease collagen synthesis.
- **Chemotherapeutic** agents inhibit the repair (cellular division) and maturation (collagen synthesis) phases.
- **Advanced** age slows cellular reparative functions.
- **Distant malignancy** may impair healing by producing cachexia, altering metabolism, and reducing inflammatory cell functions.
- **Uncontrolled diabetes** and hyperglycemia impair collagen synthesis, vascular ingrowth, and granulocyte cell functions.

13. Which factors affecting wound healing can be directly controlled by the surgeon?
Proper surgical technique by adherence to **Halsted's principles:**
- Gentle tissue handling
- Preservation of vascularity
- Surgical asepsis
- Approximation of tissues
- Obliteration of dead space
- Removal of necrotic tissue

14. Who was Halsted?
A Baltimore surgeon (1852–1922) whose name is currently associated with surgical instruments, sutures, and operations. He is considered by many to be the father of human surgical science in the United States based on the training program he established (following the example of the European schools) for surgeons at The Johns Hopkins Hospital.

15. What treatment can be used to stimulate wound healing by enhancing cellular proliferation, DNA and collagen synthesis?
Photoirradiation with low-intensity laser light.

16. What is a seroma?
A subcutaneous accumulation or pocket of protein-enriched serum in a closed wound. It serves as an excellent medium for bacterial growth and is isolated from cellular immune responses. It usually develops as a surgical failure in technique (see Halsted's principles).

17. What are characteristics of intestinal healing?
Wounds of the small intestine heal more predictably and with fewer complications than the large intestine as a result of a better vascular supply, more developed muscular layer, liquid state of contents, smaller bacterial content, and reduced tissue collagenolytic activity.

18. What is wound dehiscence?
Partial or total disruption of the operative wound layers.

19. What is evisceration?
Protrusion of viscera through a wound.

20. What is eventration?
Protrusion of the bowels through the abdominal wall.

21. What factors are associated with wound dehiscence?
- Local and systemic factors affecting wound healing (see earlier)

- Increased abdominal pressure
- Surgical technique and adequacy (suture selection, placement, knot tying) of closure

22. When does dehiscence usually occur?
Usually 3–5 days after surgery before collagen synthesis increases wound tensile strength.

23. What are the signs of wound dehiscence?
- Incisional swelling
- Pain
- Discoloration
- Tissue necrosis
- Serosanguineous discharge

24. Describe the treatments for dehiscence.
Treatments are directly related to the severity of the lesion:
- **Primary** wound closure can be performed if the injury is minor; the wound is not infected; and tissue closure is necessary to protect body cavities, joints, implants, or pressure points.
- **Second intention** healing can be permitted in cases not requiring tissue apposition.
- **Third intention** closure is performed with large defects near pressure points or to avoid subsequent excessive tissue contraction.

Evisceration or eventration require surgical intervention after immediate coverage of the wounds with moistened towels. Therapeutic antibiotics (cephalosporins, clindamycin, enrofloxacin, amoxicillin/clavulanate) are necessary in these patients. Management of wound dehiscences includes lavage, sterile dressings, and drainage.

25. What are the characteristics of bone healing?
Bone healing results from a continuum of interactions and overlapping phases; sharp demarcations or stages do not occur because of variances in lesions and repairs. Initially the fracture site is a milieu of blood clots and devitalized osseous and soft tissue structures. Within 3–4 days, a soft **fibrocartilaginous callus** forms as a collar in and around the bone to serve as an internal splint. With poor vascularity, reduced oxygenation, and reduced motion, fibrous tissue develops during the next several months. With abundant vascularity, increased oxygenation, and limited motion, endochondral ossification predominates, and a **hard callus** is formed. After bone bridging and osseous union, remodeling of the endosteal and peritoneal surfaces occurs as bone is resorbed or produced based on natural stresses and strains. These osseous changes shape the bone during the ensuing months to years.

Primary bone union is via direct osteonal healing with a small gap or end-to-end bone contact and is associated with rigid implants such as plates and screws. **Secondary bone healing** is characterized by development of a fracture callus and is associated with nonrigid implants (pins, wires).

26. What is Wolff's law?
Published in 1892, it states, "form follows function or bone develops as a structure most suited to resist the forces acting on it." This adaptive characteristic refers primarily to the cancellous trabeculae of bone and not just the cortex.

27. What are causes of abnormal bone healing?
Abnormal bone healing can be slowed (**delayed union**), nonexistent (**nonunion**), or inappropriate (**malunion**) and is associated with
- Inadequate fracture stabilization
- Decreased osteogenesis
- Impaired vascularity
- Infection

28. What are treatment options for abnormal bone healing?
Treatments are based on underlying causes and include:
- Replacement of implants
- Rigid stabilization
- Cancellous grafting
- Débridement
- Antibiotic therapy
- Bone loading by reduction of stabilizing devices

29. How does cartilage heal after injury?
In response to superficial lesions, chondrocytes proliferate and synthesize the proteoglycans and collagen of the intercellular matrix. Avascularity of cartilage limits repair, and structural defects often persist. Deep lacerations breach the subchondral bone to produce an inflammatory response, including pluripotential cells, and subsequent filling of the defect with fibrocartilage.

30. List treatment options for damaged cartilage.
- Resection of the damaged cartilage and underlying bone
- Restoration via fibrocartilage secondary to drilling or curettage of subchondral bone
- Replacement with a prosthetic device
- Arthrodesis of the joint
- Medical therapy with joint fluid modifiers (glycosaminoglycans, sodium hyaluronate) and anti-inflammatory medications (aspirin, glucocorticosteroids, carprofen, etodolac)

31. How do tendons or ligaments heal after a crush injury?
Defects heal after a sequence characterized by hematoma formation and organization, inflammatory cellular migration, matrix and cellular (fibroblasts) proliferation, and scar tissue formation. Collagen reorientation occurs through the scar and based on remodeling forces. The mechanical derangement of the tissue takes 3–4 months to subside, but the material properties of the healed tissue never equal those of an intact tendon or ligament.

32. To what does the term *one wound—one scar* refer?
After tendon injury, the amalgam of fluid, severed tissues, injured fat, and possibly bone or cartilage develops into a single viscous gel that permeates the wound. Each structure in the wound is interconnected during one phase of scar evolution.

33. What are key issues of muscle repair?
Muscle cells do not regrow by mitosis and development of new cells and tissue; old myofibrils can regenerate if not strangled by extensive fibrous tissue. Careful excision of an old scar during secondary repair may offer the best chance for maximal muscle regeneration and minimal recurrence of fibrosis. Primary repair is best performed early after injury before fibrous protein synthesis; this would be indicated for extensive, palpable gaps in the injured muscle.

CONTROVERSIES

34. Does intestinal surgery in hypoproteinemic patients result in dehiscence?
No. Intestinal biopsies of hypoalbuminemic dogs yielded uncomplicated healing during a 7-day postoperative period.

35. Do older animals heal more slowly than younger animals?
In healthy human beings, elderly volunteers had decreased epithelialization rates (2 days) and similar collagen synthesis as younger subjects after experimentally created thigh and catheter wounds.

36. Do patients receiving antineoplastic therapy develop nonhealing surgical wounds?

A definitive answer is impossible because of variable conclusions derived from a paucity of controlled clinical studies and a plethora of uncontrolled clinical studies and experimental models. In people, a combination of clinical determinants (e.g., age, concurrent disease, type of surgery, hypertension, uremia) rather than individual factors is thought to be helpful in predicting wound dehiscence.

BIBLIOGRAPHY

1. Cohen IK, Diegelmann RF, Lindblad WJ: Wound Healing, 1st ed. Philadelphia, W.B. Saunders, 1992, pp 20–129, 344–395.
2. Fowler D: Principles of wound healing. In Harari J (ed): Surgical Complications and Wound Healing, 1st ed. Philadelphia, W.B. Saunders, 1993.
3. Laing L: Effect of antineoplastic agents on wound healing. Comp Cont Educ Pract Vet 11:136–142, 1989.
4. Lucroy MD, Edwards BF: Low-intensity laser light-induced closure of a chronic wound in a dog. Vet Surg 28:292–295, 1999.
5. O'Driscoll SW: The healing and regeneration of articular cartilage. J Bone Joint Surg Am 80:1795–1805, 1998.
6. Riou JPA, Cohen JR, Johnson H: Factors influencing wound dehiscence. Am J Surg 163:324–330, 1992.
7. Swaim JF, Henderson RA: Small Animal Wound Management, 2nd ed. Baltimore, Williams & Wilkins, 1997, pp 1–12.
8. Woo SLY, Buckwalter JA: Injury and Repair of Musculoskeletal Soft Tissues, 1st ed. Park Ridge, IL, American Academy of Orthopedic Surgeons, 1988.

2. CONTROL OF INFECTION

Joseph Harari, M.S., D.V.M., Dip. A.C.V.S.

1. Define surgical wound infection.

In 1992, the Surgical Wound Infection Task Force established definitions of surgical site infections to reduce miscommunication in the medical and surgical communities. The term **surgical wound** was replaced by **surgical site** to include infections after surgery in organ spaces, such as bone and peritoneum, deep to the skin and soft tissues.

- **Superficial incisional surgical site infection**—purulence from superficial incision, microbial isolation, and local signs of inflammation.
- **Deep incisional surgical site infection**—purulence from deep incision, dehiscence, fever, local signs of inflammation, and deep abscessation.
- **Organ/space surgical site infection**—purulence from drain placed into organ/space, microbial isolation, and organ abscessation.

2. Historically, what other classification scheme has been used to predict probability of infection based on intraoperative contamination?

In 1964, the National Research Council, *Ad Hoc* Committee on trauma established the following categories of wounds:

- **Clean**—elective procedure; primary closure; no break in aseptic technique; no entrance into alimentary, respiratory, or urogenital tracts.
- **Clean-contaminated**—nonelective procedure, controlled opening of normally colonized body cavity, minimal break in asepsis, reoperative through clean incision.
- **Contaminated**—major break in asepsis, penetrating trauma < 4 hours old, chronic open wound, acute nonpurulent inflammation.

- **Dirty**—purulence, drainage, penetrating wounds > 4 hours old, rupture of colonized body viscera.

3. What rates of infection have been published for the wound categories?

Examples in Human Medicine

	CLEAN (%)	CLEAN-CONTAMINATED (%)	CONTAMINATED (%)	DIRTY (%)
Canada (1980)	1.5	7.7	15.2	40
Vermont (1986)	1.5	3.1	8.2	11.7
United States (1991)	2.1	3.3	6.4	7.1

Examples in Veterinary Medicine*

	CLEAN (%)	CLEAN-CONTAMINATED (%)	CONTAMINATED (%)	DIRTY (%)
California (1988)	2.5	4.5	5.8	18.1
Pennsylvania (1997)	4.7	5.0	12.0	10.1

*Wound infection based on purulent discharge within 14 days after surgery, dehiscence, or local signs of inflammation.

4. List the classic signs of inflammation.
- Redness (rubor)
- Swelling (tumor)
- Pain (dolor)
- Heat (calor)
- Loss of function (functio laesa)

5. Is wound contamination synonymous with wound infection?
No. **Contamination** describes microorganisms transiently present on tissue surfaces without invasion or physiologic response. **Infection** means multiplication of microbes within tissues and as subsequent host response.

6. What is the difference between disinfection and antisepsis?
An **antiseptic** is a chemical agent applied to a body surface to kill or inhibit growth of pathogenic microorganisms. A **disinfectant** is a chemical agent used to kill microorganisms on inanimate objects.

7. What is the difference between asepsis and sterilization?
Asepsis refers to the maintenance of a pathogen-free environment in biologic tissues. **Sterilization** is the complete elimination of all microorganisms from living or inanimate tissues.

8. List sources of wound infections.
- Type of wound
- Patient
- Operative procedure
- Hospital

9. Which wound factors can influence infection?
The degree of contamination, viability, and vascularity of tissues. Vascular perfusion is critical for delivery of oxygen and cellular elements necessary for metabolism, débridement, and repair in wounds.

10. Which human patient factors affect wound infection rates?

FACTOR	EFFECT
Increasing age	May be a modest risk factor
Preexisting illness	Increased ASA scores associated with increased infections
Diabetes	May be a significant factor not completely understood
Obesity	Weakly associated with certain incisions (sternotomies)
Preoperative hospitalization	Unproven association
Body site operation	Unclear association
Malignancy	Is not an independent risk factor for sepsis
Remote site infections	Catheterizations may be a concern
Malnutrition	Uncertain relationship to wound infection

ASA = American Society of Anesthesiologists.

11. Which operative factors affect wound infection?

FACTOR	EFFECT
Duration of surgery	Increasing length (>75th percentile) is a considerable risk for infection
Glove punctures	No effect
Emergency procedures	Higher rates but not statistically valid
Early morning (midnight to 8 am) surgeries	Higher rates but not statistically valid
Summer months surgeries	Higher rates but unknown significance
Airborne contamination	Conflicting data
Preoperative hair removal	Increased infection rates unless done just before surgery
Adhesive drapes	Conflicting data
Topical wound irrigation	Questionable effect
Antibiotics	Prophylaxis or therapeutic

12. Which risk factors for wound infection have been identified in veterinary patients?

HIGH RISK	LOW RISK
Surgery sites clipped before induction	Surgery sites clipped after induction
Operative procedures >90 minutes	Operative procedures <60 minutes
Animals with clean wounds receiving antibiotics >2 hours before or >24 hours after surgery	Animals with clean wounds receiving perioperative antibiotics just before and not after (>24 hours) surgery

13. Which anesthetic agent has been implicated with increased postoperative wound infections?

Propofol; the lipid-based emulsion supports rapid microbial growth secondary to external contamination.

14. What is the relationship between antibiotics, surgery, and wound infections?

As stated by Wangensteen, "Antibiotics may turn a third-class surgeon into a second-class surgeon, but never turn a second-class surgeon into a first-class surgeon." Timing is everything. Antibiotics are given in a **prophylactic** manner to prevent bacterial infection or with **therapeutic** protocols to treat an existing infection.

15. When should antibiotic prophylaxis be instituted?

Intravenous administration should be performed just **before surgery** and repeated during the operative procedure, based on the elimination half-life, to maintain levels above the minimum inhibitory concentration at the wound site. Antibiotic prophylaxis is recommended for clean procedures in which infection would be disastrous (bone implants, prosthesis, neurosurgery or cardiopulmonary surgery) or clean-contaminated wounds.

16. Which drug is most frequently used for antibiotic prophylaxis?
Cefazolin, given at 20–22 mg/kg intravenously and repeated every 90–120 minutes during surgery.

17. When are therapeutic antibiotics administered?
In contaminated or dirty wounds with existing infection, antimicrobial drugs may be given orally or parenterally based on the severity of the wound and overall patient health. Selection may be based on tissue or fluid microbiologic culture and antibiotic sensitivity testing, Gram or Wright-Giemsa staining, or be empiric based on previously known pathogens. Duration of treatment is variable (1–3 weeks) and determined by location of lesion (deep versus superficial) and signs of infection.

18. Which parameters are useful in evaluating the presence of infection?
- Clinical signs (fever depression, inappetence, limb or organ dysfunction)
- Laboratory data (leukocytosis, degenerative left shift, anemia, elevated fibrinogen, positive cultures)
- Imaging studies (bone lysis, abscessation, implant failures, increased fluid density)

19. List bacteria most often associated with surgical infections.
- *Staphylococcus intermedius* (coagulase positive)
- *Escherichia coli*
- *Pasteurella multocida*
- *Pseudomonas aeruginosa*
- β-hemolytic *Streptococcus*
- *Bacteroides* (anaerobe)
- *Klebsiella*

20. What are some useful antibiotics and their spectrum of activity for treating surgical wound infections?
- Cefazolin/cephaloxin (*Staphylococcus, Streptococcus, E. coli*)
- Amoxicillin/clavulanate (*Staphylococcus, Streptococcus, Bacteroides*)
- Enrofloxacin (*Pasteurella, Pseudomonas, Klebsiella, E. coli*)
- Clindamycin (*Staphylococcus, Streptococcus*)
- Metronidazole (*Bacteroides*)

21. What issues need to be identified with antibiotic prophylaxis or therapy?
- Likelihood of bacterial infection
- Untoward effects of the drugs in debilitated patients (i.e., metabolism and elimination)
- Development of microbial resistance
- Costs to owners

22. What are causes of antibiotic treatment failures?
- Inappropriate antibiotic selection
- Dosing errors
- Lack of delivery to affected site
- Bacterial resistance
- Polymicrobial infection
- Implant-associated conditions
- Misdiagnosis (noninfectious causes)

23. What are nosocomial infections?
Wound infections, not present or nonincubating at the time of hospital admission, that develop during hospitalization.

24. List common associations of nosocomial infections.
- Breaks in aseptic or disinfecting techniques
- Prolonged hospitalization
- Recumbency
- Catheters
- Direct contamination of wounds and bandages
- Excessive use (or misuse) of antibiotics
- Unclean hospital (wards, surgery, intensive care unit) environment

25. Which surgical preparation protocols have been found useful in operative patients?
One-step, sealed kits containing 0.5% available iodine and isopropyl alcohol, povidone-iodine, or 4% chlorhexidine gluconate rinsed with saline or isopropyl alcohol. Chloroxylenol (3%) is less effective than chlorhexidine in immediate antimicrobial activity but is associated with similar low wound infection rates.

26. Which lavage solutions are useful in reducing bacterial contamination or infection?
Chlorhexidine diacetate solutions (0.05%) have been associated with less bacterial contamination than povidone-iodine (0.1%) or saline. High volumes (500–1000 ml) can be delivered via pulsatile jet lavage, with a 19-gauge needle and 35-ml (8 psi) syringe or gravity flow. *In vitro* studies with fibroblasts reveal cytotoxic effects of normal saline and tap water compared with lactated Ringer's or phosphate-buffered saline.

27. What is the *golden period?*
4–6 hours after injury; a contaminated wound may be cleaned and primarily closed without the likelihood of infection developing. This assumes bacterial counts $<10^{5-6}$ per gram of tissue and normal host or tissue defense factors.

28. What is the relationship between sutures and infected wounds?
Multifilament, nonabsorbable sutures potentiate infection as a result of bacterial replication within the interstices of the material. Chromic catgut potentiates infection and has unpredictable absorption in infected (inflamed) tissues. Prolonged-degrading, absorbable sutures or inert, monofilament sutures are preferred in infected wounds. In general, if infected wounds are sutured, tension and large-gauge sutures and needles are avoided.

29. What parameters are used for sterilization of instruments and packs?
Although affected by pack size and content, gravity-displaced steam sterilization is performed for 10–20 minutes at 120–135°C (250–275°F). Prevacuumed sterilization is usually performed for 4 minutes at 135°C. Flash, emergency sterilization of unwrapped material is performed for 4 minutes at 135°C in a gravity-displaced autoclave. Steam sterilization causes microbial death by denaturation of cellular proteins.

30. What is ethylene oxide?
A flammable, carcinogenic gas mixture used to sterilize equipment not able to withstand steam sterilization. It destroys microbes and spores by alkylation; general guidelines include 40% humidity and 55°C (131°F) temperature for 4 hours poststerilization aeration to allow diffusion of ethylene oxide from the packs.

31. Discuss the physicians noted for their pioneering work in wound infection control.
Ignaz Semmelweis, a Hungarian surgeon, reduced puerperal sepsis by initiating handwash-

ing protocols (Vienna, 1847–1849) with hypochlorite solutions. **Joseph Lister,** in England, followed Pasteur's germ theory and developed aseptic surgical techniques (1870) using carbolic acid as a disinfectant. **John Burke** published the first conclusive data (1961) on the timing of chemoprophylaxis for dermal wounds. **Peter Cruse** (1973) and **Rosemary Ford** (1980) in Alberta, Canada, published the earliest and largest prospective studies of wound infection rates.

32. How are open, contaminated fractures classified?
   Based on the severity of the injury:
   • **Grade I**—small, external puncture wound caused by underlying bone penetration
   • **Grade II**—external wound apparent and contiguous with the fracture, moderate tissue damage
   • **Grade III**—extensive damage and loss of soft tissues and bone (high-energy wound)

33. Which factors influence infection rates in humans with open fracture wounds?

Increased Risk	No Effect
• No antibiotic treatment	• Length of antibiotic treatment
• Antimicrobial resistance	• Time between injury and surgical débridement
• Increased time from injury to antibiotic treatment	• Type of wound closure (partial or delayed)
• Extent of soft tissue damage	

CONTROVERSY

34. Are bacterial cultures and antibiotic sensitivity assays useful in the management of open contaminated wounds and fractures?
   Nearly 50% of cultures obtained at the beginning and end of fracture repair surgery yielded bacterial growth; postoperative complications were more common in dogs and cats with positive cultures than in animals with negative assays (Ohio, 1986). In 20 dogs with gunshot fractures, 19 had negative single intraoperative cultures; 3 of these dogs developed osteomyelitis (Virginia, 1995). In human patients with infections, predébridement and postdébridement cultures were rarely predictive with each other or subsequent disease (California, 1997). In all of these studies, questions abound regarding sampling techniques, effect of perioperative antibiotics, wound débridement and lavage, and a variable wound microbial population. With clean or elective orthopedic procedures, intraoperative bacterial isolation was not predictive for development of infection (Illinois, 1999).

BIBLIOGRAPHY

1. Brown DC, Conzemius MG: Epidemiologic evaluation of postoperative wound infections in dogs and cats. J Am Vet Med Assoc 210:1302–1306, 1997.
2. Culver SH, Horan TC: Surgical wound infection rates by wound class, operative procedure, and patient risk index. Ame J Med 91(3B):152S–163S, 1991.
3. Harari J: Surgical Complications and Wound Healing, 1st ed. Philadelphia, W.B. Saunders, 1993, pp 33–88, 279–306.
4. Heldmann E, Brown CD: The association of propofol usage with postoperative wound infection rate in clean wounds. Vet Surg 28:256–259, 1999.
5. Hirsh DC, Jang SS: Antimicrobial susceptibility of selected infectious bacterial agents from dogs. J Am Anim Hosp Assoc 30:487–494, 1994.
6. Leaper DJ: Prophylactic and therapeutic role of antibiotics in wound care. Am J Surg 167:155–185, 1994.
7. Lee J: Efficacy of cultures in the management of open fractures. Clin Orthol 339:71–75, 1997.
8. Page CP, Bohnan JEMA: Antimicrobial prophylaxis for surgical wounds. Arch Surg 128:79–88, 1993.
9. Patzakis MJ, Wilkins J: Factors influencing infection rate in open fracture wounds. Clin Orthol 243:36–40, 1989.
10. Sawyer RG, Pruett TL: Wound infections. Surg Clin North Amer 74:519–536, 1994.
11. Stevenson S, Olmstead ML: Bacterial culturing for prediction of postoperative complications following open fracture repair in small animals. Vet Surg 15:99–102, 1986.

12. Stubbs WP, Bellah JR: Chlorhexidine gluconate versus chloroxylenol for preoperative skin preparation in dogs. Vet Surg 25:587–494, 1996.
13. Vasseur PB, Levy J: Surgical wound infection rates in dogs and cats. Vet Surg 17:60–64, 1988.
14. Whittem T, Gaon D: Principles of antimicrobial therapy. Vet Clin North Am Sm Anim Pract 28:197–214, 1998.
15. Whittem T, Johnson AL: Effect of perioperative prophylactic antimicrobial treatment in dogs undergoing elective orthopedic surgery. J Am Vet Med Assoc 215:212–221, 1999.

3. SHOCK

Steven L. Marks, BVSc, M.S., M.R.C.V.S., Dip. A.C.V.I.M.

1. What is shock?
Loss of effective circulating blood volume leading to poor tissue perfusion and inadequate oxygen delivery. This leads to an imbalance between tissue oxygen demands and oxygen supply. Ultimately, cellular hypoxia will result in cell death and multiple organ dysfunction syndrome.

2. List the different types of shock based on pathophysiology.
• Hypovolemic
• Distributive
• Cardiogenic
• Occlusive

3. Describe each of the listed categories of shock and provide a clinical example of each.
Hypovolemic shock: Loss of volume due to vomiting, diarrhea, diuresis, third-space effusions, or hemorrhage. Traumatic hemorrhage would be an example of hypovolemic shock.
Distributive shock: Vasogenic shock due to an inappropriate distribution of blood flow. Examples include anaphylactic, septic, or traumatic shock.
Cardiogenic shock: Cardiac output is decreased due to pump failure. Animals in congestive heart failure have cardiogenic shock.
Obstructive shock: Considered by some authors to be a subset of cardiogenic shock. Primarily found with pericardial effusion and cardiac tamponade, pulmonary hypertension, and thromboembolism.

4. Which type of shock is most commonly found in small animals?
Hypovolemic shock.

5. What are the classic clinical signs associated with shock?
They include pale mucous membranes, tachycardia, weak femoral pulses, oliguria, hyperventilation, and mental depression.

6. List the organ systems most commonly affected by hypoperfusion during shock.

Cardiovascular	Gastrointestinal
Pulmonary	Central nervous system
Renal	

7. Can the clinical signs of shock be used to differentiate the etiology?
Possibly, based on physical examination; often, the clinical signs of shock are due to hypoperfusion and may be similar regardless of the underlying etiology.

8. How is shock treated?

Shock syndromes are best treated by identifying the underlying disease or problem whenever possible. In many cases, this is not possible and fluid therapy becomes the foundation of the therapeutic plan. Fluid therapy is beneficial in the majority of shock syndromes, excluding cardiogenic shock.

9. What is the fluid of choice to treat shock?

In most cases, crystalloid fluids are used to treat shock. They are rapidly and safely administered, cost-effective, and readily available. Balanced isotonic electrolyte solutions such as Normosol-R, Plasmalyte-A, and lactated Ringer's solution are common choices for fluid therapy. These fluids are similar in composition to plasma. Colloid solutions may also be used for rapid volume expansion. Products such as plasma, fresh whole blood, stored whole blood, packed red blood cells, hydroxyethyl starch, and Oxyglobin can be considered as dictated by the case.

10. What volumes of crystalloid should be administered for shock therapy?

90 ml/kg/hr intravenously for the dog
45 ml/kg/hr intravenously for the cat

11. How are these volumes best administered?

It is safe and convenient to divide the total shock volume to be administered into quarter doses. One quarter of the calculated dosage can be delivered over one quarter of the time frame. In other words, administer 1/4 of the calculated volume over 15 minutes and then reassess the pet. The full shock dosage may not need to be given. A quick formula for calculating approximate 1/4 shock volumes is to add a 0 to the body weight in pounds for the dog or the body weight in kilograms for cats.

Example: 40 lb dog. 90 ml/kg/hr = 18 kg × 90 = 1620 ml, and 405 ml is the 1/4 dose. Using the quick rule: adding a 0 to 40 gives 400 ml as the 1/4 dose.

Example: 10 lb cat. 45 ml/kg hr = 4.5 kg × 45 = 202.5 ml, and 50.6 is the 1/4 dose. Using the quick rule: adding a 0 to 4.5 gives 45 ml as the 1/4 shock dose.

12. What is a colloid solution?

Colloids are a group of solutions that are isotonic, but contain large molecules that provide increased osmolality in the intravascular space. The colloids can be divided into natural colloids such as whole blood, plasma products, and albumin products; or synthetic colloids such as hydroxyethyl starch (Hetastarch) and dextrans.

13. What is the standard dosage of colloid that can be administered during shock?

The standard maintenance dosage of colloid that can be administered is 20 ml/kg/24 hours. This can be modified and the volume given over 4–6 hours during treatment for shock syndromes. Administration to effect can also be used in critically ill patients. This volume of colloid solution can be used in combination with crystalloid solution therapy.

14. What is hypertonic saline and how is it used?

Hypertonic saline is a hypertonic (7.5%), crystalloid solution that can be used for fluid resuscitation. It is generally administered as a bolus (1–4 ml/kg cat, 4–8 ml/kg dog) and provides rapid volume expansion. The mechanism of action is based on drawing interstitial and intracellular fluid into the vascular space. The effect is short lived, but hypertonic saline can be combined with a colloid solution to prolong the effect.

15. Is oxygen therapy beneficial to patients in shock and how can it be provided?

Oxygen support may be beneficial during shock as hypoperfusion leads to poor oxygen delivery. Administration techniques include face mask, oxygen canopy, nasal cannula, and oxygen cage.

16. Are antibiotics indicated as adjunct therapy during shock?

The use of antimicrobial agents is highly recommended during therapy for shock. Certainly in septic shock it would seem intuitive that antimicrobial agents would be necessary, but, due to cellular hypoxia and depressed immune function found in all shock syndromes, antibiotics should be considered. Agents are broad spectrum and administered intravenously to provide four-quadrant (Gr± aerobes, anaerobes) coverage. Penicillins or first-generation cephalosporins, in combination with enrofloxacin or an aminoglycoside, are suggested.

17. How is shock treatment monitored?

Physical examination should be performed at least twice daily as findings can change rapidly. Although subjective assessment of the patient may provide some information, objective parameters such as central venous pressure, pulmonary capillary wedge pressure, cardiac output, arterial blood pressure, pulse oximetry, arterial blood gas analysis, ECG, blood glucose, BUN, creatinine, PCV, total protein, CBC, electrolytes, urine output, and coagulation parameters should be followed.

18. What is a Swan-Ganz catheter?

The Swan-Ganz catheter is a flexible, balloon-tipped, flow-directed catheter that is placed into the pulmonary artery. There are two ports on this catheter. Once the catheter is properly placed, one port will be in the pulmonary artery and the other in the right atrium.

19. What information can a pulmonary arterial catheter supply?

A Swan-Ganz catheter placed in the pulmonary artery can provide cardiac output, pulmonary wedge pressure, central venous pressure, mixed venous O_2, core body temperature, and pulmonary arterial pressures.

CONTROVERSY

20. Should corticosteroids be used to treat shock?

The use of corticosteroids remains controversial in the management of shock syndromes. Some studies have supported their use in septic shock, while others show no benefit at all. The suggested beneficial effects include enhanced phagocytic activity of the reticuloendothelial system, stabilization of lysosomal membranes, inhibition of vasoactive peptide release, reduction of cerebral edema, inhibition of the arachidonic acid pathway, and reduced platelet and neutrophil aggregation. Deleterious side effects include immunosuppression, gastrointestinal ulceration and hemorrhage, delayed wound healing, hepatopathy, and adrenal suppression.

BIBLIOGRAPHY

1. Cornick-Seahorn J, Marks SL: Emergency! Treating patients in shock. Vet Tech 19:355–399, 1998.
2. Kirby R, Rudloff E: Fluid and electrolyte therapy. In Ettinger SJ, Feldman EC (eds): Textbook of Veterinary Internal Medicine, 5th ed., Philadelphia, WB Saunders, 1999, pp 325–347.
3. Mathews KA. Shock. In Mathews KA (ed): Veterinary Emergency and Critical Care Manual, Ontario, Lifelearn, Inc., 1996, pp 23/1–23/8.
4. Schertel ER, Muir WW. Shock: Pathophysiology, monitoring, and therapy. In Kirk RW (ed): Current Veterinary Therapy, Vol. X. Philadelphia, WB Saunders, 1989, pp 316–330.
5. Ware WA. Shock. In Murtaugh RJ, Kaplan PM (eds): Veterinary Emergency and Critical Care Medicine. St. Louis, Mosby, 1992, pp 163–175.

4. ANESTHESIA

Leigh A. Lamont, D.V.M.

1. What are the goals of preanesthetic administration?
- Calm the patient
- Induce sedation and increase handler safety
- Provide analgesia and muscle relaxation
- Decrease airway secretion and salivation
- Obtund autonomic reflex responses
- Suppress or prevent vomiting or regurgitation
- Decrease anesthetic requirements
- Promote smooth induction and recovery from anesthesia

2. What types of cardiac dysrhythmias are most commonly associated with α_2-agonist administration?
Both **xylazine** and **medetomidine** can produce profound bradycardia with potential for sinoatrial block, first-degree or second-degree atrioventricular block, atrioventricular dissociation, and, occasionally, sinoatrial arrest.

3. Is preemptive anticholinergic administration recommended before α_2-agonist administration?
Yes. It appears that preemptive administration or coadministration of an anticholinergic is a better approach to minimizing the development of bradyarrhythmias, instead of initiating treatment after the fact. Whenever administering an α_2-agonist, heart rate and rhythm should be monitored closely.

4. What is the appropriate treatment for acepromazine overdosage?
Aggressive fluid therapy to counteract hypotension caused by α_1-receptor blockade, peripheral antiadrenergic activity, and direct vasodilatory effects. Vasopressors or catecholamines may be indicated if cardiovascular compromise is severe. Phenylephrine and ephedrine are the drugs of choice because their primary site of action is the α_1-receptor.

5. Would epinephrine be useful after acepromazine overdosage?
No. Epinephrine is **contraindicated.** In the presence of α_1-receptor blockade, epinephrine administration may lead to unopposed β_2-receptor activity, which augments vasodilation and makes hypotension more severe.

6. What preanesthetic drugs alter respiratory drive or cause apnea?
- **Opioids**
- Phenothiazines
- α_2-agonists

7. Is opioid-induced respiratory depression a common enough occurrence that it warrants withholding postoperative analgesic treatment in veterinary patients?
No. In most patients, the use of low incremental doses administered to effect minimizes potential complications. In higher-risk patients (i.e., increased intracranial pressure or preexisting respiratory disease), opioids can still be used safely if monitoring is vigilant and ventilation can be supported.

8. Is routine preoperative anticholinergic administration recommended?
No. In general, it is indicated to decrease salivary and respiratory secretions and to counteract sinus bradycardia. Its selective use is indicated when potent vagotonic preanesthetic and anes-

thetic drugs are used (e.g., α_2-agonists) or if a powerful vagal response is anticipated during the procedure.

9. How do propofol and thiopental differ in their effects on cardiopulmonary function?

There is no appreciable difference. Both cause transient dose-dependent decreases in myocardial contractility and mean arterial blood pressure, usually accompanied by a compensatory increase in heart rate. Both are potent respiratory depressants. They reduce the central stimulating effects of arterial carbon dioxide and depress peripheral chemoreceptor sensitivity at higher doses.

10. Can induction apnea be avoided when administering propofol?

Slow administration over 60–90 seconds to facilitate *dosing to effect* significantly decreases the incidence of apnea.

11. What is the treatment for thiopental-induced or propofol-induced respiratory arrest?

Secure the airway and support ventilation first, then assess the stability of the cardiovascular system. Spontaneous ventilation resumes when sufficient drug has been redistributed (usually within 5–10 minutes).

12. How does *recovery* from single bolus injections of thiopental and propofol differ?

There is no appreciable difference after a single bolus injection. Recovery occurs by drug redistribution primarily to muscle and adipose tissue, which rapidly terminates the anesthetic effects of both drugs.

13. How does *biotransformation* of thiopental and propofol differ?

Propofol is rapidly metabolized in the liver and, to a lesser degree in extrahepatic sites, to the inactive metabolite, propofol glucuronide. It is then excreted in urine and feces. The relative importance of hepatic and renal processes in thiopental clearance varies among species; however, in all cases, metabolism is much slower.

14. Why is thiopental not recommended for induction of anesthesia in sight hounds?

Sight hounds have minimal stores of adipose tissue, which rapidly become saturated with thiopental during drug redistribution. Consequently, plasma concentrations of the drug are more likely to remain high and prolong anesthetic effects.

15. What effect does ketamine have on ventilation?

Ketamine causes a respiratory pattern called *apneustic breathing,* which is characterized by a prolonged inspiratory duration and relatively short expiratory time. If administered alone, ketamine causes minimal respiratory depression. In combination with other commonly administered adjuncts, such as benzodiazepines, acepromazine, opioids, or α_2-agonists, minute ventilation is usually decreased, and arterial carbon dioxide partial pressure increases. Other respiratory effects include airway dilation and maintenance of laryngeal reflexes.

16. What effect does ketamine have on intracranial pressure (ICP)?

1. Ketamine can increase mean arterial blood pressure, which may increase cerebral blood flow leading to a passive increase in ICP in patients that are unable to autoregulate blood flow efficiently.

2. Ketamine may contribute to respiratory depression, leading to an increase in arterial carbon dioxide ($PaCO_2$). The brain responds to elevations in $PaCO_2$ by increasing cerebral blood flow, which increases ICP.

17. What type of dysrhythmia is commonly associated with the thiobarbiturates?

Ventricular bigeminy, which is usually self-limiting and transient. Thiamylal is most often associated with this dysrhythmia, although the other thiobarbiturates, including thiopental, have also been implicated.

18. What is Telazol?
A combination of equal parts by weight of the dissociative anesthetic agent, tiletamine, and the benzodiazepine, zolazepam.

19. How does recovery from Telazol anesthesia differ between dogs and cats?
The fixed ratio of dissociative anesthetic to benzodiazepine can cause different patterns of recovery among species.

In **dogs,** the zolazepam component seems to be metabolized more rapidly than the tiletamine component. Some dogs may exhibit muscle rigidity, mydriasis, vocalization, and dysphoria at recovery as a result of residual effects of the dissociative anesthetic.

In **cats,** tiletamine is typically metabolized more quickly than zolazepam, so that they often appear sedated for a prolonged period and awake more slowly and quietly.

20. Compare the cardiovascular effects of halothane and isoflurane.

Halothane	Isoflurane
• Direct myocardial depression	• Minimal myocardial depression
↓Cardiac output	• Minimal cardiac output
↓Mean arterial blood pressure	↓Systemic vascular resistance
↓Heart rate	↓Mean arterial blood pressure
• Sensitizes myocardium to catecholamines	↑Heart rate
	• No myocardial sensitization

21. Do volatile anesthetic agents possess analgesic properties?
No. With the exception of methoxyflurane, none of the commonly used volatile anesthetic agents (i.e., isoflurane, halothane, enflurane, sevoflurane) have any inherent analgesic properties.

22. Define the terms *low flow, closed,* and *semiclosed anesthesia.*
Low-flow, closed, and semiclosed refer *only* to fresh gas flow rates within a circle system. Traditional **semiclosed** circles use fresh gas flows (25–50 ml/kg/min), which significantly exceed the patient's metabolic oxygen consumption (approximately 5–15 ml/kg/min). **Low-flow** circle systems use fresh gas flows greater than the patient's metabolic oxygen consumption but less than the traditional higher flow rates noted. In a **closed circle,** the fresh gas flow matches the patient's metabolic consumption of oxygen and anesthetic (i.e., 5–15 ml/kg/min). Because oxygen consumption varies among individuals, common practice is to set a flow rate that keeps the reservoir bag approximately 75% full. Although more economical, patients anesthetized using closed circle flow rates must be monitored closely to ensure adequate oxygenation.

23. What is total intravenous anesthesia (TIVA)?
Induction and maintenance of general anesthesia using intravenous agents only. Recovery is determined by the pharmacokinetic profiles of the drugs used and, in many cases, may be faster and smoother than after inhalation anesthesia.

24. What is the most commonly used anesthetic agent for TIVA in veterinary medicine?
Propofol. Its short duration of action and rapid biotransformation to inactive metabolites make it wellsuited for this purpose in the dog. Propofol infusions of 2 hours have been successfully used to provide anesthesia for a variety of surgical procedures in dogs. For major surgical procedures, coadministration of adjunctive drugs, such as opioids, α_2-agonists, benzodiazepines or acepromazine, is recommended to decrease propofol requirements and provide preemptive and intraoperative analgesia.

25. Can propofol infusions be used in cats?
Possibly. Propofol infusions in cats have not been studied in detail, but preliminary work suggests that prolonged infusions may have toxic effects on feline red blood cells and may result in delayed recoveries.

26. When is treatment of bradycardia in anesthetized patients indicated?
When bradycardia causes an excessive decrease in cardiac output or when heart rate decreases below 50–60 beats/min in an animal with adequate circulating volume. It is helpful to quantify intraoperative bradycardia in terms of the patient's resting heart rate (i.e., has heart rate dropped by 20–30% of the preanesthetic value?). Before treatment is initiated, consideration should be given to the cause of bradycardia.

27. List the causes of bradycardia in anesthetized patients.
- Excessive anesthetic depth
- Excessive vagal tone
- Anesthetic agents that decrease sympathetic tone or directly depress depolarization
- Hypothermia
- Exogenous toxemias
- Endogenous metabolic disturbances

28. What information does pulse oximetry provide about the patient?
Pulse oximetry is an indirect, noninvasive method of measuring the percent saturation of hemoglobin (SpO_2). Normal SpO_2 readings are >95%, whereas readings <95% indicate mild hypoxemia. Readings <90% indicate serious hypoxemia, and readings <75% indicate life-threatening hypoxemia. Although patients that are intubated and are breathing 100% oxygen are at much less risk of developing hypoxemia, pulse oximetry provides early warning of potentially dangerous desaturation. Cyanosis, the cardinal clinical sign of hypoxemia, is not apparent until severe desaturation has already occurred.

BIBLIOGRAPHY

1. Andress JL, Day TK, Day DG: The effects of consecutive day propofol anesthesia on feline red blood cells. Vet Surg 24:277–282, 1995.
2. Lemke KA, Tranquilli WJ, Thurmon JC, et al: Alterations in the arrhythmogenic dose of epinephrine after xylazine or medetomidine administration in halothane-anesthetized dogs. Am J Vet Res 54:2132–2138, 1993.
3. Paddleford RR: Manual of Small Animal Anesthesia, 2nd ed. Philadelphia, W.B. Saunders, 1999.
4. Quandt JE, Robinson EP, Rivers WJ, et al: Cardiorespiratory and anesthetic effects of propofol and thiopental in dogs. Am J Vet Res 59:1137–1143, 1998.
5. Thurmon JC, Tranquilli WJ, Benson GJ (eds): Lumb and Jones Veterinary Anesthesia, 3rd ed. Baltimore, Williams & Wilkins, 1996.
6. Wright B, Hellyer PW: Respiratory monitoring during anesthesia: pulse oximetry and capnography. Comp Cont Educ Pract Vet 18:1083–1096, 1996.
7. Zoran DL, Riedesel DH, Dyer DC: Pharmacokinetics of propofol in mixed-breed dogs and Greyhounds. Am J Vet Res 54:755–760, 1993.

5. PERIOPERATIVE PAIN MANAGEMENT

Leigh A. Lamont, D.V.M.

1. How do we know if an animal is in pain?
Veterinarians must rely on behavioral and physiologic parameters to assess pain. Because there are inherent limitations in all pain scoring systems, it is important to **anticipate** the level of pain associated with a particular trauma or surgical procedure and focus on **proactive pain management**. In most cases, the benefits of analgesic administration greatly outweigh the risks; if an animal's pain status is uncertain, anthropomorphism is appropriate in guiding analgesic therapy.

2. Describe the pathophysiology of acute postoperative pain.

The surgical insult activates a specialized set of peripheral nerve endings (**nociceptors**), which trigger transmission of the signal to the dorsal horn of the spinal cord. Other neurons can intervene at this level and modulate the afferent information. Spinal tracts then carry the impulse to higher brain stem and cortical structures. Pain is the end result of the integration, modulation and perception of noxious stimuli by the nervous system. Neurons can become *sensitized* by the release of inflammatory mediators from damaged tissue or by sustained noxious input to the dorsal horn. Sensitization reduces the stimulus threshold required to produce pain and causes an exaggerated response to noxious stimuli at the site of injury and in nearby noninjured tissue.

3. What are the adverse physiologic effects associated with postoperative pain?

- The release of stress hormones (**catecholamines**) secondary to pain can cause tachycardia and hypertension, which increase cardiac work and myocardial oxygen consumption.
- Increased sympathetic tone decreases gastrointestinal motility and may prolong recovery.
- Muscle splinting, arising from abdominal or thoracic pain, impairs chest wall excursions and may decrease alveolar ventilation and promote atelectasis.
- Metabolic processes are shifted into a catabolic state, immune function may be impaired, and behavioral patterns are affected.
- Animals experiencing postoperative pain often suffer from disruptions in their normal sleep cycle and may be unwilling to eat or drink, both of which can further delay recovery.

4. What is preemptive analgesia?

Administration of analgesic drugs before the initiation of painful stimuli. Acute postoperative pain is associated with altered processing of pain information by the nervous system, a phenomenon referred to as *sensitization*. Preemptive analgesia is based on the premise that these changes can be minimized, resulting in a better response to postoperative pain treatment and an earlier return to function.

5. What is multimodal analgesia?

Administration of a combination of different classes of analgesic drugs to achieve optimal pain control in the perioperative period. The rationale is based on targeting several points along the pain pathway, resulting in additive or synergistic analgesic effects, while minimizing adverse side effects seen with the administration of larger doses of a single analgesic drug.

6. What preanesthetic drug combinations are commonly used to provide preemptive analgesia?

An **opioid** in combination with a **sedative/tranquilizer** such as acepromazine, medetomidine, or midazolam, administered intramuscularly before anesthesia. In geriatric or debilitated patients, the opioid may be administered alone. A variety of local and regional analgesic techniques may also be employed preemptively depending on the type of surgical procedure.

7. What drugs can be used to provide supplemental analgesia intraoperatively?

Supplemental doses of **opioids,** such as oxymorphone and fentanyl. The incorporation of local and regional techniques, such as epidural analgesia/anesthesia, greatly diminishes intraoperative requirements for additional analgesics, often resulting in a more stable plane of anesthesia with a lower inhalant anesthetic vaporizer setting. In very painful procedures, low doses of ketamine or medetomidine in combination with opioids may be administered intraoperatively.

8. In addition to intramuscular or subcutaneous injections, what other routes are available for administration of postoperative analgesic agents?

A **constant rate infusion** may be administered by adding morphine or fentanyl to the patient's intravenous fluids. **Transdermal** opioid delivery is also available in the form of a fentanyl patch. Once the patient is awake, **oral administration** of a nonsteroidal anti-inflammatory drug

(NSAID), such as carprofen or ketoprofen, provides effective postoperative analgesia for a variety of orthopedic procedures.

9. List the commonest classes of analgesic drugs in veterinary medicine.
- Opioids
- NSAIDs
- Local anesthetics

10. In addition to opioids, NSAIDs, and local anesthetics, what other drugs can be used for perioperative pain management?
The dissociative agent, ketamine and the α_2-agonists, such as **medetomidine** and **xylazine,** can be used in low, subanesthetic dosages in combination with other traditional drugs to enhance analgesia.

11. What is the mechanism of ketamine-induced analgesia?
Although ketamine has multiple binding sites, it is believed that N-methyl-D-aspartate (NMDA) receptor blockade is responsible for most of the drug's analgesic actions. Ketamine diminishes NMDA receptor–mediated *wind-up* and subsequent sensitization of dorsal horn neurons and may even abolish hypersensitivity once it is already established.

12. How do α_2-agonists produce analgesia?
α_2-agonists bind α_2-receptors located in the dorsal horn of the spinal cord, which inhibits the release of substance P, calcitonin gene–related peptide, and various other neurotransmitters involved in transmission of pain impulses. Binding of α_2-receptors located supraspinally in the locus coeruleus, thalamus, and cerebral cortex inhibits norepinephrine release, producing profound sedation, which diminishes the conscious perception of pain.

13. What are analgesic adjuncts?
Drugs that have primary indications other than pain but have analgesic actions in some painful conditions. **Tranquilizers** such as acepromazine and the benzodiazepines, have little or no inherent analgesic effect when administered alone but may enhance analgesia produced by other drugs and minimize patient anxiety. **Corticosteroids** contribute to analgesia through their local anti-inflammatory effects at the site of tissue injury.

14. What is the difference between opioid agonists and agonist-antagonists?
Pure opioid agonists, such as morphine, oxymorphone, and fentanyl, bind to and activate opioid receptors to produce analgesia. Opioid antagonists, such as naloxone, bind to and inhibit opioid receptors and may be used to reverse the effects of pure agonists. Drugs such as butorphanol and buprenorphine have agonist and antagonist actions at various subpopulations of opioid receptors.

15. Why is this difference clinically significant?
Mixed agonist-antagonist drugs have a **ceiling effect.** That is, once the maximal effect is achieved, further increases in dosage are not accompanied by additional analgesia. The interactions between opioid agonists and agonist-antagonists are complex, and the effect produced by combinations of such drugs may vary among species, with different dosages, and with different types of pain.

16. List the side effects of opioid therapy.
- Urinary retention
- Nausea
- Vomiting
- Respiratory depression
- Bradycardia
- Sedation
- Dysphoria
- Histamine release (with urticaria, hypotension, erythema, pruritus)

17. What is the difference between opioid potency and efficacy?

Potency refers to the number of milligrams of drug required to produce an effect, whereas **efficacy** measures the capacity of the agonist-receptor complex to produce a response in an appropriate clinical setting. The potencies of commonly administered opioids relative to morphine are as follows: oxymorphone, 10; fentanyl, 75–125; butorphanol, 3–5; and buprenorphine, 300. If dosed appropriately, morphine, oxymorphone, and fentanyl are considered to be equally efficacious for moderate-to-severe pain, whereas butorphanol and buprenorphine are effective for only mild-to-moderate pain.

18. Can cats be treated with pure opioid agonists?

Yes. Cats are more likely to experience opioid-induced excitement and dysphoria than are dogs. By avoiding intravenous bolus dosing and using lower doses combined with a tranquilizing agent, such as acepromazine or medetomidine, opioid agonists can be used preemptively in a preanesthetic protocol or postoperatively at regular dosing intervals to manage pain.

19. What is a fentanyl patch?

Fentanyl is a highly lipid-soluble opioid agonist that can be effectively absorbed through the skin. Fentanyl transdermal patches have been developed for use in humans and have been successfully used for perioperative pain management in dogs and cats, although they are not currently approved for use in these species. Plasma fentanyl concentrations usually peak within 24 hours of patch application in the dog and remain stable for 3 days, whereas plasma concentrations can peak as early as 4–8 hours in the cat and remain stable for 5 days. For perioperative use, the patch should be applied 12–24 hours before surgery, and additional opioids may be required postoperatively to treat breakthrough pain.

20. What are complications of fentanyl patch usage?

In addition to side effects associated with any type of opioid administration, accidental human exposure and the potential for abuse are significant concerns. For this reason, many recommend that fentanyl patches be reserved for hospitalized patients only.

21. What are the onset and duration of action of local anesthetic agents commonly used in small animal patients?

DRUG	ONSET OF ACTION	DURATION OF ACTION
Lidocaine	5–10 min	1–2 h
Bupivacaine	20 min	4–6 h

22. What are the toxic doses of lidocaine and bupivacaine in dogs and cats?

In **dogs,** toxic side effects occur at intravenous doses of approximately 10 mg/kg of lidocaine and 3–5 mg/kg of bupivacaine. In **cats,** total doses should not exceed 2.5 mg/kg of lidocaine and 1.0 mg/kg of bupivacaine.

23. List the toxic side effects of lidocaine and bupivacaine.

- Restlessness
- Muscle tremors
- Seizures
- Cardiopulmonary depression
- Coma
- Death

24. List the commonest local and regional analgesic techniques used in small animal patients.

- Surgical site infiltration
- Interpleural administration
- Regional nerve blocks (including dental nerve blocks and intercostal nerve blocks)
- Brachial plexus blocks
- Intra-articular blocks
- Epidural anesthesia/analgesia

25. What is epidural anesthesia/analgesia?

Analgesic agents are placed into the epidural space, located between the dura mater and the intervertebral ligament. The lumbosacral junction is the most commonly used site for accessing the epidural space in dogs and cats.

26. What types of drugs can be administered into the epidural space?

In small animal veterinary patients, **local anesthetics** and **opioids** are commonly used in epidural techniques, although other agents, such as α_2-agonists and ketamine, are occasionally added to standard drug combinations.

27. Which opioids are most commonly administered in the lumbosacral epidural space?

DRUG	LIPID SOLUBILITY	DURATION OF ANALGESIA (h)	USES
Morphine	Low	18–24	Hindlimb, thoracic, and forelimb procedures with lumbosacral injection
Oxymorphone	Intermediate	8–10	Hindlimb procedures only with lumbosacral injection
Fentanyl	High	0.5–1	Infusion or repeated boluses through epidural catheter

28. For what types of procedures is epidural analgesia/anesthesia beneficial?

- Hindlimb orthopedic procedures
- Tail amputations
- Perineal hernia or perianal fistula repairs
- Cesarean sections or other painful abdominal procedures
- Forelimb orthopedic procedures (opioids only)
- Thoracotomies (opioids only)

29. Which NSAIDs are commonly used for pain management in veterinary patients?

- Carprofen
- Ketoprofen
- Etodolac
- Meloxicam
- Meclofenamic acid
- Aspirin

30. What types of pain can be effectively managed with NSAIDs?

Aspirin and the newer NSAIDs are the drugs of choice for management of mild-to-moderate inflammatory pain (musculoskeletal pain, including bone pain and arthritis) and are less effective for pain of visceral origin. Although traditionally used on an outpatient basis for the management of chronic pain syndromes, carprofen and ketoprofen may be used in the perioperative period in combination with other analgesics as part of a balanced pain management protocol.

31. What are the adverse side effects associated with NSAID use?
- Gastrointestinal irritation and ulceration
- Renal insufficiency
- Bleeding resulting from inhibition of platelet function

BIBLIOGRAPHY

1. Basbaum A: Anatomy and physiology of nociception. In Kanner R (ed): Pain Management Secrets. Philadelphia, Hanley & Belfus, 1997.
2. Kyles AE: Transdermal fentanyl. Comp Cont Educ Pract Vet 20:721–726, 1998.
3. Matthews KA: Nonsteroidal antiinflammatory analgesics to manage acute pain in dogs and cats. Comp Cont Educ Pract Vet 18:1117–1123, 1996.
4. Papich MG: Principles of analgesic drug therapy. Semin Vet Med Surg Sm Anim 12:80–93, 1997.
5. Pascoe P: Local and regional anesthesia and analgesia. Semin Vet Med Surg Sm Anim 12:94–105, 1997.
6. Quandt JE, Rawlings CR: Reducing postoperative pain for dogs: Local anesthetic and analgesic techniques. Comp Cont Educ Pract Vet 18:101–111, 1996.
7. Raffe M: Recent advances in our understanding of pain: How should they affect management? Semin Vet Med Surg Sm Anim 12:75–79, 1997.
8. Thurmon JC, Tranquilli WJ, Benson GJ: Perioperative pain and distress. In Thurmon JC, Tranquilli WJ, Benson GJ (eds): Lumb and Jones Veterinary Anesthesia, 3rd ed. Baltimore, Williams & Wilkins, 1996.
9. Tranquilli WJ, Thurmon JC: Perioperative pain and its management. In Thurmon JC, Tranquilli WJ, Benson GJ (eds): Essentials of Small Animal Anesthesia and Analgesia. Baltimore, Lippincott Williams & Wilkins, 1999.
10. Woolf CJ, Chong MS: Preemptive analgesia—treating postoperative pain by preventing the establishment of central sensitization. Anesth Analg 77:362–379, 1993.

6. ACUPUNCTURE

Andrea L. Looney, D.V.M.

1. What is acupuncture?
The stimulation of specific predetermined points on the body to achieve a therapeutic effect.

2. What is traditional Chinese medicine (TCM)?
Empiric knowledge that has been accumulated over many centuries based on astute, detailed, and subtle observations of patients, their symptoms, and their reactions. TCM is divided into many specialties, including:
- Herbal medicine
- Nutrition
- Spinal and cranial manipulation
- Massage and exercise therapy
- Acupuncture

3. Contrast Western medicine with TCM.
TCM and acupuncture employ a whole body systems view of health and disease. Euroamerican medical thinking tends to be linear (A leads to B, and B causes C). In TCM, there are no causal relationships, but rather *patterns* of health and disease. TCM stresses recognition of the

complex relationships involved in the manifestation of a disease (imbalance) and rebalance of an unhealthy individual. Euroamerican medicine and veterinary medicine stress identification of specific causative factors, riddance of these factors, and repair of the signs of illness.

4. What is integrative acupuncture?

Most veterinary acupuncturists use their typical Western biomedical and veterinary education *and* TCM training together; acupuncture is not used as one of many *alternative* treatments but rather as a *complement* to scientifically proven diagnostic and therapeutic regimens.

5. What are the goals of Western and Chinese therapies?

The goals of Western medicine and acupuncture are to **restore homeostasis.**
- Western medicine uses conventional medical and surgical means (from fluid therapy to H2 antagonists to transfusion to renal transplant) to treat forms of renal disease.
- Acupuncture, as part of TCM, uses point stimulation to support the body's intrinsic healing mechanisms (encourage blood flow, decrease gastric acidity, promote urine output) and to support other organs while the kidneys begin to heal.

6. What does the half-black and half-white circle symbolize in veterinary and human acupuncture?

There exists a life energy force known as Chi, Qi, or Ki (the circle). Qi consists of two aspects, **Yin** (negative, black half of circle) and **Yang** (positive, white half of circle). Yin and Yang are depicted as part of a constantly evolving circle of life energy and are often symbolized by the black and white flowing symbols within the continuous circle diagram.

7. What are meridians according to TCM?

Pathways through which the energy or chi flows within the body. Each meridian corresponds to an individual body system, usually named after a chief organ in the system.

8. What are meridians according to neurophysiologic and biomedical principles?

Pathways along which bioelectric and biochemical changes occur. Meridians are a gathering or grouping of acupuncture points, a collection of points having related functions.

9. What are the major meridians?

- Heart (HT)
- Lung (LU)
- Small Intestine (SI)
- Large Intestine (LI)
- Gallbladder (GB)
- Liver (LV)
- Spleen (SP)
- Stomach (ST)
- Kidney (KI)
- Bladder (BL)

The **Bladder meridian** is a major meridian of importance for diagnostic and therapeutic purposes in veterinary and human acupuncture. Both major and minor (collateral) meridians exist within the body. There are 12 bilaterally distributed meridians, and 8 extra channels that are not directly associated with organs or organ systems.

10. What do the meridians have to do with the organ for which they were named?

Sometimes, very little. In traditional Chinese acupuncture, the concept of the organ rarely corresponds with what we know as the physiologic accumulation of cells and tissues having a similar function.

11. Define an acupuncture point.

A region of decreased electric resistance or increased electric conductivity within the skin. Research has demonstrated that, anatomically, acupuncture points correspond to one of four known neural structures or areas.

12. What are the types of points?
- **Type I** points correspond to motor points localized with electromyography. Motor points are areas of the muscle that produce maximum contractions with minimal intensity of stimulation.
- **Type II** points are located along dorsal and ventral midlines where bilateral superficial nerves meet.
- **Type III** points are located at high-density foci of major superficial nerves or plexi.
- **Type IV** points are located at muscle-tendon junctions, where Golgi tendon organs are abundant.

13. Describe the anatomy and histology of the acupuncture point.
Histologic studies have shown acupuncture points to be neurovascular bundles, sites within or above the fascia where nerves and vessels penetrate toward the skin surface. Nerves and blood vessels within these bundles are enveloped by concentric laminae of collagen fibers. The spaces between these fibers are filled with sheets of loosely arranged connective tissue containing increased extracellular water content in addition to fat and mast cells.

14. How are points located?
Most acupuncture points have much lower electric resistance than that of surrounding skin. Many have increased temperature compared with surrounding skin. Local tenderness on palpation is common. Many can be palpated, especially in large animals, because they lie in true anatomic depressions or because the perforations in the fascia where they appear are grossly palpable. Points can also be located by proportional measurements using anatomic descriptions (acupuncture *maps*). Electronic point finders work via finding areas of higher conductance along the skin surface associated with known acupuncture points.

15. How are points named?
All acupuncture points have traditional Chinese names but are more commonly designated in the United States and Europe by an alphanumeric code indicating the particular meridian on which the point is located and the number of the point on the meridian. For example, BL-60 designates the 60th point on the Bladder meridian. Points are further classified as source, connecting, association, alarm, master, trigger, and sedation points based on their actions when stimulated.

16. Discuss the neurophysiologic basis for acupuncture's beneficial effects.
Numerous mechanisms of action have been proposed and identified:
- The **gate theory of acupuncture** is based on the same theory of pain postulated by Melzack and Wall in the late 1950s. In short, acupuncture's effects are transmitted via certain sensory nerve fibers to the dorsal horn of the spinal cord, where synapse with inhibitory neurons occurs, closing the gate to further cranial transmission of pain impulses.
- The **neural opiate theory of acupuncture** is based on evidence that acupuncture stimulates the release of endogenous opiates, endorphins, and enkephalins, chemicals that act at various levels peripherally and centrally to inhibit pain perception in higher centers of the central nervous system and to inhibit autonomic activation, which results from pain transmission.
- The **hormonal theory of acupuncture** is based on the interaction of neurons (secondary to peripheral stimulation) with the subsequent release of humoral factors—β-endorphin, serotonin, and norepinephrine. These neurochemicals are known to exert multiple effects throughout the body via their actions with endocrine, neural, and gastrointestinal end-organ receptors, yet most of these actions seem to be mediated via β-endorphin.

17. Is a medical workup required before acupuncture treatment?
Yes. The workup should consist of physical examination, history, specialist examination, ancillary testing (blood work, radiographic procedures, ultrasonography, electromyography), and

point and body system examination: The acupuncturist observes the skin color, hair texture, eyes, ocular and nasal discharges, and tongue. The acupuncturist palpates the pulse, auscultates the breathing pattern, and palpates several diagnostic points along the bladder meridian and along the thorax.

18. **What are the indications of acupuncture in clinical small animal veterinary practice?**
    - Musculoskeletal conditions, such as chronic degenerative joint disease, disk disease, spondylopathies, and hip dysplasia
    - Chronic pain, hyperalgesia, neurapraxias
    - Canine and feline neurologic disorders, including epilepsy, cerebrovascular accidents, geriatric vestibular disease, and certain nerve paralyses
    - Gastrointestinal motility conditions, including megaesophagus
    - Dermatologic conditions, including lick granulomas and contact and atopic dermatitis

19. **Is increasing patient age a contraindication for acupuncture therapy?**
    No. Many geriatric patients are already polypharmacy cases that may have become nonsurgical candidates because of anesthetic risk. Acupuncture can readily be incorporated into a comprehensive approach to optimal health care, improving geriatric energy levels, circulatory function, appetite, and attitude as well as strengthening the owner-patient bond.

20. **List the contraindications to acupuncture therapy in small animals.**
    - Problems with no diagnosis
    - Last-ditch effort in dying patient
    - Neoplastic conditions
    - Acute life-threatening traumatic or infectious conditions
    - Following a heavy meal or exertion
    - Pregnancy
    - Coagulation disorders

21. **What is a common side effect of acupuncture?**
    Geriatric animals often become fatigued after an acupuncture treatment. Causes are speculated to be relaxation from sudden release of chronic pain or multiple local muscle spasms and sympathetic deactivation resulting from endogenous opioid release during the treatment. Relaxation or fatigue may be seen in any patient with any chronic condition and usually lasts 24–48 hours.

22. **List rare sequelae of acupuncture.**
    - Fractured needles
    - Systemic infection
    - Nausea
    - Vomiting
    - Hematomas
    - Pneumothorax
    - Syncope (one case)
    - Cardiac arrest (one case)

23. **How does an aspiring acupuncturist decide on which points to use in treatments?**
    Two major theories used to return balance to body systems in TCM are the **five element theory** and the **eight principle theory.** Most American veterinary acupuncturists use treatment of a combination of points derived from these theories along with empiric point selection (based on so-called major point theory). The latter involves locating points on the body via diagnostics (palpation, observation, owner questioning) where stimulation produces a beneficial change in the local tissue and peripheral and central nervous system by modulating ongoing physiologic activity. Many of these points are special acupoints termed *alarm, association, tonification, sedation, master,* and *source* points. Most acupuncturists learn and memorize these points in an effort to has-

ten treatment protocols individualized for each patient's points. Acupuncturists use simple alarm and association points, trigger points (points located over intensely painful muscle areas), or ting points (points located on distalmost aspect of each meridian).

24. What are some useful guidelines for treatments?
- Treat the main condition or add one to two points more to treat for the most serious sign of this condition (symptomatic, major points).
- For musculoskeletal conditions, choose points according to the innervation or in the same dermatome as the problem area.
- Treat trigger, myalgic, and hyperalgesic areas first. Think in terms of referred pain, prior injury, and chronic muscular response to injury. In Chinese, these are referred to as *ah-shi* (tender) points.
- Choose local points for local problems or points on major meridians that traverse the lesion. Choose distant points on the same meridian for systemic problems that originate from the local lesions.
- Initially, choose points well known for their symptomatic effects.
- The more acute the condition, the more dramatic the effect if the correct meridian is chosen.
- Combination of local and distant points results in slow strengthening and improvement of chronic conditions.
- Chronic conditions (e.g., scars, nonhealing wounds) seem to respond well to encircling of the lesion or area (use of many local points).

25. What are the common treatment modes of stimulation used with veterinary acupuncture?
- **Dry needling** is the term often associated with simple acupuncture. Solid stainless steel needles, 0.5–2 inches in length, 25–32 gauge, with coiled insertion handles are most commonly used.
- **Acupressure** is a form of transdermal pressure therapy applied to the body surface in a general pattern at designated points or locations.
- **Moxibustion** uses heat to stimulate acupoints, either directly or indirectly.
- **Sonipuncture** involves the use of small ultrasound probes to assist in stimulating points.
- **Aquapuncture** involves the injection of solutions (e.g., electrolytes, vitamins) into acupuncture points.
- **Electroacupuncture** is the use of electronic devices to augment the stimulation given to acupuncture points.
- **Laser acupuncture** uses cold, low-intensity lasers (gallium arsenide diodes, infrared lasers) to stimulate acupuncture points.
- **Implantation acupuncture** involves surgical placement of gold or stainless steel beads or wire pieces into acupuncture points.

26. Describe acupuncture analgesia?
By stimulating certain acupoints, pathways within the brain and spinal cord, specifically within the periaqueductal gray matter, afford some inhibition of incoming pain information at the level of the dorsal horn of the spinal cord and above. These pathways involve many neurotransmitters, including serotonin, endogenous opiates, and norepinephrine. The term *acupuncture analgesia* has classically been reserved to refer specifically to the use of acupuncture to induce a plane of surgical analgesia comparable to barbiturate or general anesthetic use.

27. What are some indications for acupuncture analgesia?
Avoidance of respiratory depression, decreased blood pressure, and decreased cardiac output produced by injectable or inhalant anesthetics. If patients have known anesthetic adverse reactions, acupuncture analgesia may be a useful adjunct to surgical anesthesia. Another use for acupuncture is to assist treatment or prevent postoperative pain. Acupuncture analgesia may be extremely beneficial in cases of geriatric surgery, cesarean section, or animals having known drug sensitivities (brachycephalics and opioids).

28. What are some techniques for acupuncture analgesia?

Traditional needling and electroacupuncture, used near the ears and head (auriculo-acupuncture) or on one to two main meridians (depending on surgical site).

29. What are some problems of acupuncture analgesia?

- Lack of restraint
- Lengthy induction periods
- Appropriate point selection has not been researched well enough to provide practitioners with a formula to produce analgesia specific to any surgery.

30. Describe a typical acupuncture treatment.

In **acute** cases, treating the animal every 2–3 days (with short treatment times of 1–5 minutes) usually causes steady improvement until the desired results are achieved.

In more **chronic** cases, improvement is achieved more slowly and may vary in response. Animals are treated less frequently (about once every 7–10 days to begin with) and for longer durations of treatment (approximately 20–30 minutes per treatment). These sessions usually continue for 3–6 weeks, then treatments are tapered to schedule as few as possible to maintain a pattern of health and effect, which varies a great deal.

31. What if acupuncture doesn't work?

The response of the patient may be revised by changing the selection of points, type of stimulation, or duration of treatment to produce the desired effect. Several questions should be asked:

1. Is the diagnosis correct?
2. Would other conventional surgical or medical techniques benefit this patient in addition to acupuncture?
3. Is acupuncture appropriate for this problem and patient?
4. Is the technique appropriate (i.e., should laser acupuncture be used instead of needling)?
5. Is the time interval correct?
6. Could the selection of points be changed?
7. Are nutritional, daily exercise, and rest factors coming into play (i.e. consider the animal's emotional [psychologic] and social environment)?
8. Could other therapies assist the animal at home (e.g., massage, interaction, physical therapy)?

32. What is GV 26?

An extremely powerful and important point for the stimulation of cardiovascular and respiratory function (Governing Vessel 26 or the 26th point on the Governing Vessel meridian). It is located at the **philtrum** in most animals, and its use has been well documented in cases of respiratory and cardiac arrest in the dog, horse, and human. Stimulation of this point seems to cause massive sympathomimetic output related to endogenous epinephrine and norepinephrine release. These, in turn, cause an increase in cardiac output, systemic vascular resistance, and bronchodilation in patients with respondent cardiorespiratory systems.

33. How is GV 26 used?

This point is often stimulated in cases of shock, resuscitation, or anesthetic emergency by inserting a small-gauge hypodermic or acupuncture needle perpendicular to the philtrum, at a point located in the dorsal midline of the animal parallel with the lower canthi of the nares.

BIBLIOGRAPHY

1. Altman S: Acupuncture therapy in small animal practice. Comp Cont Educ Pract Vet 19:1233–1245, 1997.
2. Janssens LA: Trigger points in 48 dogs with myofascial pain syndromes. Vet Surg 20:274–278, 1991.
3. Lewith GT, Kenyon JN: Physiological and psychological explanations for the mechanism of acupuncture as a treatment of chronic pain. Soc Sci Med 19:1367–1378, 1984.

4. Looney AL, Rothstein E: Use of acupuncture to treat psychodermatosis in the dog. Canine Prac 23:18–21, 1998.
5. Rosted P: Literature survey of reported adverse effects associated with acupuncture treatment. Am J Acupunct 24:27–34, 1996.
6. Smith FWK: Neurophysiologic basis of acupuncture. Prob Vet Med 4:34–45, 1992.
7. Still J: A clinical study of auriculotherapy in canine thoracolumbar disc disease. J South Afr Vet Assoc 61:102–105, 1990.

7. PHYSICAL THERAPY

Lin McGonagle, M.S.P.T.

1. What is physical therapy?

Alleviation of impairment and functional limitation by design, implementation, and modification of therapeutic interventions. Prevention of injury and disability is also part of physical therapy.

2. Is physical therapy a replacement for traditional veterinary medicine?

No. Physical therapists work in collaboration with veterinarians using a team approach to examination and intervention. Acquiring a veterinary referral before client evaluation is the preferred model of practice.

3. What are the educational and licensure requirements for physical therapists?

Most physical therapists enter the profession with a master's degree and many further their education by attaining a doctoral degree. There are 159 physical therapy programs, graduating approximately 4,500 therapists each year in the U.S. The core curriculum requires 2–2½ years. Each student completes 4–6 months of clinical internships prior to graduation. Every therapist must pass a national licensure examination. Additional requirements vary from state to state.

4. List the benefits of physical therapy for animals.

Improved recovery from injury or surgery	Minimized side effects of injury or surgery
Return to typical performance or work	Improved biomechanics and posture
Enhancement of natural healing processes	Increased flexibility
Reduced pain	Prevention of future injury through owner/trainer education
Increased speed and quality of movement	
Improved strength and endurance	Positive psychologic effects for pet and owner

5. List the common conditions addressed by physical therapist intervention.

Postsurgical: orthopedic, neurologic	Pain management
Soft tissue injury	Overuse injuries
Spinal dysfunction	Edema and circulation deficiency
Gait abnormality or lameness	Wound healing
Joint injury	Respiratory complications
Contractures	Peripheral nerve injury
Managing performance in the canine athlete	Critical care recovery
Rehabilitation for degenerative disease	Geriatric issues — hospice

6. List common physical therapy interventions.

Massage	Physical agents — heat, cold, ultrasound, electric stimulation
Manual therapy, including joint mobilization and manipulation	Electric stimulation — FES, transcutaneous electrical nerve stimulation (TENS)

Range of motion and stretching
Individualized conditioning and
    strengthening programs
Hydrotherapy
Magnetic field therapy
Postural drainage and percussion
Acupressure

Home care instruction
Functional training

Neuromuscular facilitation and reeducation
Wound care
Relaxation techniques

7. Describe a typical physical therapy session.
   After the initial visit for evaluation, a follow-up session may last 30–60 minutes. A brief discussion of responses to past treatment and new concerns occurs. The therapist assesses function and takes any objective measurements relative to the injury. The treatment protocol may include several techniques within one session. Measurements are documented after the intervention as needed. Modifications might be made to the home program. Client education and recommendations for future treatment are discussed.

8. What equipment is recommended for a rehabilitation clinic?
Portable, adjustable-setting electric
    stimulator
Ultrasound that offers 1 and 3 MHz,
    pulsed and continuous
Hot and cold pack
Stethoscope
Accustim for acupressure points
Tape measure with pressure gauge
Goniometer
Reflex hammer
Leash with collar
Muzzle
Blood pressure cuff to measure
    weight bearing in dogs

Clipper
Straps for electrodes
Conducting gel
Jumps for canine obstacle course
Physioball
Access to stairs
Treadmill
Video camera
Laser
Dog treats, carrots, corn
Hydrotherapy tank with underwater
    treadmill
Gait analysis system

9. What might be a *low-tech* approach to rehabilitation in the intensive care unit?
   • Massage and heat for relaxation
   • Ice packs to decrease edema
   • Pressure stockings to decrease edema
   • Range of motion: 2–3 times/day to prevent joint contractures
   • Postural drainage and percussion to improve ventilation
   • Positioning changes every 2 hours to prevent pressure sores and urine scald

10. What would a rehabilitation plan include for geriatric patients, especially in cases dealing with osteoarthritis?
Individualized exercise programs
Functional training
Change environment (ramps, remove
    rugs, avoid slippery surfaces)
Elevate food bowls
Mobility sling or towel walking
Massage
Range of motion
Heat and ice to decrease pain
Restrict jumping

Swimming
Education in positioning and lifting
Underwater treadmill
Pain management using TENS and
    acupressure
Wound care

11. What measurements are useful in a rehabilitation program?
- Limb circumference
- Range of motion
- Gait analysis
- Pain scale
- Functional skill inventory

12. What is the function of massage?
To stimulate circulation, reduce edema, improve muscle and tendon mobility, decrease muscle spasm, minimize scar tissue formation, and relax the patient through use of the hands to mobilize soft tissue (muscle, tendons, ligaments, and fascia).

13. Describe traditional massage techniques.
Swedish massage includes the traditional strokes: effleurage, petrissage, and friction.
- **Effleurage** is gentle stroking over large areas of the body using slight-to-moderate pressure. It can have a stimulating or calming effect depending on the pressure and speed of the strokes.
- **Petrissage** is kneading and a deeper technique directed at specific muscles to decrease spasms and increase circulation.
- **Transverse friction** decreases scar tissue and prevents adhesions. The stroke consists of small circular strokes across muscle and tendon fibers using firm pressure.

14. What is the standard protocol for a cranial cruciate ligament repair?
There is **no standard rehabilitation** protocol for any surgical procedure—all intervention is tailored to the individual patient. A variety of approaches are summarized:
Day 1—crate confinement, ice for 10–15 minutes every 2–4 hours, compression bandages, range of motion 2–3 times-day, leash walks for toileting only.
Day 2—electric stimulation to quadriceps or biceps femoris and hamstrings once per day for 15 minutes for 4–5 days, then every other day for 4–5 weeks; active movement; joint approximation; laser for pain relief and to decrease edema.
Day 7–10—begin hydrotherapy: underwater treadmill or free swimming in a pool 2–3 minutes, then work up to 10–15 minutes; leash walks 5–10 minutes on flat surfaces, no hills, ramps, or stairs; continue with electric stimulation.
Week 2—add ultrasound (pulsed); add functional training.
Week 3–4—add inclines, walks 10–15 minutes.
Week 5–6—add stairs, leash walks 15–20 minutes, add *dancing* (walking on back legs while holding front legs off floor), balance activities.
Add running, jumping, and agility exercises as directed by the veterinarian.

15. List physical therapy interventions for acute back pain.
- Ice to painful area
- Electric stimulation for pain
- Ultrasound
- Laser
- Massage
- Myofascial release
- Acupressure

16. Should acute musculoskeletal injuries be treated with cold and chronic injuries with warmth?
Cold therapy should be used for the first 24–72 hours after an injury. Light pressure bandages to prevent further edema are also recommended. In the presence of swelling or heat, even in a chronic injury, it is advisable to use cold therapy initially. Warm compresses (moist hot packs) or continued cold can be effective. Alternating warm and cold baths are also used in clinical practice.

17. What rehabilitation approaches can improve postoperative care?
- Immediate and frequent use of ice and lightweight pressure bandages to reduce edema
- Early passive range of motion and stimulation of involved musculature
- Pain management interventions

- Early weight bearing through use of an underwater treadmill
- Postural drainage and percussion as appropriate to prevent respiratory complications
- Functional training to address individual patient goals

18. What strategies are useful to encourage postoperative weight bearing?
- Wheelbarrow walk or dancing (forelimb/hindlimb usage)
- Slow walks on stairs, over obstacles, on sand, inclines and declines
- Syringe cap under contralateral foot

19. List methods to enhance recovery from fracture repairs.

Superficial heat and cold therapies	Electric stimulation
Massage	Pressure bandages
Exercise	Range-of-motion
Hydrotherapy	Controlled weight bearing

20. Define active and passive exercises.

Passive exercises are movements to the joints or muscles performed without the patient's participation. Range of motion and stretching are two common passive exercise methods used to increase flexibility. Range of motion involves cycling of a joint through all planes of movement. Each joint can be moved individually, or a total limb technique addressing several joints at the same time can be used. Stretching involves moving the muscle into an elongated position and holding it for several seconds to several minutes.

Active exercises involves the participation of the patient. The techniques of stimulating active movement in animals are aimed at improving strength, coordination, balance, and functional skills. Active exercise includes walking in a figure eight, using stairs and inclines, repeated sit-to-stand movements, underwater treadmill, and an agility obstacle course with jumps.

21. What can be done for pulmonary complications?

A rehabilitation program might include positioning, postural drainage, percussion, vibration, tracheal suctioning, rib springing, induced cough, massage, passive and active exercise, compression bandages, and standing frames or carts. Precautions to physical therapy intervention are pain, open wounds or burns, unstable cardiovascular conditions, recent skin graft, thoracotomy within the previous 24 hours, pneumothorax, coagulopathy, and rib fractures.

22. What functional skills would a physical therapist address in the dog?
- Ambulation in or on a straight line, circles, inclines, stairs, and curbs
- Arising, running, jumping, rolling, crouching, climbing
- Head and neck movements
- Performance of "work" related skills, e.g., sled dogs, police/rescue dogs

BIBLIOGRAPHY

1. Chambers JN: Postoperative care of the orthopedic patient. In Olmstead ML (ed): Small Animal Orthopedics. St. Louis, Mosby, 1995, pp 164–167.
2. Bromily M: Physiotherapy in Veterinary Medicine. Blackwell Scientific Publications, 1991.
3. Hodges CC, Palmer RH: Postoperative physical therapy. In Harari J (ed): Surgical Complications and Wound Healing. Philadelphia, W.B. Saunders, 1993, pp 389–405.
4. Manning AM, Ellis D: Physical therapy for critically ill veterinary patients: Part I. Chest physical therapy. Comp Cont Educ Pract Vet 6:675–685, 1997.
5. Millis DL, Levine D: The role of exercise and physical modalities in the treatment of osteoarthritis. Vet Clin North Am Sm Anim Prac 4:913–930, 1997.
6. Moore M, Rasmussen J: Physical therapy in small animal medicine—Part I. Comp Cont Educ Pract Vet 4:199–203, 1981.
7. Moore M, Rasmussen J: Physical therapy in small animal medicine—Part II. Comp Cont Educ Pract Vet 5:262–266, 1981.

8. Tangner CH: Physical therapy in small animal patients: Basic principles and application. Comp Cont Educ Pract Vet 10:933–936, 1984.
9. Taylor R: Postsurgical physical therapy: The missing link. Comp Cont Educ Pract Vet 12:1583–1594, 1992.
10. Bloomberg R, Dee J, Taylor R: Canine sports medicine and surgery. In Taylor R (ed): Physical Therapy in Canine Sporting Breeds. Philadelphia, W.B. Saunders, 1998, pp 265–274.

8. PERIOPERATIVE NUTRITION

Sheila M. McCullough, D.V.M., M.S., Dip. A.C.V.I.M.

1. What role does nutrition play in the perioperative patient?
- Enhances wound healing
- Enhances immunocompetence
- Speeds onset of therapeutic effects from other treatments
- Serves to meet the metabolic demands of the patient
- Improves survival rate of critical care patients

2. What are the goals of providing perioperative nutrition?
- Provide enough calories to aid the body in healing from surgery and underlying disease
- Prevent atrophy of the gut, which predisposes the patient to ulceration, bacterial translocation, and potential for sepsis
- Ensure adequate glucose levels and avoid large fluctuations
- Maintain neutral pH
- Provide organs with nutritional support to prevent organ failure as a result of malnutrition

3. Describe the pathophysiology of starvation in the critically ill patient.
Demands on the body place the patient in a hypermetabolic and catabolic state. Hypermetabolism results from the increasing hormonal response (e.g., glucagon, epinephrine, norepinephrine, and cortisol) to maintain normal glucose levels and the production of inflammatory mediators, such as cytokines (e.g., tumor necrosis factor-α, also known as cachectin; interleukin-1, interleukin-6; prostaglandins). Increased oxygen consumption, hypoglycemia, and acidosis can progress rapidly.

4. How can the anorectic patient be fed with minimal invasiveness?
Force feeding is an option, although it may lead to food aversion and a belligerent behavior. The initial approach is to test the appetite by small amounts of canned food in a flat dish. Sense of smell is enhanced by clearing nasal discharge, removing nasal tubing, using beef or chicken bouillon with food, making homemade recipes, or hand feeding. Often clients are involved in hospital feeding schedules. Appetite stimulants, such as cyproheptadine, oxazepam, and diazepam, are useful but not completely reliable and may cause inappropriate sedation. Hepatic failure in feline patients resulting from diazepam therapy has been reported.

5. What are the approaches to feeding the surgical patient?

Enteral
- Force feeding/appetite stimulation
- Nasoesophageal tube
- Nasogastric tube
- Percutaneous endoscopic gastrostomy tube

Parenteral
- Partial parenteral nutrition (PPN)
- Total parenteral nutrition (TPN)

- Gastrostomy tube
- Jejunostomy tube

6. What is parenteral nutrition?
TPN

A mixture of dextrose, amino acids, and lipid solution providing 100% of the patient's nutritional requirements in a central vein.

PPN

- Dextrose solutions that provide minimal calories to the patient
- Free amino acid solutions (FreeAmine, Aminosyn, Travasol) with balanced electrolytes added
- Amino acid and dextrose solutions (Clinimix, Quick Mix, ProcalAmine)
- Dextrose, amino acids, and lipid mixtures that provide 50% of the patient's caloric requirements

7. List the advantages and disadvantages of PPN.

Advantages	Disadvantages
• Peripheral vein	• Sepsis potential
• Noninvasive	• Partial nutrition
• Easy to obtain	• Dedicated line
• Cost-effective	• Must be rehydrated
• Can feed immediately	

8. List the advantages and disadvantages of TPN.

Advantage	Disadvantages
• Full nutrition	• Expensive
	• Central vein
	• Dedicated line
	• Sepsis potential
	• Increase feedings gradually
	• Must be rehydrated

9. List the advantages and disadvantages of enteral nutrition.

Advantages	Disadvantages
• Most physiologic	• Invasive
• Inexpensive	• Infection
• Prevents gut atrophy and ulcers	• Expensive
• Decreases bacterial translocation	• Slow feeding

10. List the advantages and disadvantages of nasoesophageal and nasogastric tubes.

Advantages	Disadvantages
• Easy to place and care for	• Must use liquid enteral solution
• Immediate nutrition	• Nasogastric tubes cross the lower esophageal sphincter (with or without reflux esophagitis)
• Bolus feeding or constant rate infusion	
• Does not require general anesthesia for placement	• Chronic vomiting may displace tube
	• May require Elizabethan collar

11. What are the benefits of an esophagostomy or pharyngostomy tube?

An **esophagostomy** is the preferred choice because of fewer surgical complications. Properly placed esophagostomy or pharyngostomy tubes can be maintained for months if needed, are large enough to give pureed canned foods, and are easily managed by the client.

12. What are the indications for percutaneous endoscopic gastrostomy tubes?
- Bypass oral, pharyngeal, and esophageal dysfunctions
- Long-term hospital or home feedings
- Supplemental nutrition for hyporexic patient

13. What are the indications for jejunostomy tubes?
- Patients with gastroesophageal, pancreatic, and proximal intestinal dysfunctions
- Nutritional support and avoidance of aspiration pneumonia
- Open abdominal procedures and need for extended nutritional support

14. When is aggressive nutritional support indicated for a surgical patient?
- Patients present with anorexia, protracted vomiting, or diarrhea for a few days
- Patients have poor body condition scores or have not eaten for at least 3 days
- Patients with sustained illnesses, such as neoplasia, severe infection, or trauma

15. When are TPN and PPN indicated?
- Patients cannot tolerate enteral feeding
- As a supplement to enteral feeding

16. What is nutritional pharmacology?

The study of the importance of particular nutrients in the diet and their trophic effects on the gut.

17. Discuss the importance of glutamine to the diet.

Glutamine is a free amino acid that has been shown to be significant in maintenance of a functional gastrointestinal lining and local immune function. Glutamine is important in gluconeogenesis, nitrogen transport, nucleotide synthesis, renal ammonia genesis, and as an energy source for dividing cells. In stressed animals, glutamine levels are low and may prove to be an essential requirement for enteral and parenteral nutrition formulations.

18. Define RER, IER, and PER.

   RER: Resting energy requirement = amount of calories to maintain minimal metabolism; $30 \times$ body weight (kg) $+ 70 =$ kcal/day (for patients weighing 2–35 kg)

   IER: Illness energy requirement = amount of calories required to feed an ill patient; IER $=$ RER $\times$ illness factor (illness factors = cage rest [1.25], postsurgery [1.30], trauma [1.5])

   PER: Partial energy requirement = amount of calories required to supply 50% of the IER

19. What are the major complications in enteral and parenteral nutrition delivery?

   Mechanical: Blocked enteral tubes and kinked catheters can present physical difficulties

   Metabolic: Alterations in electrolyte balances, hyperglycemia, acid-base disturbances, and hyperlipidemia occur. It is not uncommon to see diarrhea or soft stool from enteral nutrition.

   Septic: Parenteral solutions are an ideal growth medium for bacteria (aseptic technique is essential when administering parenteral solutions).

20. How is a patient monitored during nutritional support?

Patients should be weighed daily. **Temperature, pulse,** and **respiration** can be monitored four times a day. A minimum database of packed cell volume, total protein, glucose, and blood urea nitrogen should be performed twice a day. Monitoring electrolyte imbalances, albumin, hypertriglyceridemia, hypercholesterolemia, hyperammonemia, and urine dipstick for glucosuria and ketones is recommended. The patient should be monitored for volume overload.

21. What is refeeding syndrome?
Occasionally, when a debilitated patient is started on nutritional support, severe electrolyte disturbances, such as hypokalemia, hypophosphatemia, and hypomagnesemia, may occur. Severe hypophosphatemia may result in red blood cell hemolysis.

22. How is refeeding syndrome managed?
It may be necessary to give a blood transfusion. The main directive is to continue supportive care, correct electrolyte imbalances, and maintain perfusion.

23. Why is nutritional assessment critical for patients?
"All deaths are hateful to miserable mortals, but the most pitiable death of all is to starve" (Homer, *Odyssey* XII:341).

BIBLIOGRAPHY

1. Layton CE: Nutritional support of the surgical patient. In Harari J (ed): Surgical Complications and Wound Healing. Philadelphia, W.B. Saunders, 1993, pp 89–124.
2. Michel KE: Interventional nutrition for the critical care patient. Clin Tech Sm Anim Pract 13:204–210, 1999.
3. Remillard R, Martin R: Nutritional support in the surgical patient. Semin Vet Med Surg 5:197–207, 1990.
4. Zsombor-Murray E, Freeman LM: Peripheral Parenteral Nutrition. Compendium on Continuing Education 21(6):512–523, 1999.

9. DRESSINGS AND EXTERNAL COAPTATION

Joseph Harari, M.S., D.V.M., Dip. A.C.V.S.

1. What are the functions of bandages?
- Cover and protect open wounds
- Promote wound healing
- Reduce edema, hemorrhage, and dead space
- Immobilize osseous and soft tissue structures

2. What are the components of a bandage?
- Inner, **primary (contact)** layer
- Middle, **secondary (intermediate)** layer
- Outer, **tertiary (external)** layer

3. What are the types of and indications for dressings used in the contact layer?
Adherent
- Wet or dry gauze used to absorb exudate or mechanically débride necrotic tissue
Nonadherent
- Semiocclusive dressings that retain moisture and promote epithelialization; used during reparative stages (healthy granulation, minimal tissue necrosis)
- Occlusive dressings, completely impermeable to air and promote epithelialization and collagen synthesis

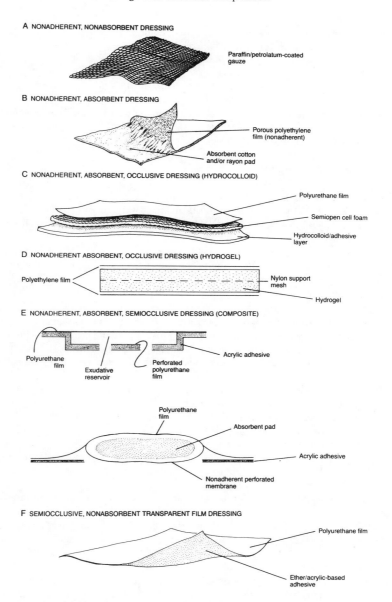

Composition of various nonadherent dressings. (Adapted from Cohen IK, Diegelmann RF, Lindblad WJ [eds]: Wound Healing, 1st ed. Philadelphia, W.B. Saunders, 1992, p 568, with permission.)

4. List examples of nonadherent, semiocclusive dressings.
- Commercial preparations (Telfa, Release)
- Petrolatum-impregnated (with or without antibiotics) autoclaved gauze sponges
- Polyurethane foam (Hydrasorb)

5. List examples of nonadherent, occlusive dressings.
- Hydrocolloids (DuoDerm)
- Hydrogels (BioDres)
- Silicone membrane (BioBrane)
- Natural products such as seaweed fibers (Curasorb)

6. What biologic tissues have been used as primary wound dressings in veterinary medicine?
- Autogenous skin grafts
- Equine amnion
- Feline greater omentum

7. Who declared, "I dressed the wound (him) and God healed it."
Ambroise Paré (1510–1590), the most celebrated surgeon of the Renaissance; famous for abolishing boiling oil treatment of gunshot wounds and using ligatures during limb amputation.

8. What are the functions and composition of the intermediate bandage layer?
To absorb wound exudate, blood, and debris away from the wound, and inner bandage layer; secure the contact layer to the wound; reduce tissue swelling; and provide limb support. Materials used for this layer include cast padding, combine or cotton roll, and disposable diapers.

9. What are the functions and composition of the outer bandage layer?
To secure the other bandage layers in place, provide pressure support, and protect the middle layer from external contamination. Materials used include porous, elastic, or waterproof adhesive tape. Conforming stretch bandage, stockinette, and cling are also used in combination with tape.

10. Which lavage solutions have been used in contaminated or infected wounds?
- Tap water (severe contamination, cytotoxic)
- Saline (mechanical flushing, acidic pH)
- Lactated Ringer's (mechanical flushing)
- 0.05% chlorhexidine (antimicrobial)
- 0.1–1% povidone-iodine (antimicrobial activity inactivated by purulence, irritating)
- Tris-EDTA (increased susceptibility of gram-negative bacteria)

11. What volume of lavage solutions should be used to treat contaminated or infected wounds?
Difficult, if not impossible, to determine from the medical literature. General recommendations (500 ml-1.0 L) are to reduce gross contamination, while avoiding tissue edema and discoloration.

12. What rate of delivery is recommended for lavage solutions?
Various systems have been described: pulsatile lavage, gravity flow, or manual (8 psi) delivery via a 35–60 gauge syringe with an 18–19 gauge needle. Caution is always expressed for dispersal of contaminants into and through diseased tissues.

13. List topical dressings that have been used in veterinary patients.
- Antimicrobials (bacitracin/neomycin/polymyxin, gentamicin, nitrofurazone, chlorhexidine, and silver sulfadiazine)
- Hydrophilic agents
- Enzymatic debridement agents
- Hydrogels
- Yeast derivatives
- Aloe vera

14. Which agents are useful in burns?
- Silver sulfadiazine (antimicrobial activity permeates eschar)
- Hydrogels (enhanced healing)
- Aloe vera (antithromboxane activity)

15. Is topical antibiotic lavage useful in reducing wound infections?
Not likely; some surgeons are convinced a reduction of bacterial contamination in the suction units may be the major benefit.

16. What are some general guidelines for applying bandages to small animals?
- Animals often require chemical restraint.
- Limbs and joints should be placed in near-normal positions, unless elimination of weight bearing is required.
- Joints above and below the injury need to be stabilized.
- Bandages and splints should be evaluated weekly for damage, soiling, or constriction of tissues.
- Postsplintage radiographs are useful in confirming adequacy of bone alignment.

17. What is a Robert Jones bandage?
A bulky and compressive cotton roll applied to injuries below the elbow and stifle joints. In general, 1 lb of cotton is used per 20 lb of body weight; correctly applied, it should sound like a ripe watermelon when tapped. Named after the British surgeon, **Sir Robert Jones** (1858–1933).

18. What is a modified Robert Jones bandage?
Similar to a **Schanz** (German orthopedist, 1868–1931) **padded limb bandage;** cast padding is used instead of cotton roll and often supported with metal, aluminum, wooden, or cast splint.

19. What is a spica splint?
A lateral bandage (often supported with splints) applied over the shoulder and hip joints, adjacent vertebrae, and trunk. Used to immobilize proximal limb injuries; the name is derived from the Latin term, *spica,* meaning "ear of wheat" (i.e., the bandage crosses on itself).

20. What is a Velpeau sling?
A padded bandage applied to a flexed forelimb held in close apposition to the thorax used to treat shoulder luxation and scapular fracture injuries; name is derived from a French surgeon, **Alfred Armand Louis Velpeau** (1795–1867).

21. What is an Ehmer sling?
Tape and bandaging material applied to a pelvic limb to produce non–weight bearing, internal rotation, and abduction; used to treat coxofemoral fractures and luxations. Named after **Anton Emerson Ehmer,** a Washington State University veterinary alumnus (1918).

22. What is a Schroeder-Thomas splint?
A traction device composed of bandages, tape, and aluminum rods used for treatment of minimally displaced forelimb and hindlimb fractures. Named after a veterinarian, **E. F. Schroeder,** who described traction (1933) and modification of a splint developed by a British surgeon (**Hugh Owen Thomas,** 1834–1891).

23. What is a pelvic limb sling?
A combined limb and abdominal wrap used to control weightbearing after hindlimb or pelvic injuries (surgery). It permits modified joint motions to prevent fibrosis and was developed by **Louis McCoy,** a veterinary technician, at the Henry Bergh Memorial Hospital in New York City during the 1970s.

24. Which factors determine the ultimate strength of a cast?
The tensile and compressive strengths of the material as well as the degree of adhesion (lamination) between the cast layers. The latter is affected by the amount and distribution of resin and efficiency of application.

25. What are some differences between plaster of Paris and fiberglass casts?
Plaster of Paris is stronger in compression than tension because of its crystalline structure, whereas fiberglass casting tapes are stronger in tension. Synthetic casts are lightweight, radiolucent, easy to apply, and more expensive than plaster casts.

BIBLIOGRAPHY

1. Brockman DJ, Pardo AD: Omentum-enhanced reconstruction and chronic nonhealing wounds in cats. Vet Surg 25:99–104, 1996.
2. Fossum TW: Small Animal Surgery, 1st ed. St Louis, Mosby-Year Book, 1997, pp 91–107.
3. Harari J: Small Animal Surgery, 1st ed. Baltimore, Williams & Wilkins, 1996, pp 53–60.
4. Lozier SM: Topical wound therapy. In Harari J (ed): Surgical Complications and Wound Healing, 1st ed. Philadelphia, W.B. Saunders, 1993.
5. Morgan WP, Binnington AG: The effect of occlusive and semi-occlusive dressings on the healing of acute full-thickness wounds. Vet Surg 23:494–502, 1994.
6. Swaim SF, Henderson RA: Small Animal Wound Management, 2nd ed. Baltimore, Williams & Wilkins, 1997, pp 53–86.
7. Wilson DG, Vanderby R: An evaluation of fiberglass cast application techniques. Vet Surg 24:118–121, 1995.

10. MONITORING THE POSTOPERATIVE PATIENT

Steven L. Marks, B.V.Sc., M.S., M.R.C.V.S., Dip. A.C.V.I.M.

1. What parameters should be evaluated postoperatively?
Parameters are based on the underlying disease process or the surgical procedure performed.
- Heart rate
- Pulse quality
- Respiratory rate
- Capillary refill time
- Body weight
- Body temperature
- PCV
- Total protein
- Serum glucose
- Activated clotting time (ACT)

2. List techniques used to monitor the respiratory system.
- Visual assessment of respiratory rate and pattern
- Thoracic auscultation
- Thoracic percussion
- Pulse oximetry
- Blood gas analysis
- Thoracic radiographs

3. What is pulse oximetry?
A noninvasive technique that provides continuous estimation of arterial oxyhemoglobin saturation. A light source and photodetector are used to measure a difference in light absorption between pulsatile blood and background absorption to calculate a percentage of hemoglobin saturation (SaO_2). It does not correlate directly with PaO_2 but is an indicator of tissue perfusion. The pulse oximeter also provides a pulse rate.

4. What information does arterial blood gas analysis provide?
- pH
- PaO_2
- $PaCO_2$
- Sodium bicarbonate
- Base excess
- Hemoglobin saturation

5. What is the A-a gradient?

The **alveolar-arterial** gradient is calculated using arterial blood gas analysis in hypoxemic patients.

$$A = (BP - 47).21 - PaCO_2/.8$$
$$a = PaO_2$$

BP is barometric pressure.
47 is the vaporization pressure of water.
.21 is the approximate concentration of O_2 in room air.
.8 is the respiratory exchange ratio and is a constant.
A-a should be < 10 mm Hg.
Abnormal values indicate a significant oxygen transport problem.
At sea level (barometric pressure = 760 mm Hg), the formula can be simplified to 150−$PaCO_2/.8$.

6. How is thoracic percussion performed?

Running the middle finger of one hand along the intercostal space and striking this finger with the middle finger of the opposite hand allows thoracic percussions to be heard. Change in resonance assists in detecting pulmonary or pleural space disease.

7. List techniques used to monitor the cardiovascular system.
- Thoracic auscultation
- Palpation of peripheral arterial pulses
- Capillary refill time
- Electrocardiography
- Echocardiography
- Thoracic radiographs
- Cardiac output

8. Does the ECG provide information about cardiac function?

No. The ECG provides information concerning electric activity of the heart and conduction of this activity. The morphology of the complexes suggests chamber size.

9. What is central venous pressure?

Central venous pressure is measured by placing a large-bore catheter via the jugular vein into the intrathoracic cranial vena cava. The catheter is connected to a fluid-filled line creating a continuous fluid column between the right atrium and a manometer. The manometer is zeroed at the approximate level of the right atrium with the animal in lateral or sternal recumbency. The monitoring of this parameter can be used to assess right atrial pressures and correlate well with hydration status. **Normal values for the dog and cat are 0–5 cm H_2O.**

10. What is a pulmonary artery catheter?

A flexible, balloon-tipped, flow-directed catheter placed into the pulmonary artery (also called **Swan-Ganz catheter**). This catheter has two ports. When placed correctly, the proximal port is in the right atrium and the distal port in the pulmonary artery. The information provided includes cardiac output, pulmonary artery pressure, mixed venous O_2, central venous pressure, pulmonary wedge pressure, and core body temperature.

11. Name three techniques for obtaining blood pressure measurements in the dog and cat.
1. **Direct**—catheterization of peripheral artery and connection to pressure transducer.
2. **Indirect**—Doppler crystal with inflatable cuff.
3. **Indirect**—oscillometric.

12. List the laboratory tests used to evaluate the coagulation system.
- ACT
- Prothrombin time (PT)
- Partial thromboplastin time (PTT)
- Buccal mucosal bleeding time (BMBT)

13. What do the tests measure?
- The ACT and the PTT evaluate the intrinsic and common pathways.
- The PT evaluates the extrinsic and common pathways.
- The BMBT evaluates platelet function and Von Willebrand's factor.

The intrinsic pathway can be remembered by the pneumonic **"Kmart is in."** At Kmart, the price is not $12, but rather $11.98 (intrinsic pathway contains factors 12, 11, 9, and 8). The extrinsic pathway only has one factor (7). The tests with more letters (ACT and PTT) evaluate the pathway with more factors (intrinsic). The test with fewer letters (PT) evaluates the pathway with fewer factors (extrinsic).

14. What is the normal urine output for a dog and cat?
1–2 ml/kg/hr. This is measured by an indwelling urinary catheter with a closed collection system.

15. What are ins and outs?
Ins and outs describe a technique for calculating fluid requirements based on measurement of urine output in the dehydrated patient with oliguria or diuresis. Initially a fluid rate based on the patient's hydration status is administered for 4 hours. When using this technique, fluid administration can be divided into six, 4-hour periods. At the end of the first 4 hours, urine output is measured, and this is the sensible portion of the fluid requirement for the next 4 hours. The insensible portion of the fluid requirement is calculated based on 20 ml/kg/24 h (one third of maintenance, which is 60 ml/kg/24 h) divided by 6. By calculating the insensible requirements and measuring the sensible requirements, the clinician meets the fluid requirements of the patient without overhydrating the patient.

16. List techniques for evaluating the neurologic system.
- Evaluate mentation
- Cranial nerve examination
- Complete neurologic examination

17. List monitoring techniques that can be used to assess the abdominal cavity.
- Abdominal palpation
- Abdominal paracentesis
- Diagnostic peritoneal lavage
- Abdominal radiographs
- Abdominal ultrasound

18. How does one monitor for pain in postoperative patients?
Signs of pain:
- Tachycardia
- Tachypnea
- Hypertension
- Cardiac arrhythmias
- Dilated pupils
- Salivation
- Vocalization
- Restlessness
- Behavior changes—aggression or depression
- Abnormal body postures
- Bruxism (teeth grinding)

BIBLIOGRAPHY

1. Haskins SC: Monitoring the critically ill patient. Vet Clin North Am Small Anim Pract 18:1059–1078, 1989.
2. Kaplan PM: Monitoring. In Murtaugh RJ, Kaplan PM (eds): Veterinary Emergency and Critical Care Medicine. Chicago, Mosby-Year Book, 1992, pp 21–39.
3. Kolata RJ: Monitoring the surgical patient. In Slatter D (ed): Textbook of Small Animal Surgery. Philadelphia, W.B. Saunders, 1993, pp 212–224.

11. MINIMALLY INVASIVE SURGERY

Timothy C. McCarthy, D.V.M., Ph.D., Dip. A.C.V.S.

1. What are the main advantages of minimally invasive surgery?
- Exploratory examination and surgery performed in the chest and abdomen through 5–10 mm diameter portals without painful and traumatic laparotomy or thoracotomy.
- Direct visualization of abdominal and thoracic structures and pathology.
- Submacroscopic lesions can be easily visualized with laparoscopy or thoracoscopy.
- The visual field is moved into the area of the operative site.

2. List the most common indications for minimally invasive abdominal and thoracic surgery.
- Thoracic and abdominal neoplasia
- Ovarian remnant syndrome
- Cushing's disease (adrenal hyperplasia and neoplasia)
- Cryptorchidism
- Cholecystectomy
- Pancreatic biopsy and partial pancreatectomy
- Gastric volvulus prevention (gastropexy)
- Spontaneous pneumothorax
- Pericardial effusions (pericardial window)
- Pleural effusions (thoracic duct occlusion)
- Abdominal hemorrhage, hemothorax, pneumothorax
- Ovariohysterectomy

3. Can minimally invasive surgery be cost-effective (and profitable) in small animal practice?
Yes. The time savings in some common minimally invasive procedures are dramatic and can make minimally invasive surgery a profitable endeavor. The most significant deterrents (cost of the equipment and time spent on the learning curve) are easily overcome.

4. How long do minimally invasive surgical procedures take compared with traditional surgery?
An accomplished minimally invasive surgeon can expect to complete procedures in a time similar to the intraabdominal or intrathoracic portion of open surgery, without having to perform an open approach or closure.

5. What instrumentation is needed for minimally invasive surgery?
- Metzenbaum scissors
- Tissue graspers (two)
- Dissectors
- Suture scissors
- Knot pusher
- Suction and irrigation cannula
- Hemostatic clip applicators
- Pretied suture loops
- Additional instrument cannulas

6. Is a video camera required for performing minimally invasive surgery?
Yes. A good-quality endoscopic video camera is an absolute necessity for performing minimally invasive surgery, whereas diagnostic laparoscopy and thoracoscopy can be performed using direct visualization without a video camera.

7. Is an insufflator required for performing minimally invasive abdominal surgery?

Yes. An insufflator is necessary for performing minimally invasive surgery, whereas diagnostic laparoscopy can be performed without an insufflator using manual control from a flow valve, such as the nitrous oxide flowmeter on an anesthetic machine.

8. Is electrosurgery needed for most currently performed minimally invasive surgical procedures?

No.

9. Can the same instrumentation and techniques be used for minimally invasive thoracic surgery as are used for minimally invasive abdominal surgery?

Yes. The major differences in equipment for thoracoscopy are an abdominal insufflator is not needed, an anesthetic ventilator is required, cannula designs are different, 30° telescopes have advantages, and double-lumen endotracheal tubes may be needed for selective bronchial intubation when one-lung ventilation is required.

10. What telescope size and configuration are best for minimally invasive surgery in small animal practice?

The most common telescopes used for minimally invasive abdominal and thoracic surgery are 10- and 5-mm diameter laparoscopes. Another important telescope factor is the visual angle. Zero degree telescopes, which view straight ahead, with the axis of the visual field centered on the axis of the telescope, provide the most accurate image orientation, least distortion, and least operator disorientation and are optimal for minimally invasive surgery. In the chest, a 30° angle of view, in which the axis of the visual field is angled 30° from the axis of the telescope, has advantages because the ribs of the rigid chest wall can interfere with positioning of the telescope.

11. Is more than one telescope needed?

No. A 5-mm-diameter, 0° visual angle telescope can be applied effectively for most currently performed thoracic and abdominal, diagnostic and minimally invasive surgical procedures in small animal patients.

12. How much of an investment in equipment is required?

Total cost for a basic minimally invasive surgery system is $20,000–50,000. Addition of minimally invasive surgery capability to an already existing diagnostic laparoscopy and thoracoscopy system could cost $5000–15,000.

13. Can this equipment be used for anything else?

The video system and light source can be used for all diagnostic and operative endoscopic procedures. A 5-mm diameter 0° degree laparoscope can be used for diagnostic laparoscopy and thoracoscopy, bronchoscopy in small dogs, and transurethral or percutaneous cystoscopy in large female dogs.

14. Which insufflation gases and pressures are recommended for minimally invasive abdominal surgery?

Carbon dioxide and nitrous oxide are readily available, inexpensive, colorless, and eliminated through the lungs. Carbon dioxide is the standard for minimally invasive human surgery and has the major advantage of not supporting combustion. The major disadvantages of carbon dioxide are that it forms carbolic acid, which is irritating to visceral surfaces, and absorption can cause hypercarbia with acidosis and subsequent deleterious physiologic consequences. Advantages of nitrous oxide are that it is not irritating, has analgesic properties that augment anesthetics and postoperative pain management, and does not contribute to hypercarbia. The major disadvantage of nitrous oxide is that it can support combustion and, in the presence of methane gas from the large bowel, can be explosive; it cannot be used in procedures employing electrosurgery or lasers. Insufflation pressures (10–20 mm Hg) recommended for minimally invasive abdominal surgery are the same as for diagnostic laparoscopy.

15. Is insufflation used for minimally invasive thoracic surgery?

Pleural insufflation is used only for the case with stiff noncompliant lungs that do not collapse with simple pneumothorax.

16. Is one-lung ventilation necessary for minimally invasive thoracic surgery?

One-lung ventilation, the procedure of choice in human thoracoscopy, is not necessary for diagnostic thoracoscopy or for basic operative thoracoscopy. Single-lung ventilation produces complete collapse of the lung on the side of the invaded hemithorax. This greatly facilitates performing surgical procedures by improving visualization through reduced lung volume and reduced tissue movement with ventilator excursions.

17. What is VATS?

Video-assisted-thoracic surgery; synonymous with minimally invasive thoracic surgery.

18. How is patient positioning and preparation relative to preparation for open surgery?

Preparation of patients for minimally invasive surgery is essentially the same as for open surgery. Anesthetic considerations are similar to those for open surgery, but one must consider the anesthetic consequences of abdominal insufflation and selective intubation with single-lung ventilation.

19. How does postoperative recovery from minimally invasive surgery compare with open surgery?

Postoperative recovery is much faster with minimally invasive surgery than with an open laparotomy or thoracotomy. Patients are typically fully recovered, pain-free, and acting like nothing was done within a few hours after the procedure. Many patients can be released from the hospital on the day of or day after surgery (assuming no severe underlying disease processes).

20. Are there are contraindications for performing minimally invasive surgery?

Inadequate level of minimally invasive surgical skills.

21. Discuss the most common complications of minimally invasive surgery.

Most complications of diagnostic laparoscopy and minimally invasive abdominal surgery are associated with abdominal wall penetration and with insufflation. Severe complications associated with insufflation include:

- Laceration of solid organs with the Veress needle or with trocar placement
- Perforation of a hollow viscus with a trocar
- Perforation or laceration of major abdominal vessels
- Overinsufflation causing cardiorespiratory compromise or abdominal wall or diaphragm injury
- Pneumothorax from inadvertent penetration of the diaphragm
- Gas embolism

With proper care, attention to detail, and adequate training, the incidence of significant complications with minimally invasive thoracic and abdominal surgery is low.

22. Where can one receive training on minimally invasive surgery in animals, and are there any good references available?

Courses are available that cover instrumentation, indications, and technique with wet laboratories to provide initial exposure and experience. The definitive publication on minimally invasive surgery in veterinary medicine is *Veterinary Endosurgery* edited by Lynn Freeman.

23. What is the learning curve for minimally invasive surgery, and is it worth the effort?
Basic minimally invasive surgery, even with the difficulties of becoming proficient, is within the reach of anyone who is willing to make the effort and time to learn.

BIBLIOGRAPHY

1. Faunt KK, Cohen LA, Jones BD: Cardiopulmonary effects of bilateral hemithorax ventilation and diagnostic thoracoscopy in dogs. Am J Vet Res 59:1491–1498, 1998.
2. Faunt KK, Jones BD, Turk JR: Evaluation of biopsy specimens obtained during thoracoscopy from lungs of clinically normal dogs. Am J Vet Res 59:1499–1502, 1998.
3. Freeman LJ (ed): Veterinary Endosurgery. St. Louis, Mosby, 1999.
4. Remedios AM, Ferguson J: Minimally invasive surgery: Laparoscopy and thoracoscopy in small animals. Comp Cont Educ Pract Vet 18:1191–1198, 1996.
5. Twedt DC: Laparoscopy of the liver and pancreas. In Tams TR (ed): Small Animal Endoscopy. St. Louis, Mosby, 1999, pp 409–426.
6. Walton RS: Thoracoscopy. In Tams TR (ed): Small Animal Endoscopy. St. Louis, Mosby, 1999, pp 471–488.

12. ARTHROSCOPY

Timothy C. McCarthy, D.V.M., Ph.D., Dip. A.C.V.S.

1. What are the indications for arthroscopy in small animals?
Whenever a history, physical finding, radiographic change, or laboratory result suggests **joint disease.**

2. What are the major advantages of arthroscopy over conventional surgery?
1. Arthroscopy can provide more information about intraarticular pathology than any other diagnostic technique, including postmortem examination.
2. Arthroscopes magnify intra-articular structures, allowing visualization of anatomic details and pathologic changes that are beyond the resolution of radiographs, computed tomography, and magnetic resonance imaging.
3. Submacroscopic lesions missed with open surgical exploration can be easily visualized with arthroscopy.
4. The small sizes of telescopes allow placement into the deepest parts of joints and, combined with angulation (30°), provide visual access to areas not seen with open surgery.
5. Arthroscopy is a minimally invasive technique with less tissue trauma compared with arthrotomy.

3. Are there any disadvantages?
Equipment cost and the long, difficult learning process.

4. How much does arthroscopy equipment cost?
A basic arthroscopy setup with one telescope, hand operative instruments, and a video camera costs approximately $15,000. A complete setup with multiple telescopes, a power cartilage shaver, and a complete video system costs greater than $40,000.

5. Which joints can be examined with arthroscopy in dogs and cats?
In **dogs,** most commonly, the shoulder, elbow, and stifle joints, much less commonly, the carpus, hip, and hock joints.
Arthroscopy has been performed on the **stifle** of **cats,** but its use is largely unexplored in cats.

6. List the most common diagnoses with arthroscopy according to joints.

Shoulder
- OCD
- Bicipital tendinitis and ruptures
- Medial glenohumeral ligament and subscapularis tendon injuries
- Lateral glenoid labial separations
- Chondromalacia
- Ununited supraglenoid tubercle
- Neoplasia

Elbow
- Coronoid processes fragmentation
- OCD of the humerus
- Ununited anconeal process
- Joint incongruity
- Intracondylar fractures
- Synovitis and villus synovial proliferation

Radiocarpal
- Radial carpal bone fractures
- Chip fractures of the dorsal margin of the distal radius
- Dorsal joint capsule tears
- Immune-mediated arthropathies

Hip
- Hip dysplasia
- Dorsal joint capsule tears

Stifle
- Cruciate ligaments rupture
- Meniscal injuries
- OCD of the femoral condyles
- Medial patellar luxation
- Degenerative joint disease
- Intracapsular surgical failures
- Neoplasia

Hock
- OCD of the talus
- Intraarticular fractures
- Immune-mediated arthropathies

7. List the most common surgical procedures performed according to joints.

Shoulder
- OCD cartilage flap removal and lesion débridement
- Bicipital tendon transection
- Osteophyte and joint mouse removal

Elbow
- Coronoid processes fragment removal
- Coronoid process revision for incongruity
- OCD cartilage flap removal and lesion débridement
- Anconeal process removal
- Osteophyte removal

Radiocarpal
- Carpal chip removal

Stifle
- Cruciate ligament débridement and removal
- Meniscectomy—partial
- OCD cartilage flap removal and lesion débridement
- Meniscal release
- Osteophyte removal

Hock
- OCD cartilage flap removal and lesion débridement
- Joint mouse removal
- Tarsal chip removal

8. What additional equipment is required for arthroscopy?

1. **Telescope cannulas** ($3,700): Arthroscopes must be used with a cannula or sheath that protects the telescope and provides a channel for fluid flow.

2. **Egress cannulas** ($500–700): A site is required for outflow of fluid from joints to maintain a clear visual field during arthroscopy.

3. **Operating cannula** ($400): Access for instrumentation is established and maintained by placing a cannula into the joint at the operative portal site.

4. **Operative hand instruments** ($1,800–3,600): Rongeurs, forceps, curets, probes, knives.

5. **Light source** ($3,000–3,500): A light source and fiberoptic light guide cable are required for arthroscopy.

6. **Power shaver** (optional; $8,000): Used to remove cartilage, bone, and soft tissues and to smooth surfaces after tissue removal.

7. **Fluid pumps** (optional; $2,500–8,000): Mechanical pumps maintain constant pressures and flows (such as gravity).

8. **Video system** ($10,000–30,000): Camera, monitor, printer and recorder.

9. **Does one need a power shaver to get started with arthroscopy?**
No. The potential for excessive joint damage is greatly increased when an inexperienced surgeon attempts to use a power shaver.

10. **What is the optimum fluid for joint irrigation during arthroscopy?**
There are no proven clinical disadvantages or adverse effects of using either **lactated Ringer's solution** or **saline.**

11. **Where are the portals for the commonly examined joints?**
   A. Shoulder joint portals
   Telescope: Lateral portal placed distal to the tip of the acromion process and cranial to the acromion portion of the deltoid muscle.
   Egress: An outflow portal is established on the cranial aspect of the joint medial to the greater tubercle and lateral or medial to the bicipital tendon.
   Operative: A caudolateral (similar to surgery) portal is used for removing OCD treatments. A cranial operative portal site is employed for transecting the bicipital tendon.
   B. Elbow joint portals
   Telescope:
   - **Medial:** Located 1–1.5 cm directly distal and caudal to the tip of the medial humeral epicondyle.
   - **Craniolateral:** At the intersection of the cranial margin of the radial head and cranial aspect of the capitulum.
   - **Caudal:** The telescope can also be inserted into the olecranon fossa from medial, from lateral, or through the triceps tendon. This portal allows visualization of the anconeal process and olecranon fossa and provides access to the lateral coronoid process.
   - **Operative:**
   - **Craniomedial:** Caudal to the medial collateral ligament and 1.0 to 1.5 cm cranial and slightly proximal to the cameral portal.
   - **Lateral:** Access to the lateral coronoid process of the ulna and capitulum can be obtained by entering the joint on the lateral surface distal to the epicondyle.
   - **Craniolateral:** An operative portal can also be established at the craniolateral camera portal site.
   - **Egress:** A caudal portal with the cannula positioned in the olecranon fossa.
   C. Radiocarpal joint portals
   All portals for the radiocarpal joint are on the cranial or dorsal aspect of the joint.
   D. Hip joint portals
   All portals for the hip joint are on the dorsal aspect of the joint.
   E. Stifle joint portals
   Telescope: Cranial aspect of the joint medial or lateral to the patellar tendon approximately halfway between the distal end of the patella and the tibial crest.
   Operative: Placed on the side of the patellar tendon not used for the telescope and at the same level as the telescope.
   Egress: Suprapatellar pouch.
   F. Hock joint portals
   Telescope: All four quadrants of the tibiotarsal joint can be entered for arthroscopy.

Dorsal: Telescope and operative portals are interchangeable and are either medial or lateral to the long digital extensor tendon and the tendon of the cranial tibial muscle on the dorsal aspect of the joint.

Plantar: Medial or lateral, at the junction of the plantar margin of the distal tibial articular surface and the plantar portion of the trochlear ridge of the talus.

Operative: Access to OCD lesions on the medial ridge of the talus can be achieved through a medial operative portal distal to the medial malleolus and immediately caudal to the collateral ligament.

Egress: The tibiotarsal joint is small, and in many cases there is not enough room for all three portals.

12. How is the patient positioned for arthroscopy on the different joints?
Most commonly, in a similar manner to what would be used for an open arthrotomy.

13. How long do typical arthroscopic procedures take compared with conventional surgery?
For the experienced arthroscopic surgeon, commonly performed procedures (OCD lesion or coronoid process fragment removal) take considerably less time than an open arthrotomy. Times are dramatically longer for the beginner. Speed is not the most important criterion or the most important advantage of arthroscopy over open arthrotomy.

14. How does postoperative recovery differ from that of open arthrotomy?
Recovery is much faster after arthroscopy than after an open arthrotomy. Most dogs recover to their preoperative status of lameness and pain within a few hours after arthroscopy.

15. What are the complications of arthroscopy?
Clinically significant complications are uncommon.
Potential complications include:
- Failure to enter the joint
- Articular cartilage damage
- Periarticular fluid accumulation
- Neurovascular injury (**rare**)
- Infection (**rare**)

16. What are the contraindications for arthroscopy?
To date, none.

17. How does one learn arthroscopy?
Courses are available that cover instrumentation, indications, and technique with hands-on wet laboratories to provide initial exposure and experience. Additional learning can be obtained on cadavers and by performing arthroscopy, initially as a diagnostic procedure, then as an operative procedure, on every joint that is going to have an open arthrotomy.

18. How difficult is arthroscopy to learn?
Arthroscopy is the most difficult of all the endoscopic techniques to master.

19. If arthroscopy is this difficult, is it worth learning?
Yes, because of its significance in small animal orthopedics.

20. Is the fragmented coronoid process syndrome a surgical or a medical disease?
Neither. It is an **arthroscopic disease**. Results after arthroscopic revision of the elbow joint for coronoid process fragmentation are superior to those with surgical or medical management.

CONTROVERSY

21. Which is the best arthroscope for small animal arthroscopy?

Commonly used telescopes include a long 2.7-mm arthroscope (universal telescope), a short 2.7-mm arthroscope, a 2.4-mm arthroscope, and a 1.9-mm arthroscope. Each has advantages, disadvantages, and applications. A practical answer to this question is based on practice type more than the attributes of individual telescopes. If the telescope is to be used exclusively for arthroscopy, the short 2.7-mm or the 2.4-mm arthroscope is the best choice. If the telescope is to be used for multiple applications (rhinoscopy and cystoscopy), the long 2.7-mm arthroscope is the best choice.

BIBLIOGRAPHY

 1. McCarthy TC: Arthroscopy. In Freeman LJ (ed): Veterinary Endosurgery. St. Louis, Mosby, 1999, pp 237–250.
 2. Taylor RA: Arthroscopy. In Tams TA (ed): Small Animal Endoscopy. St. Louis, Mosby, 1998, pp 461–470.
 3. van Bree HJ, Van Ryssen B: Diagnostic and surgical arthroscopy in osteochondrosis lesions. Vet Clin N Am Sm Anim Pract 28:161–189, 1998.

13. SUTURES AND STAPLES

Bradley R. Coolman, D.V.M., M.S.

1. What are functions of sutures?

To facilitate healing (approximation of divided tissues) and control hemorrhage (ligation of severed vessels).

2. Do sutures have any negative effects on healing wounds?

Yes. Suture materials are foreign bodies in the wound, can delay healing, and can lead to the development of infection. Cutaneous wounds held together with tape heal faster than sutured wounds, suggesting that sutures may delay healing. In a classic study of human subjects, the number of *Staphylococcus* required to cause a subcutaneous infection decreased 10,000-fold by adding a single silk suture to the wound.

3. What guidelines should be used when placing sutures in surgical wounds?

The fewest number of the smallest diameter, least reactive sutures required to give adequate support to the wounded tissues should be used.

4. List the characteristics of an *ideal suture material.*
   - Adequate tensile strength
   - Good knot security
   - Easy to handle
   - Nonreactive, nonelectrolytic, noncapillary, nonallergenic, nontoxic
   - Does not promote bacterial adherence or growth
   - Absorbable at a dependable rate after healing is complete
   - Readily available
   - Easily sterilized
   - Inexpensive

5. Does the ideal suture material exist?
No. Some of the currently available synthetic suture materials come close.

6. How are suture materials classified?
- Natural origin versus synthetic
- Absorbable versus nonabsorbable
- Multifilament versus monofilament

7. What is the difference between natural and synthetic sutures?
- **Natural** origin sutures are derived from plant (e.g., cotton) or animal (e.g., catgut, silk) sources.
- **Synthetic** origin sutures are polymers from man-made sources.

8. What is the difference between absorbable and nonabsorbable sutures?
- **Absorbable** sutures undergo degradation and rapid loss of tensile strength within 60 days of implantation.
- **Nonabsorbable** sutures retain tensile strength for > 60 days after implantation.

9. What is the difference between multifilament and monofilament sutures?
- **Multifilament** sutures are made by twisting or braiding multiple smaller strands of a material into a larger suture. These sutures have an irregular surface, which increases the friction (drag) during placement and can harbor bacteria away from the patient's immune system.
- **Monofilament** sutures are a single, smooth strand of suture material made by extrusion. These materials have less tissue drag and decreased bacterial adherence.

10. How are some commonly used suture materials classified?
- Chromic catgut—natural, absorbable, multifilament
- Silk—natural, nonabsorbable, multifilament
- Polyglactin 910 (Vicryl), Polyglycolic acid (Dexon)—synthetic, absorbable, multifilament
- Polydioxanone (PDS), Polyglyconate (Maxon), Poliglecaprone 25 (Monocryl)—synthetic, absorbable, monofilament
- Polypropylene (Prolene), Nylon (Ethilon)—synthetic, nonabsorbable, monofilament

11. What is the origin of catgut suture material?
Not from the feline intestinal tract. Catgut is derived from the submucosal layer of **sheep intestine** or the serosa of **bovine intestine** and is composed of formaldehyde-treated collagen fibers.

12. How is catgut degraded and absorbed?
Catgut is absorbed in a two-staged process involving macrophages (**phagocytosis**). First, molecular bonds are broken by acid hydrolysis and collagenolysis. Then, the protein is digested and absorbed by proteolytic enzymes. Because catgut is a foreign protein, it stimulates a significant inflammatory reaction after implantation.

13. How are synthetic absorbable sutures degraded?
Synthetic absorbable sutures are broken down by **hydrolysis** through esterase enzyme activity. These materials are associated with a significantly decreased inflammatory process when compared with catgut and have a more consistent rate of absorption and a more constant rate of tensile strength loss after implantation in surgical wounds.

14. List commonly used absorbable suture materials from highest to lowest initial tensile strength.
- Poliglecaprone 25 (Monocryl) (**strongest**)
- Polyglyconate (Maxon)

- Polydioxanone (PDS)
- Polyglactin 910 (Vicryl)
- Polyglycolic acid (Dexon)
- Chromic catgut (**weakest**)

15. Which absorbable suture material retains its tensile strength the longest after implantation in a surgical wound?
Polydioxanone sulfate (PDS). It takes PDS approximately 6 weeks to lose half of its original tensile strength.

16. List commonly used nonabsorbable suture materials from highest to lowest initial tensile strength.
- Stainless steel (**strongest**)
- Polyester (Ethibond, Mersilene)
- Polymerized caprolactum (Vetafil, Braunamid)
- Nylon (Ethilon)
- Polypropylene (Prolene)
- Silk (**weakest**)

17. What determines the strength of a freshly closed surgical wound?
Sutured wounds are only as strong as the **tissue** anchoring the sutures. The strength of a closed wound depends on content and orientation of the collagen fibers in the sutured tissue (not the strength of the suture material).

18. What are the relative holding strengths of soft tissues?
- **Strongest**—ligaments, tendons, fascia, skin
- **Intermediate**—muscle, hollow organs (stomach and small intestine > colon and urinary bladder)
- **Weakest**—fat, parenchymal organs (liver, kidney, spleen)

19. What is *knot security?*
The ability of a suture to hold without slipping when tied with a square knot. Knot security is a relative measurement and an inherent property of the suture material.

20. How many throws are needed to tie a secure knot?
The **minimum** number of throws required depends on the suture material and suture pattern.
- **Simple interrupted pattern:**
  Stainless steel—2 throws (one square knot)
  Polyglactin 910, polyglycolic acid, surgical gut, polypropylene—3 throws
  Polydioxanone, nylon—4 throws
- **Starting continuous patterns:** add one additional throw for minimum security.
- **Ending continuous patterns:**
  Polyglycolic acid, surgical gut, polypropylene—5 throws
  Polyglactin 910, nylon—6 throws
  Polydioxanone—7 throws

21. What is the most frequent cause of dehiscence for beginning surgeons?
Improperly tied knots.

22. What are the advantages and disadvantages of interrupted suture patterns?
- **Advantages:**
  Greater security
  Allow for precise adjustment of tension at each point of suturing

- **Disadvantages:**
  Use more suture material (poor suture economy)
  Leave greater amounts of foreign material in the wound
  More time-consuming to place compared with continuous patterns.

23. What is capillarity?
Ability of a suture material to act as a *wick* and transport contaminated fluid along the suture to adjacent sterile tissues.

24. Which suture materials have the greatest degree of capillary action?
Multifilament suture materials such as chromic catgut, silk, coated caprolactum, polyester, and cotton, have the most capillarity and should be avoided in contaminated and infected wounds. Multifilament suture materials have a large surface area and interstices to harbor bacteria.

25. List some principles for selection and use of suture needles.
- Swaged needles are less traumatic and are preferred to eyed needles.
- Suturing deeper tissues requires a needle with a greater curvature.
- Taper point needles should be used whenever possible because they are less traumatic and make a smaller hole in the tissue.
- Cutting point needles should be used for skin, tendons, ligaments, and dense fascia.

26. What are the advantages and disadvantages of using surgical stapling devices in small animal surgery?
- **Advantages:**
  Speed
  Consistency of application
  Security of hemostasis
  Utility in areas that are difficult to access (i.e., deep cavity ligation)
- **Disadvantages:**
  Increased cost
  Lack of availability of stapling equipment in many practices
  Lack of familiarity with stapling techniques
  Potential for failure if used improperly

27. What are some surgical stapling instruments used in small animal surgery?
- **Skin staplers** have been used for a wide variety of surgical applications, including skin closure, fixation of drains and surgical drapes, securing mesh for hernia repairs, fashioning colostomies, closure of gastrointestinal wounds, intestinal anastomoses, fixation of gastropexies, and emergency closure of penetrating cardiac wounds.
- **Vascular clips** are V-shaped metallic staples that are useful for rapid hemostasis or vessel ligation.
- **Ligating-dividing staplers (LDS)** apply two U-shaped vascular clips and simultaneously divide the vessel (useful for rapid splenectomy).
- **Thoracoabdominal (TA)** stapling instruments (United States Surgical Corporation, USSC) and the **proximate linear stapler** (Ethicon) are useful for lung lobectomy, division of large vascular pedicles, resection of atrial appendage tumors, typhlectomy, liver lobectomy, partial splenectomy, and closure of gastrointestinal incisions.
- **Gastrointestinal anastomoses (GIA)** staplers (USSC) and **proximate linear cutters** (Ethicon) can perform many of the same functions as the TA and linear staplers and are useful for partial gastrectomy, intestinal anastomoses, cholecystojejunostomy, and resection of esophageal diverticulum.
- **End-to-end anastomosis (EEA)** stapler is used for esophageal anastomosis, gastroduodenostomy (Bilroth I), and colorectal anastomosis (subtotal colectomy in cats).

BIBLIOGRAPHY

1. Boothe HW: Suture materials, tissue adhesives, staplers, and ligating clips. In Slatter D (ed): Textbook of Small Animal Surgery, 2nd ed. Philadelphia, W.B. Saunders, 1993, pp 204–212.
2. Booth HW: Selecting suture materials for small animal surgery. Comp Cont Educ Pract Vet 20:155–63, 1998.
3. Pavletic MM (ed): Surgical stapling. Vet Clin North Am Sm Anim Pract 24:225–429, 1994.
4. Smeak DD: Selection and use of currently available suture materials and needles. In Bojrab MJ (ed): Current Techniques in Small Animal Surgery, 4th ed. Baltimore, Williams & Wilkins, 1998, pp 19–26.

14. LASER SURGERY

Thomas R. Fry, D.V.M., M.S., Dip. A.C.V.S., and Kenneth E. Bartels, D.V.M., M.S.

1. What is a laser?

A device that emits a high-intensity, narrow spectral width, highly directional or near-zero divergent beam of light (electromagnetic radiation) by stimulating electronic, ionic, or molecular transitions to higher energy levels and allowing them to fall to lower energy levels.

2. What is the derivation of the term *laser*?

Light **A**mplification by **S**timulated **E**mission of **R**adiation.

3. Do all lasers emit radiation in the same region of the electromagnetic spectrum?

No. The electromagnetic spectrum relevant to lasers consists of invisible ultraviolet (short wavelength) radiation, visible light, and infrared (long wavelength) radiation. Medical lasers may be in all portions of the spectrum. Wavelength is most often measured in nanometers or 10^{-9} m. The most commonly used lasers in veterinary medicine include the **diode (635–980 nm)** and **neodymium: yttrium-aluminum-garnet (Nd:YAG) (1,064 nm) lasers** in the near-infrared spectrum, and the **carbon dioxide (CO_2) (10,600 nm)** laser in the far-infrared spectrum (see figure).

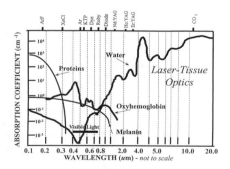

4. What are the components of a generic laser?

- **Optical resonator:** a chamber containing the active medium. CO_2 lasers contain CO_2 gas and small amounts of nitrogen (serves as an *excitor*) and helium (serves as a *buffer*) inside the optical resonator as the active medium.
- Total and partially **reflective mirrors** at each end of the optical resonator allow laser energy (light) to bounce back and forth within the chamber and generate more light, a process known as *amplification*. The partially reflective mirror lets part of the light escape around

its edge, through a hole, or through a partially transparent section. The light that leaks out of the laser cavity is the **laser beam**.

- **Power source:** electricity, another laser, or a flash/arc lamp. The power source causes the molecules of the lasing medium to reach higher energy levels, releasing photons, a process called *stimulated emission.*

5. What are the three types of laser delivery systems?

1. **Articulated arms** are a series of hollow tubes and mirrors that deliver the beam to the laser tip. Older-generation CO_2 lasers, excimer lasers, and ruby lasers all use this system. These are often bulky, easily damaged, and expensive to maintain.

2. **Fiberoptic systems** are thin-diameter quartz fibers capable of delivering laser energy through small-diameter fibers and are extremely useful in endoscopic or relatively inaccessible surgical sites. They are the most economical of the delivery systems. Nd:YAG, potassium titanyl phosphate (KTP), holmium:YAG, and diode lasers all use quartz fiber delivery.

3. **Hollow wave guides** are a refinement of articulated arm systems. They are small-diameter, flexible metal, plastic, or ceramic tubes lined with thin metal as a reflective surface. They are much more flexible than articulated arms, have lower maintenance, and have many of the advantages of quartz fiber systems. Newer-generation CO_2 lasers use this technology.

6. How may the surgeon vary the output of the laser beam or alter the tissue interaction?

- Power density (watts/cm^2 of target tissue) may be changed by varying the power input.
- Changing the mode of gating mechanism. CO_2 and Nd:YAG lasers may be continuous wave, pulsed, superpulse (CO_2), or Q-switched (Nd:YAG).
- Varying the diameter or characteristics of the tip.
- Distance from the tissue plays a significant role, not in beam output but in tissue effects.

7. What are the unique characteristics of laser light?

- Monochromatic—single color (wavelength)
- Coherent—a single wavelength that is spatially and temporally stable
- Nondivergent or collimated—light travels in parallel lines

8. How are lasers named?

Based on the active medium in the optical resonator or determined by the material stimulated by an energy source. Laser pointers (helium neon lasers) have helium and neon gases as the active medium. Diode lasers are composed of wafers of a semiconductor material, such as gallium aluminum arsenide (GaA1As).

9. How do lasers differ from electrocautery devices?

Laser radiation does not stimulate nerve and muscle causing movement in the patient as does electrocautery. Lasers seal nerve endings and lymphatic vessels, in contrast to cautery. Appropriate laser use results in reduced inflammation and lessens postoperative edema and discomfort. Depth of penetration is more reliable with lasers, which increases safety in applications next to vital structures. Coagulation ability differs tremendously between laser types. CO_2 lasers are ineffective at coagulating vessels > 0.5 mm diameter, whereas Nd:YAG lasers are quite effective. Lasers may be used to incise, vaporize, coagulate, and sterilize.

10. What are the minimum standards for laser safety?

Standards are based on the American National Standards Institutes document: *Safe Use of Lasers in Health Care Facilities,* ANSI Z 136.3—1993. General considerations for safety should avoid a **burn and learn** attitude and include:

- Shielding patient corneas and using wavelength-specific goggles for the OR team.
- Using a smoke evacuator to minimize exposure to the laser plume (smoke). Laser plumes may contain carcinogens, toxins, viable bacteria, and viable viruses.
- Using gloves and gowns; saline moistened sponges over any patient tissues at risk.

- Shielding or moistening anything (hair) at risk with drapes. Placing a moistened sponge into the rectum (of the patient) to minimize risk of gas ignition. Avoiding flammable preparations (isopropyl alcohol) on the skin.
- Avoiding polyvinyl chloride endotracheal tubes, which may ignite; use special laser tubes, which are commercially available.
- Using the laser in a closed room with appropriate warning signs.
- Using instruments with antireflective coatings if they will come in contact with the beam.
- Completing a training course specific to the type and manufacturer of laser being used.
- Observing state and Occupational Safety and Health Administration (OSHA) regulations applicable for lasers in veterinary medicine.

11. What are the types of laser tissue interaction?

Laser tissue interaction occurs when laser energy is converted to heat, chemical, or acoustic energy. These reactions are termed **photothermal, photochemical,** and **photomechanical** (photodisruptive) reactions. All of these reactions are representative of absorption, which is the conversion of one energy form to another. Absorption is the desired effect of a laser on the target tissue.

12. What is meant by a cold laser and how are they used?

Low-energy laser radiation is thought by some to stimulate wound repair, regenerate tissues, or decrease painful stimuli. Most data regarding these properties are currently anecdotal.

13. Discuss undesirable laser tissue interactions.

Reflection, scatter, and **transmission** are not desired reactions; absorption is the desired effect. Reflection of laser energy may injure the patient or operator. Scatter damages tissue adjacent to the intended target tissue, and transmission penetrates deep to the desired target tissue. Vaporization of the surgeon's own tissues is also undesirable. As laser technology and the concept of photonics (use of different types and aspects of radiant energy) advance, transmitted, absorbed, back-scattered, and reflective light energy will be used for diagnostic and therapeutic purposes.

14. What are typical soft tissue responses in photothermal laser tissue interaction?

Photothermal tissue responses to laser light are similar to burns. A superficial zone of vaporization (ablation) is adjoined by an intermediate zone of hyperthermia, coagulation, and necrosis and finally a deep zone of cellular edema, thermal injury, and repair. Tissue in the superficial and intermediate zones is ablated, whereas tissue in the deep zone is retained. Depth of this damage depends on laser type and wavelength, tissue characteristics, and laser settings.

15. What are some examples of lasers that work by different methods of absorption?

- **Photothermal** reactions are typical of CO_2 and Nd:YAG lasers. Both cause vaporization of tissues high in water content. Both are examples of infrared lasers in which water is heated by the laser beam, and indirectly other components of the tissue are heated. Depth of penetration for the CO_2 laser is superficial (0.1 mm), whereas penetrance of the Nd:YAG laser may be 5 mm.
- **Photochemical** reactions are typical of dye lasers or new-generation diode lasers in which laser light is applied to affected tissue that is pretreated with photosensitizing agents. Laser application results in singlet oxygen production at the mitochondrial level leading to tissue death. This process is known as **photodynamic therapy** and is useful in the treatment of certain tumors.
- **Photomechanical** or **acoustic** reactions occur with holmium:YAG lasers used at high-energy settings for lithotripsy of urinary tract and gallbladder concretions. The holmium laser may also have photothermal effects similar to Nd:YAG and CO_2 lasers when used at similar settings. This effect is due to the wavelength, water absorption differences, and pulsed energy delivery system inherent to most holmium lasers.

16. Why choose one laser over another for a given task?

Absorption characteristics of the target tissue must be considered as well as the desired depth of ablation, which may be illustrated by the following examples (see figure with Question 3).

- CO_2 lasers are highly absorbed by water with little variability because of tissue pigments. CO_2 lasers would be a poor choice for tissue ablation if the tissue has low water content (i.e., bone).
- **Ruby lasers** are highly absorbed by dark pigment but minimally absorbed by hemoglobin. They are an excellent tool for tattoo removal in humans.
- Because of their greater depth of penetration, **Nd:YAG** lasers are useful for large resections, particularly if coagulation of a rich blood supply is needed. Nd:YAG energy is also readily absorbed by proteins in addition to water. As a result, extensive adjacent thermal damage is possible if too aggressive of an approach is made.

17. Discuss some uses for lasers in small animal surgery.

- Treatment of **brachycephalic airway syndrome** with CO_2, Nd:YAG, diode, and KTP lasers
- Nd:YAG palliation of **meningioma** and subtotal **prostatectomy;**
- Ablation of numerous **neoplasms** using Nd:YAG, CO_2, diode, and KTP lasers
- **Eosinophilic granuloma, feline stomatitis, perianal fistula** resection with CO_2 and Nd:YAG modalities
- Feline **onychectomy** with CO_2 and diode lasers
- Treatment of **nasal squamous cell carcinomas** in cats with Nd:YAG, CO_2, and photodynamic therapy laser applications
- **Pulpotomy** as well as other dental procedures in dogs with the CO_2 laser
- Holmium:YAG laser for prophylactic ablation of canine intervertebral **disks**.

The authors have used lasers for chronic wound treatment (tissue sterilization), ear canal ablation, salivary mucocele resection, nasopharyngeal stenosis treatment, tumor resections in pocket pets, oral mass resections, treatment of feline fibrosarcoma, anal sacculectomy, rectal polyp and neoplasia resections, feline thyroidectomy, orbital mass resections, acral lick lesions, lingual masses in dogs and cats, and ear tumor cytoreduction. Diode laser treatments in ophthalmology are now commonplace in the treatment of retinopathy and glaucoma. These same conditions have also been treated with Q-switched Nd:YAG lasers. The CO_2 laser was used to treat epibulbar melanomas in dogs as well as a variety of eyelid tumors.

BIBLIOGRAPHY

1. Bartels KE: Laser Surgery. In Bojrab MJ (ed): Current Techniques in Small Animal Surgery. Baltimore, Williams & Wilkins, 1998, pp 45–52.
2. Dickey DT, Bartels KE, Henry GA: Percutaneous thoracolumbar intervertebral disc ablation in the dog using the holmium laser. J Am Vet Med Assoc 208:1263–1267, 1996.
3. Ellison GW, Bella JR, Stubbs WP: Treatment of perianal fistulas with the Nd:YAG laser: Results in twenty cases. Vet Surg 24:140–147, 1995.
4. Feder BM, Fry TR, Kostolich M: Nd:YAG laser cytoreduction of an invasive intracranial meningioma in a dog. Prog Vet Neurol 4:3–9, 1993.
5. Fry TR, Bartels KE: CO_2 laser excision of lingual masses in dogs and cats. Lasers Surg Med Suppl 11:59, 1999.
6. Hardie EM, Stone EA, Spaulding KA, et al: Subtotal canine prostatectomy with the neodymium:yttrium aluminum garnet laser. Vet Surg 19:348–355, 1990.
7. Lucroy MD, Magne ML, Peavy GM, et al. Photodynamic therapy in veterinary medicine: Current status and implications for applications in human disease. J Clin Laser Surg Med 14:305–310, 1997.
8. Nassisse MP, Davidson MG, English RV: Treatment of glaucoma by use of transcleral neodymium:yttrium aluminum garnet laser cyclocoagulation in dogs. J Am Vet Med Assoc 197:350–353, 1990.
9. Sapienza JS, Miller TR, Gum GG: Contact transcleral cyclophotocoagulation using a neodymium:yttrium aluminum garnet laser in normal dogs. Prog Vet Comparative Ophthalmol 2:147–153, 1993.
10. Shelley BA, Bartels KE, Ely RW: Use of the neodymium:yttrium aluminum garnet laser for treatment of squamous cell carcinoma of the nasal planum in a cat. J Am Vet Med Assoc 201:756–758, 1992.
11. Sherk HH (ed): Laser in Orthopaedics. Philadelphia, J.B. Lippincott, 1990.

15. RECONSTRUCTIVE MICROSURGERY

David Fowler, D.V.M., M.V.Sc., Dip. A.C.V.S.

1. What is microsurgery?
Any surgical procedure performed with the aid of an operating microscope.

2. What is reconstructive microsurgery?
The application of microsurgical techniques to the reconstruction of wounds.

3. Are there synonyms for the term reconstructive microsurgery?
- Microvascular surgery
- Free tissue transfer
- Microvascular free tissue transfer

4. What is meant by microvascular free tissue transfer?
The distant transfer of a tissue or composite of tissues from a donor site to a recipient site for wound reconstruction. The transferred flap must be nourished by a single dominant angiosome. During dissection, the vascular pedicle feeding the flap is transected. The flap is revascularized at the recipient site by performing microvascular anastomosis of the flap artery and vein to a suitable artery and vein located at the recipient site.

5. What is an angiosome?
A region of tissue nourished by a single source artery and vein.

6. How are free flaps classified?
According to the type of tissues forming the flap and the anatomic source of those tissues. Examples of classification according to **tissue type:**
- Cutaneous flaps
- Muscle flaps
- Microvascular bone transfers
- Myo-osseous flaps
- Myocutaneous flaps
- Osteomusculocutaneous flaps
- Myoperitoneal flaps

Examples of classification according to **anatomic source of the tissue:**
- Trapezius muscle flap
- Cranial abdominal myoperitoneal flap
- Medial tibial osteocutaneous flap

7. When should microvascular free tissue transfer be considered for wound reconstruction?
Whenever local tissues are not available or appropriate for wound reconstruction and for wounds requiring early reconstruction.
Examples:
- Grade III open fractures of the distal extremities
- Rehabilitation of irradiated wound beds
- Oral or cranial reconstruction after ablative cancer surgery
- Reconstruction of the weight-bearing portions of the paw

8. List advantages of microvascular reconstruction.
- Ability to select the most appropriate tissue for the reconstructive problem, without geographic limitations
- Facilitation of early wound reconstruction
- Provision of robust tissues that enhance wound healing
- One-stage wound reconstruction

9. List disadvantages of microvascular reconstruction.
- Technically more difficult than local procedures
- Longer operative times
- Potential for catastrophic failure

10. Is it preferable to reconstruct traumatic wounds early or late?
Traumatic open wounds that are not associated with deep tissue injury to critical structures, such as bone or joints, can be managed open for extended periods with little associated risk. Traumatic wounds that are associated with extensive vascular disruption, exposed fractures, or open joints benefit from early reconstruction using well-vascularized tissues. Early reconstruction, in such instances, is associated with decreased infection rates, more rapid bone healing, and fewer wound complications.

11. With a poorly vascularized wound bed, what type of flap is preferable for the provision of vascular augmentation?
Muscle (although somewhat poorly documented)

12. What other factorĭs should be considered in selecting an appropriate flap?
- Tissue types lost at the recipient site
- Vascular integrity of tissues at the recipient site
- Size of recipient site defect
- Need for structural support (e.g., bone, footpads) at the recipient site
- Familiarity of the surgeon with the proposed donor flap

13. How long can flaps survive without blood flow (how long to transfer the flap)?
This is called the **critical ischemia time** of the flap and varies according to the type of tissue:

    1. Bowel has a relatively short critical ischemia time and should be revascularized within 1 hour.

    2. Muscle and bone are intermediate in their tolerance to warm ischemia but appear to survive with little compromise for 2 hours and with marginal tissue injury for 4 hours.

    3. Skin can tolerate extended warm ischemia times of 6 hours or more.

14. What is the typical ischemia time during free tissue transfer?
30–120 minutes. The ischemia time can be minimized by dissecting and preparing the recipient artery and vein before transection of the donor artery and vein. Flaps should be stabilized at the recipient site before microvascular anastomosis but only to the point that the ultimate position of the flap and its vascular pedicle are determined.

15. Can electrocautery be used during flap dissection?
Cautery can be used but should be limited to **bipolar cautery**. It is necessary to skeletonize the vascular pedicle of the flap to its greatest possible length. Small vascular branches encountered during this process are best managed by application of small hemostatic clips, rather than by application of cautery, which can cause thermal injury to the intima of the parent vessel.

16. What are the uses of washout solutions?
- To clear the vasculature of blood
- To provide a temporary source of nutrition
- To limit tissue injury during many organ transplantation procedures

17. Can washout solutions be used for free flaps?
Not recommended. Many studies have demonstrated that washout does not extend critical ischemia times and is potentially damaging to the microvasculature.

18. Will the blood that remains in the flap clot?
No, provided that the endothelium is healthy and intact.

19. Should systemic anticoagulation be considered before flap transfer?
Not unless systemic factors are present that place the patient in a hypercoagulable state. Systemic anticoagulation increases the risk of significant blood loss, without improving the chance of flap survival.

20. Are any antithrombotic or anticoagulation strategies recommended?
Many microsurgeons routinely use low-dose aspirin to inhibit platelet aggregation for 1 to 2 weeks after surgery. Topical washout of vessel ends, using heparinized saline, is routinely recommended before vascular anastomosis.

21. List specialized instrumentation required for microvascular free tissue transfer.
   • Specialized microvascular clamps
   • Microvascular dissecting scissors
   • Vessel dilators
   • Microneedle drivers
   • Fine jeweler's forceps
   • Suture manufactured specifically for microvascular repair
   • Operating microscope

22. Can free tissue transfer be performed without an operating microscope?
Many accomplished microsurgeons perform free tissue transfer using only loupe magnification. Surgeons performing such procedures generally have a great deal of previous microsurgical experience using the operating microscope.

23. How does one select an appropriate recipient artery and vein?
Recipient vessels must
   • Be free from previous trauma
   • Be located outside the zone of trauma of the wound
   • Have sufficient length and diameter to permit microvascular anastomosis to the donor artery and vein

24. What can be done if the donor artery and vein do not physically reach the recipient artery and vein after inset of the flap?
An interpositional vein graft can be used to facilitate reconstruction.

25. Is any risk involved with use of a vein graft?
Slightly increased risk of postoperative thrombosis.

26. Which is better — end-to-end or end-to-side microvascular arterial anastomosis — and why?
End-to-side anastomosis. End-to-end anastomosis is technically easier to perform but requires a relatively close match between the donor and recipient vessel diameters. A mismatch of approximately 1.5:1 is generally tolerated. End-to-end anastomosis has the disadvantage of *stealing* the vessel from its normal function at the recipient site. This is not a significant problem for most veins but can result in arterial compromise to distal extremities in the case of a major recipient artery.

27. What factors place microvascular free flaps at risk for failure?
   • **Systemic,** or patient-related, factors:
     Pre-existing peripheral vascular disease
     Diseases that induce a hypercoagulable state

- Operative factors
  Traumatic flap dissection
  Iatrogenic injury to donor or recipient vascular pedicles
  Poor anastomotic technique
  Exposed subendothelial collagen
  Adventitial infolding at the anastomotic site
- Postoperative factors
  Excessive pain
  Hypotension
  Reduced vascular volume
  Hypothermia
  Positional compression of vascular pedicles

28. At what point is thrombosis from a faulty anastomosis evident?
Typically, within 30 minutes of reestablishing blood flow through the anastomosis.

29. What should be done if thrombosis occurs?
Cut it out and start over. Do not try to salvage a faulty anastomosis.

30. How are free flaps monitored?
Visual inspection assessing color and capillary refill. Arterial flow through a superficially located vascular pedicle can be assessed using a Doppler flow probe. Brisk hemorrhage of bright red blood after pinprick indicates adequate flap perfusion. Nuclear scintigraphy can be used to evaluate vascularized bone transfers within the first 5 days after surgery.

31. What is the success rate of microvascular free flaps in veterinary surgery?
A retrospective analysis of 57 microvascular procedures revealed a success rate of 93%.

BIBLIOGRAPHY

1. Basher AWP, Fowler JD, Bowen CV, et al: Microneurovascular free digital pad transfer in the dog. Vet Surg 19:226–231, 1990.
2. Degner DA, Walshaw R, Lanz O: The medial saphenous fasciocutaneous free flap in dogs. Vet Surg 25:105–113, 1996.
3. Degner DA, Lanz OI, Walshaw R: Myoperitoneal microvascular free flaps in dogs: an anatomical study and a clinical case report. Vet Surg 25:463–470, 1996.
4. Fowler JD, Degner DA, Walshaw R, et al: Microvascular free tissue transfer: Results in 57 consecutive cases. Vet Surg 27:406–412, 1998.
5. Moens NMM, Fowler JD: The microvascular carpal footpad flap: Vascular anatomy and surgical technique. Vet Comp Orthop Traum 10:183–186, 1997.
6. Philibert D, Fowler JD, Clapson JB: The anatomic basis for a trapezius muscle flap in dogs. Vet Surg 21:429–434, 1992.
7. Philibert D, Fowler JD: The trapezius osteomusculocutaneous flap in dogs. Vet Surg 22:444–450, 1993.
8. Szentimrey D, Fowler D: The anatomic basis of a free vascularized bone graft based on the canine distal ulna. Vet Surg 23:529–533, 1994.

II. Soft Tissue Surgery

16. SKIN GRAFTS

Steven F. Swaim, D.V.M., M.S.

1. What is the difference between a skin graft and skin flap?
"A graft is a piece of detached skin which is dead when you put it on and comes to life later. A flap is a partly attached piece of skin which is alive when you put it on and may die later."[1]

A **skin graft** is a piece of skin taken away from its blood supply and placed on a recipient wound, where it develops a new blood supply. A **skin flap** is a piece of skin that remains attached to a blood supply when it is placed over a recipient wound.

2. Where are skin grafts primarily used?
Repair of wounds on the distal aspects of limbs.

3. Considering wound size, when are skin grafts indicated?
- Large wounds where the edges could never be apposed, either by wound contraction or use of skin stretching techniques.
- Wounds on or near the paws where wound contraction would result in malalignment of the paw pads and weight bearing on skin not designed for that purpose.

4. What skin stretching and relaxing technique can be used to close limb wounds so that a graft is not necessary (or reduce wound size so that only a small graft is needed)?
An **adjustable horizontal mattress suture.** This is a continuous, monofilament, intradermal, horizontal mattress suture. The tension on the suture can be modified periodically by an adjustment apparatus on either end of the suture.

5. What type of tissue must be present in a wound for a skin graft to heal?
Healthy granulation tissue or vascularized tissue that can produce granulation tissue.

6. What are three primary reasons grafts do not heal well?
1. Movement of the graft on the wound
2. Hematoma or seroma formation beneath the graft
3. Infection beneath the graft

7. What are three types of skin grafts that help alleviate the reasons grafts do not heal well?
1. Mesh grafts
2. Strip grafts
3. Pinch/punch grafts

8. How should a traumatic wound be treated in the early period of management to prepare it for grafting?
- Staged débridement and lavage with a 0.05% chlorhexidine solution
- Application of a topical water-soluble antibiotic/antibacterial (e.g., silver sulfadiazine, or nitrofurazone ointment) compound
- Daily bandage change

9. How should a wound be treated the day before skin graft application?
- Gentle scraping of the surface with a surgical blade to help remove surface coagulum and resident bacterial flora
- Application of 0.1% gentamicin sulfate ointment on a sterile, open-mesh, gauze sponge
- Application of outer bandage layers

10. On the day of surgery, what should be done to prepare the wound for grafting?
Nothing, but protection from surgical preparation soaps and solutions used on the skin around the wound.

11. Where is skin harvested for grafts?
Lower craniolateral thoracic area because the skin is thin and contains hair. The thinness of the skin is beneficial for quick revascularization, and the hair provides a functional and cosmetic graft.

12. How should the donor site be prepared for surgery?
It is important to clip the hair **widely** on the donor site. As the donor site is closed, haired, unprepared skin is not pulled from under the drapes as wound edges are advanced and apposed. Routine scrub and antiseptic applications are used for skin preparation.

13. If a wound has granulation tissue and a rim of epithelium at its edge, what is the first thing to be done to prepare it for mesh grafting?
A No. 15 scalpel blade and thumb forceps are used to remove the rim of epithelium. The first incision is perpendicular to the wound surface at the junction between haired skin and epithelium (step 1 in figure). The second incision is parallel to the wound surface under the epithelium (step 2 in figure).

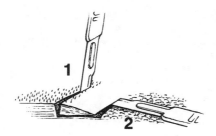

Removing epithelium from the wound edge prior to grafting.

14. How is a pattern made of the wound to be used to obtain the graft?
A piece of sterile towel is cut to a size slightly larger than the wound and placed over the wound. A blood imprint of the wound edge is made because the edge has a hemorrhagic surface (from epithelium removal). Using scissors, the towel is cut to the shape of the imprint to provide a pattern for the graft.

15. How is the towel pattern of the wound placed on the donor site?
The pattern is placed on the donor site so that the direction of hair growth on the graft, after it is placed on the wound, is the same as the hair growth of the skin around the wound.

16. What happens if the towel pattern is accidentally turned over as it is transferred from the wound to the donor site?
After the graft is harvested, it fits on the wound only if it is placed epidermal (haired) side against the wound, obviously not a good situation.

17. To insure accurate shape to the graft, what should be done?

Trace around the pattern with a skin marking pen. Alternatively a sterile toothpick or a cotton-tipped applicator stick, broken to a splintered end, can be dipped in sterile methylene blue for tracing. The traced graft is then incised with a No. 15 scalpel blade.

18. How should the wound be managed while the graft is being harvested and prepared?

The wound should be covered with a sterile, saline-moistened sponge.

19. How is the dermal surface of the graft prepared for placement on the wound?

Using hypodermic needles, the graft is fixed dermal-side up on a piece of autoclaved corrugated cardboard. The graft is stretched in all directions as needles are placed. Thumb forceps and sharp-sharp scissors are used to remove *all* cutaneous trunci muscle and subcutaneous tissue from the dermis. The dermal surface should have a cobblestone appearance after this tissue is removed. The *cobblestones* are bulbs on hair follicles.

20. What is a simple, inexpensive way to mesh a skin graft?

Mesh holes about 1 cm long can be cut with a No. 11 scalpel blade in parallel, staggered rows 0.5 cm apart.

21. Describe the closure technique of the donor site.

- While a graft is being prepared by one clinician, another clinician can be closing the donor site.
- "Walking" sutures of 2–0 or 3–0 absorbable suture material are used to advance the wound edges together.
- A simple continuous subcutaneous suture of 2–0 or 3–0 absorbable suture material is placed near the wound edge.
- Simple interrupted 2–0 or 3–0 nonabsorbable sutures or skin staples are used for final skin apposition.

22. After removing the graft from the cardboard and properly orienting it on the wound, what needs to be done immediately?

Application of a simple interrupted suture to affix one point of the graft to the wound edge to avoid inadvertent loss of the graft (on the floor).

23. What should be done if a graft does fall on the floor?

Lavage it thoroughly with sterile physiologic saline, and proceed with graft placement. Administer **antibiotics.**

24. What are some ways to affix a graft to the wound edges?

Simple interrupted or simple continuous 2–0 or 3–0 monofilament nonabsorbable sutures (polypropylene or nylon) or skin staples.

25. After affixing the graft edges, what is the next important step?

Placement of tacking sutures follows graft edge fixation. These are placed *between* mesh holes, deep into underlying tissue to help immobilize the graft on the wound surface.

26. Is it necessary to place tacking sutures between all mesh holes?

No; however, they should especially be placed in areas where there may be potential movement that would interfere with graft immobilization. They should also be placed in areas of wound concavity to pull the graft against the underlying wound surface.

27. What materials and medications should be used in bandaging the grafted area?

- **Primary layer**—semiocclusive nonadherent bandage pad with a *thin* coat of 0.1% gentamicin sulfate ointment

- **Secondary layer**—soft absorbent bandage wrap
- **Tertiary layer**—surgical adhesive tape

28. How often should bandages be changed?

For dogs, daily for the first week, every other day the second week, and twice the third week. Bandages are usually discontinued after 3 weeks. A bandage may be left in place for 1 more week, however, if the dog shows signs of hyperesthesia of the graft because of reinnervation. Bandage changes may be less frequent and for a shorter time for cats because of more rapid healing.

29. What shape and location of wound lends itself to strip grafting?

Wounds that are parallel to the long axis of the limb.

30. What type of wound bed is necessary for strip grafting?

A granulation tissue bed must be present so that grooves can be cut in it to place the grafts.

31. What are the dimensions for the grooves to accommodate strip grafts and the dimensions for the strip grafts?

Grooves for the grafts are parallel and approximately 2 mm deep and 3 to 5 mm apart. The grafts are measured 5 mm wide.

32. What is the most expedient way to remove subcutaneous tissue from a strip graft?

Cut the long dimensions and one end of the grafts; leave the other end temporarily attached. Grasp the free end of each graft with thumb forceps and apply tension to stretch the graft because the remaining end is still attached to skin. Run scissors down the dermal side of the graft to remove subcutaneous tissue.

33. How are strip grafts sutured in place?

One simple interrupted 3-0 polypropylene or nylon suture is placed at each end of the graft and, where needed, along the edges of the graft to anchor it in the groove.

34. How do strip grafts heal in place?

With the grafts setting in grooves, they revascularize from the bottom and edges of the grooves. Myofibroblasts, from the granulation tissue between grafts, attach to the graft edges and contract so grafts widen as they heal. Epithelium from the graft edges covers the granulation tissue between grafts.

35. What are advantages and disadvantages of strip grafts?

- **Advantages:**
  They require no special instruments
  They heal quickly.
- **Disadvantage:**
  They may not be cosmetic mesh grafts or skin flaps.

36. What are ways that pinch/punch grafts can be harvested?

- The point of a suture needle can be placed in the donor skin. Upward tension is placed on the needle to tent the skin. A No. 15 scalpel blade is used to cut the tip off of the tent to provide a pinch graft (see figure). Alternatively, fine-toothed thumb forceps can be used to tent the skin.
- A dermal biopsy punch (4–6 mm diameter) can be used to cut a punch graft. By angling the biopsy punch parallel to the angle of the hair follicles in the skin, more intact hair follicles are obtained with each graft (see figure).

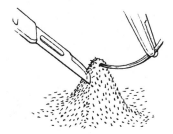

A suture needle tents the skin while a No. 15 scalpel blade cuts the tip off of the "tent."

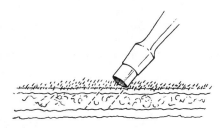

A dermal biopsy punch is angled parallel to the direction of hair follicles to cut a punch graft so it has the greatest number of viable hair follicles possible.

37. How is a recipient site prepared for a pinch/punch graft?
- A No. 15 scalpel blade can be inserted into the granulation tissue of the wound almost parallel to the wound surface to make pockets that are 2–4 mm deep and 5–7 mm apart. After the pocket is made, a graft is placed in the pocket. A pocket and graft placement are done sequentially and immediately.
- A dermal biopsy punch 1 size smaller than the punch used to harvest the skin graft is used to cut a plug from the wound granulation tissue. After attaining hemostasis in the resulting hole with a cotton-tipped applicator stick, a pinch/punch graft is placed in the hole, being certain the graft is below the level of the wound surface.

38. How is bandaging of pinch/punch grafts different from bandaging mesh grafts?
Bandages are not changed daily, but every 3rd to 5th day. Because these grafts are not sutured in place, bandages are not changed as often to prevent disruption of the grafts.

BIBLIOGRAPHY

1. Gillies H, Millard DR: The principles and art of plastic surgery. Boston, Little Brown, 1957, p 113.
2. Pavletic MM: Atlas of Small Animal Reconstructive Surgery, 2nd ed. Philadelphia, W.B. Saunders, 1999, pp 275–296.
3. Scardino MS, Swaim SF, Henderson RA, Wilson ER: Enhancing wound closure on the limbs. Comp Cont Educ Pract Vet 18:919–933, 1996.
4. Swaim SF: Surgery of Traumatized Skin: Management and Reconstruction in the Dog and Cat. Philadelphia, W.B. Saunders, 1980, pp 423–475.
5. Swaim SF: Skin grafts. In Slatter DH, (ed): Textbook of Small Animal Surgery, 2nd ed. Philadelphia, W.B. Saunders, 1993, pp 325–340.
6. Swaim SF, Henderson RA: Small Animal Wound Management, 2nd ed. Baltimore, Williams & Wilkins, 1997, pp 295–370.

17. SKIN FLAPS

David Fowler, D.V.M., M.V.Sc., Dip. A.C.V.S.

1. What is a skin flap?

The elevation of a skin region with a vascular attachment at the donor site.

2. How are skin flaps classified?

By their vascular supply:

- **Axial pattern skin flaps** incorporate a direct cutaneous artery and vein in the flap design.
- **Subdermal plexus flaps** are harvested without consideration of their inherent vascular supply. Blood reaches the flap via the subdermal vascular plexus, which is maintained at the cutaneous attachment. Also called **random pattern** or **local flaps.**

3. Is there a difference between axial flaps and subdermal plexus flaps in terms of size or reliability?

Yes. Axial flaps have a consistent and reliable vascular supply, whereas subdermal plexus flaps have an inconsistent vascular supply. As a result, extensive areas of skin can be elevated in an axial flap design.

4. Why would one use a subdermal plexus flap, if axial flaps are more consistent and reliable?

Subdermal plexus flaps are useful primarily for the local redistribution of tension around a wound. They are particularly helpful when reconstructing wounds located adjacent to critical structures, such as the eyelid, prepuce, or anus.

5. How are subdermal plexus flaps classified?

According to the type of movement used to transfer the flap from donor to recipient site:

- **Advancement flaps** are advanced in a linear direction parallel to the length of the flap.
- **Rotation flaps** are elevated using an arcuate incision extending away from the wound.
- **Transposition flaps** are elevated approximately 90° from the orientation of the wound.

6. What factors determine the choice of subdermal plexus flap design?

- Location, shape, and size of the wound
- Elasticity of surrounding skin

7. Is there a reliable method to determine the size of subdermal plexus flap that can be harvested relative to the size and location of the attached cutaneous border?

No.

8. What size subdermal plexus flap is generally considered safe?

Length-to-width ratios of less than 2:1 are quite safe. Longer and narrower flaps are at increased risk of partial flap necrosis.

9. At what tissue depth should subdermal plexus flaps be elevated?

To preserve the vascular supply to the flap, dissection should be carried out in deep subcutaneous tissue. Larger flaps located in areas where superficial cutaneous musculature exists should be dissected deep to the cutaneous muscle layer.

10. Should sutures be used to obliterate dead space underlying the flap?

No. Sutures placed into the deep surface of the flap compromise blood supply and increase the risk of partial flap necrosis. A drain should be used, if necessary.

11. What is a pouch flap?

A two-stage technique used for transfer of a single-pedicle or bipedicle flap from the body wall to a distal extremity.

12. Describe the pouch flap procedure.

In the first stage, a flap is elevated from the thoracic or abdominal wall. The distal extremity wound is placed beneath the flap, and the flap margins are sutured to wound margins as completely as possible. The limb is then bandaged such that it is stabilized onto the body wall for 10–14 days. During this period, vascular ingrowth occurs from the recipient wound bed into the overlying flap. During the second stage, the flap pedicle is transected, and the remaining margins between the wound and the flap are sutured. The donor site is débrided and closed.

13. When should pouch flaps be used?

Perhaps never, because a pouch flap is nothing more than a delayed skin graft. Skin grafts can be used with equal success and without the disadvantages of a staged surgical procedure and extended periods of immobilization in an unnatural and uncomfortable position.

14. When should axial pattern flaps be used?

For reconstruction of large defects located on the face or on the proximal to midextremities.

15. How many axial pattern flaps exist in the dog and the cat?

As many as there are direct cutaneous arteries and veins.

16. How is an axial pattern flap selected for clinical use?

The vascular territories (or angiosomes) that are supplied by direct cutaneous vessels vary considerably in size. Only the largest of the axial pattern flaps are used clinically. This reduces the number of clinically useful flaps to four or five. The flap that is chosen is the one that will reach the recipient wound after elevation.

17. How are axial pattern flaps defined?

According to the direct cutaneous vessels that support the flap.

18. What are the most useful axial pattern flaps?

- Superficial cervical (omocervical)
- Thoracodorsal
- Caudal superficial epigastric

19. How can the vascular pedicle be identified with certainty before dissection?

The general location of the vascular pedicle can be determined using **anatomic landmarks.** Precise localization can be achieved by locating the arterial signal using a **Doppler flow probe.**

20. What preoperative planning is necessary to ensure adequate flap dimensions?

The location of the vascular pedicle must be determined precisely because this forms the point of fixation for the flap. The distance from the vascular pedicle to the most distant point of the wound should be slightly less than the distance from the vascular pedicle to the most distant point of the flap.

21. Can inadequate length be compensated by excess width?

Yes, if the flap is not quite long enough to reach the most distant aspect of the wound comfortably. In this situation, the excess width of the flap can be translated into additional length without creating undue tension.

22. At what depth should axial pattern skin flaps be elevated?

Dissection should be performed to include all underlying subcutaneous tissue and superficial cutaneous musculature. This dissection ensures preservation of the flap's microvasculature.

23. Does a cutaneous attachment need to be maintained?

No. It is easier to transpose axial flaps into position if they are dissected as island flaps. The only attachment that should be preserved at the donor site is that of the vascular pedicle.

24. Can the flap be rotated without obstructing the vascular pedicle?

Yes. Flap rotation of 180° is well tolerated, as long as there is no tension placed on the vascular pedicle.

25. What should be done if intact skin is interposed between the donor and the recipient site?

An access incision should be made extending from the vascular pedicle to the recipient site. Skin edges can be undermined and the axial pattern flap placed into the resulting defect. The formation of tube flaps extending over intact skin between the donor and recipient sites is not recommended.

26. What is a reverse saphenous conduit flap?

A flap based on the cranial and caudal branches of the medial saphenous artery and vein. The saphenous vessels are ligated and transected as they arise from the femoral artery. Flap elevation is extended distally, raising the skin from the medial aspect of the crus with the branches of the saphenous vessels maintained with the elevated skin flap. The distal extension of the medial saphenous vessels is maintained, as is a distal cutaneous attachment. Vascular perfusion of this flap is provided by retrograde flow through the branches of the saphenous artery and vein, with arterial flow extending from distal to proximal and venous return flowing from proximal to distal. Anastomotic connections between the saphenous vessels and other arterial and venous systems in the foot are necessary to ensure flap perfusion.

27. What are the applications of a reverse saphenous conduit flap?

Reconstruction of wounds located on the tarsus and metatarsus.

BIBLIOGRAPHY

1. Fowler D, Williams JM: Manual of Canine and Feline Wound Management and Reconstruction. Cheltenham, British Small Animal Veterinary Association, 1999.
2. Pavletic MM: Atlas of Small Animal Reconstructive Surgery, 2nd ed. Philadelphia, W.B. Saunders, 1999, pp 237–273.
3. Swaim SF, Henderson RA: Small Animal Wound Management, 2nd ed. Baltimore, Williams & Wilkins, 1997, pp 320–330.

18. MANAGEMENT OF BURN WOUNDS

David Fowler, D.V.M., M.V.Sc., Dip. A.C.V.S.

1. What are some common causes of burn wounds?

- Extreme temperature (**thermal burns**)
- Chemicals (**caustic**)
- Electricity
- Irradiation

2. How are burn wounds classified in small animals?

According to cause, depth of injury, or surface area involved. Burns are further classified as either **partial-thickness** or **full-thickness** injuries.

3. **What is the *rule of nine*?**
   A rapid method to estimate the percentage of affected surface area:
   - Each forelimb represents 9% of the total body surface area.
   - The dorsal and ventral surfaces of each hind limb represent 9%.
   - The head and neck represent 9%.
   - The dorsal and ventral surfaces of the trunk each represent 18%.

4. **Is there a critical temperature at which thermal injury occurs?**
   No. Tissue injury depends on temperature and time of exposure. Thermal injury can occur at temperatures as low as 44°C (111°F) with prolonged exposure.

5. **What patient factors predispose an anesthetized animal to thermal injury?**
   The ability of the animal to dissipate heat from an area of local application can affect the extent of injury. Dehydrated animals or animals with poor peripheral perfusion are at increased risk when exposed to relatively low-temperature heating devices (>42°C) for prolonged periods of time.

6. **List actions that can be taken to minimize the risk of iatrogenic thermal injury in anesthetized patients.**
   - Do not use electrical heating sources.
   - Use circulating warming devices—either air or water.
   - Avoid prolonged application of heat over pressure points.
   - Maintain the patient's hydration, blood pressure, and peripheral perfusion.

7. **How are burn wounds recognized?**
   Not easily in small animals because of an absence of blistering and a covering hair coat. Within the first few hours after injury, thermal wounds are characterized by erythema, transudation of fluid, and easily epilated hair follicles. A full-thickness burn has three concentric zones of injury:
   1. Central coagulative necrosis
   2. Middle vascular stasis
   3. Outer hyperemia

   The ultimate depth and extent of tissue injury may not be readily apparent for 24–72 hours, at which time obvious margins of demarcation between healthy and nonviable tissue usually develop.

8. **What causes fluid shifts after burn injury?**
   Thermal damage causes direct vascular injury, resulting in a breakdown of the semipermeable vascular wall. Large-molecular-weight compounds escape into surrounding tissues, and oncotic pressure becomes ineffective in maintaining intravascular volume. Massive loss of plasma albumin accompanies moderate-to-severe burns.

9. **How are red blood cells damaged during burn wounds?**
   In severe injuries, many red blood cells are directly destroyed by heat. Red blood cell membranes can be damaged such that cells are removed prematurely from the circulating pool in the first 5–7 days. Red blood cell loss can be significant after thermal injury, necessitating whole-blood transfusion.

10. **Which electrolytes must be monitored during the treatment of severe burn wounds?**
    Sodium and potassium.

11. **How is sodium affected?**
    - Sodium loss directly accompanies intravascular fluid loss after injury.

- Sodium has a high affinity for denatured collagen in burn wounds.
- The sodium pump in damaged cells becomes inefficient.

12. How is potassium affected?
- Potassium is released from damaged red blood cells and other tissue cells immediately after injury and may cause a transient hyperkalemia.
- In the presence of adequate renal function, urinary potassium excretion increases, resulting in the potential development of hypokalemia.
- Intravenous fluid therapy can further aggravate hypokalemia.

13. Are there other systemic effects of burn wounds?
Yes. **Immune competence** is adversely affected by severe thermal injury and can predispose the patient to burn wound infection and septicemia. Nutritional demands increase in direct proportion to the severity of injury.

14. Discuss the immediate treatment of dogs and cats with severe burn wounds.
Fluid support using a balanced electrolyte solution is critical. Acute reduction of intravascular fluid volume must be offset to maintain cardiac output and peripheral tissue perfusion. Colloid and plasma replacement therapy is generally not indicated for the first 24 hours after injury because continued escape of large-molecular-weight compounds through damaged vessel walls can exacerbate ongoing fluid shifts. Analgesia (opioids) must also be provided. Nonsteroidal anti-inflammatory drugs may have a beneficial action in reducing the extent of ongoing tissue injury, but adequate renal function should be clearly established before their administration. Topical cooling is also effective in reducing pain associated with burn wounds.

15. Should systemic antibiotic therapy be initiated?
Probably not. Although burn wounds are susceptible to the development of infection, the prophylactic administration of antibiotics does not appear to decrease infection rates. Antibiotic therapy should be reserved for the management of established wound infection or septicemia, to avoid the risk of resistant bacterial infection.

16. How aggressively should nutritional support be provided?
Burn patients should be fed at least 1.5 times their resting energy requirement. Many animals do not eat, especially if oropharyngeal edema is present. Esophagostomy or gastrostomy tube placement is indicated in these patients.

17. Can respiratory tract injury occur subsequent to thermal injury?
Yes. Direct thermal injury is uncommon and is generally limited to the nasal cavity, pharynx, and larynx because of efficient heat exchange in these tissues.

18. What is the mechanism of injury to lower airways and lung?
Inhalation injury occurs secondary to toxic agents in smoke. The severity of inhalation injury depends upon the extent and duration of exposure as well as the source of the smoke. Wood fires are particularly damaging because of their elevated levels of carbon monoxide and aldehyde gases such as acrolein.

19. Is the severity of inhalation injury apparent at initial presentation?
No.

20. Over what time period do respiratory complications progress?
The first 24–36 hours are most crucial in predicting the severity of inhalation injury. Animals that do not develop severe respiratory complications within the first 24 hours generally make an

uncomplicated recovery. Progressive respiratory compromise over the first 24 hours indicates a relatively poor prognosis for uncomplicated recovery.

21. How should inhalation injury be managed?

Delivery of supplemental oxygen is beneficial in improving oxygen delivery to tissues and in reducing carbon monoxide levels. Tracheostomy may be required if pharyngeal or laryngeal edema causes obstruction to air flow. Adequate intravenous fluid support reduces the risk of pulmonary edema and pneumonia.

22. When is débridement indicated for treatment of burn wounds?

Full-thickness injuries should be aggressively débrided as soon as areas of nonviable tissue are established. Maintaining the eschar over a burn wound is contraindicated and is associated with increased risk of infection and wound complications. Débridement can be conservative (hydrotherapy, wet dressings) or aggressive via surgery.

23. What bandaging techniques are indicated for the management of open burn wounds?

This depends on the size of the wound and complicating systemic factors.
- Smaller burn wounds in systemically healthy patients can be managed using a traditional wet-to-dry contact dressing to assist in wound débridement.
- Larger wounds in debilitated patients should receive a nonadherent contact dressing that provides a moist wound environment.
- Biologic dressings, such as freeze-dried porcine xenografts, can be considered for severe wounds to help reduce ongoing fluid losses.
- A topical nonirritating antimicrobial (water-miscible) agent, such as silver sulfadiazine, is useful.

24. How frequently should the wound be evaluated?

In most cases, daily assessment is required for the first several days because progressive tissue injury can occur during this period. Débridement is repeated to remove all nonviable tissue.

25. When should the wound be reconstructed?

In general, **full-thickness** burn wounds should be reconstructed as soon as
- There is no ongoing tissue necrosis.
- All nonviable tissue has been débrided from the wound.
- There is no complicating wound sepsis.
- In many cases this may be as early as 2–3 days after injury.

26. How should the wound be reconstructed?

Location, size, availability of regional tissues, and inherent vascularity of tissues in the wound bed should be considered in selecting an optimal method for reconstruction. Options include the following:
- Mesh grafts
- Axial pattern flaps
- Skin advancement

BIBLIOGRAPHY

1. Drobatz KJ, Walker LM, Hendricks JC: Smoke exposure in dogs and cats. J Am Vet Med Assoc 215:1306–1316, 1999.
2. Pavletic M: Burns. In Pavletic M (ed): Atlas of Small Animal Reconstructive Surgery, 2nd ed. Philadelphia, W.B. Saunders, 1999, pp 70–84.
3. Williams JM: Special considerations in wound management. In Fowler D, Williams JM (eds): Manual of Canine and Feline Wound Management and Reconstruction. Cheltenham, British Small Animal Veterinary Association, 1999, pp 123–136.

19. EAR CANAL RESECTION, ABLATION, AND BULLA OSTEOTOMY

Elizabeth J. Laing, D.V.M., D.V.Sc., Dip. A.C.V.S.

1. Lateral ear canal resection, vertical canal resection, and total ear canal ablation are all treatments for what common condition?

Otitis externa. Each procedure removes a progressively greater amount of tissue.

2. What are other indications for these surgical treatments?

They also provide access to the deeper regions of the ear canal and tympanic bulla for removal of tumors, polyps, and foreign bodies.

3. When might a simple ear infection benefit from lateral ear canal resection?

When it has not responded to or has recurred after appropriate medical management. The goal of lateral resection is to provide drainage and ventilation to the horizontal ear canal, improving the efficacy of future medical treatment.

4. When should lateral resection not be performed in favor of a more radical procedure?

With chronic and diffuse hyperplastic otitis externa. Also, because most dogs require some degree of ear care after surgery, it is not the surgery of choice for aggressive dogs. For both of these reasons, it rarely is the best choice for cocker spaniels.

5. What is the overall success rate for lateral ear canal resection?

1/3 of patients are cured.
1/3 are better but require regular ear cleaning and medication.
1/3 continue to have recurrent and progressive ear disease.

6. What is the difference between a Zepp and Lacroix procedure?

These two terms are often used synonymously, albeit incorrectly, to describe the **lateral ear canal resection.** Although both procedures involve removal of the lateral wall of the vertical ear canal, only in the Zepp is that tissue used to form a ventral drain board.

7. What are the indications for a vertical ear canal resection?

- To remove disease (usually tumors) confined to the vertical ear canal
- To relieve stenosis of the ear canal secondary to traumatic cartilage separation

8. What are the commonest surgical complications of lateral and vertical ear resections?

- Wound dehiscence
- Stenosis of the canal opening

9. Can surgical complications of lateral and vertical ear resections be avoided?

Wound dehiscence and **stenosis of the canal opening** can be minimized (but not entirely avoided) by meticulous tissue handling, accurate apposition of epithelial margins, and appropriate antibiotic therapy.

10. What are the most common ear canal tumors?

- Benign tumors
   Inflammatory polyps
   Papillomas
   Sebaceous and ceruminous gland adenomas
   Basal cell tumors

- Malignant tumors
  Ceruminous gland adenocarcinoma
  Squamous cell carcinoma
  Carcinoma of undetermined origin

11. Do malignant tumors look different than benign or inflammatory masses?
Only under a microscope.

12. From the surgeon's viewpoint, what are some of the characteristics of end-stage otitis?
Severe calcification or rupture of the ear cartilages
- Occlusion of the ear canal by hyperplastic tissue unresponsive to antibiotics
  glucocorticoids, or both
- Antibiotic-resistant bacterial infections of the external or middle ear
- Noncompliant patients and owners

13. What is the treatment of choice for end-stage otitis externa?
Total ear canal ablation with lateral bulla osteotomy.

14. Can dogs still hear after total ear canal ablation–lateral bulla osteotomy?
Maybe. Most studies show hearing loss after surgery, with any remaining auditory function resulting from bone conduction rather than air conduction. Because most dogs with chronic otitis already have diminished hearing, however, owners frequently do not notice any deterioration postoperatively.

15. How is such a radical procedure justified to the client?
Tell owners their pet will have less pain and odor.

16. What is the purpose of a lateral bulla osteotomy during total ear canal ablation?
To remove debris and epithelial remnants, decreasing (it is hoped) the incidence of postoperative fistula formation and improving middle ear drainage. Creating a wide opening to the tympanic bulla encourages granulation tissue ingrowth and provides the immune system with direct vascular access to any residual pathogens.

17. Should a lateral bulla osteotomy always be performed during total ear canal ablation?
Yes.

18. What nerve crosses the base of the ear canal and must be avoided during ear ablation–lateral bulla osteotomy?
The **facial nerve**. A prudent and meticulous surgeon can expect a 10% incidence of postoperative transient neurapraxia. Overzealous dissection or retraction may result in permanent nerve damage.

19. How would one diagnose postablation facial nerve injury?
The ipsilateral blink reflex is weak or absent.

20. How is this condition treated?
Artificial tears or ophthalmic lubricants for 4–6 weeks.

21. What other structures may be injured during total ear ablation–lateral bulla osteotomy?
- Parotid salivary gland
- Greater auricular artery and vein

- External carotid artery
- Auditory ossicles
- Vestibular apparatus
- Hypoglossal nerve
- Oculosympathetic trunk

22. What is the recommended treatment for postablation fistulas?

If due to residual infection, systemic antibiotics (based on bacterial culture and sensitivity) may be helpful. Usually, however, fistulas result from residual epithelial tissue and require surgical exploration. There is no consensus as to whether a lateral or ventral bulla osteotomy is a better approach in these cases.

23. What are middle ear polyps?

Benign growths that arise from the mucous membranes lining the tympanic cavity, auditory canal, and nasopharynx. They occur primarily in younger cats and probably develop secondary to chronic inflammation and tissue irritation, although the exact cause is not known.

24. How are middle ear polyps treated?

Polyps extending along the auditory canal into the nasopharynx are removed through an oral approach, retracting the soft palate rostrally. Polyps within the middle ear are removed via a ventral bulla osteotomy, remembering that cats have a bipartite bulla divided by a bone septum and that both chambers must be explored. Alternatively the polyp can be removed via traction through the external ear canal, with the aid of a rigid fiberoptic scope. This approach is not recommended for cats with advanced middle ear disease. In any case, if excision is incomplete, expect recurrence.

CONTROVERSY

25. Should a drain be placed after total ear ablation and bulla osteotomy?

Conventional wisdom may suggest yes; however, a report showed no significant difference in treatment outcome between dogs having a passive drainage system and those without drains. The drainage group required a longer hospital stay. A drain may be useful in cases with preoperative clinical signs of otitis media, especially if associated with antibiotic-resistant bacterial infections. Otherwise, it probably is not necessary.

BIBLIOGRAPHY

1. DeVitt DM, Seim HB, Willer R: Passive drainage versus primary closure after total ear canal ablation-lateral bulla osteotomy in dogs: 59 dogs (1985–1995). Vet Surg 26:210–216, 1997.
2. Henderson JT, Radasch RM: Total ear canal ablation with lateral bulla osteotomy for the management of end-stage otitis in dogs. Comp Cont Educ Pract Vet 17:157–164, 1995.
3. Holt D, Brockman DJ, Sylvestre AM: Lateral exploration of fistulas developing after total ear canal ablations: 10 cases (1989–1993). J Am Anim Hosp Assoc 32:527–530, 1996.
4. Krahwinkel DJ: External ear canal. In Slatter D (ed): Textbook of Small Animal Surgery. Philadelphia, W.B. Saunders, 1993, pp 1560–1567.
5. Krahwinkel DJ, Pardo AD, Sims MH: Effect of total ablation of the external acoustic meatus and bulla osteotomy on auditory function in dogs. J Am Vet Med Assoc 202:949–952, 1993.
6. McAnulty JF, Hattel A, Harvey CE: Wound healing and brain stem auditory evoked potentials after experimental total ear canal ablation with lateral tympanic bulla osteotomy in dogs. Vet Surg 24:1–8, 1995.
7. McCarthy RJ, Caywood DD: Vertical ear canal resection for end-stage otitis externa in dogs. J Am Anim Hosp Assoc 28:545–552, 1992.
8. Smeak DD, Crocker CB, Birchard SJ: Treatment of recurrent otitis media that developed after total ear canal ablation and lateral bulla osteotomy in dogs: Nine cases (1986–1994). J Am Vet Med Assoc 209:937–942, 1996.
9. Trevor PB, Martin RA: Tympanic bulla osteotomy for treatment of middle-ear disease in cats: 19 cases (1984–1991). J Am Vet Med Assoc 202:123–128, 1993.

20. SALIVARY GLAND DISEASES

Marie-Eve Nadeau, D.V.M., M.S.

1. Name the four pairs of salivary glands.
1. Parotid
2. Mandibular
3. Sublingual
4. Zygomatic

2. Which important neurovascular structures lie in proximity to the parotid gland?
- Internal maxillary artery courses through the gland.
- Palpebral, auriculotemporal, and buccal nerves lie underneath the rostral portion of the gland.
- Facial nerve lies underneath the dorsomedial aspect of the gland in close proximity to the external ear canal.

3. What is the course of the parotid duct?
It arises from the rostral border of the gland and courses rostrally with the masseter muscle. It terminates by a small **papilla** opposite the caudal aspect of the **fourth premolar.**

4. Which important vascular structures lie in proximity to the mandibular gland?
The gland lies between the maxillary vein ventrally and the linguofacial vein dorsally.

5. Which salivary gland is closely associated with and shares the same fibrous capsule as the mandibular gland?
The monostomatic portion of the sublingual gland adjoins the rostroventral portion of the gland. Both glands share a common thick fibrous capsule that originates from the deep cervical fascia.

6. What is the course of the mandibular duct?
It arises from the medial surface of the gland and runs rostrally in close association with and medially to the sublingual gland. It courses with the major sublingual duct and opens on a small **papilla** located lateral to the rostral end of the **frenulum.**

7. Describe the two parts of the sublingual gland.
1. The **monostomatic** part is flat, truncated, and darker than the mandibular gland. It is composed of lobules that are loosely arranged around the mandibular duct near the root of the tongue. Its secretions are emptied in the major sublingual duct.
2. The **polystomatic** portion is formed by 6–12 small lobules that secrete directly into the oral cavity.

8. Do the sublingual and mandibular glands have a common opening into the oral cavity?
Yes, in 20–34% of dogs.

9. Where is the zygomatic gland located?
Ventral to the zygomatic arch against the ventral portion of the periorbita.

10. Where is the zygomatic duct opening in the oral cavity?
The major zygomatic duct opens 1 cm caudal to the **parotid papilla;** several other small ducts open caudally to the major duct along the same plane.

11. What are the major diseases of the salivary system?

DISEASE	CLINICAL SIGNS
Zygomatic sialoadenitis	Epihora, painful swelling below the eye, exophthalmos, swelling lateral to the last maxillary molar
Parotid gland neoplasia	Generally nonpainful swelling in the area of the affected gland
Sublingual mucocele	Cervical: nonpainful, inframandibular fluid-filled swelling
	Pharyngeal: respiratory distress, dysphagia
	Oral cavity: oral bleeding
Parotid sialoliths	Painful swelling in the parotid gland area
Mandibular gland necrosis	Severe pain during swallowing or palpation of the head and neck

12. What is a ranula?

A mucocele on the floor of the mouth.

13. Which salivary disease is most common?

Mucocele: accumulation of saliva in the subcutaneous tissue subsequently causing tissue reaction to the saliva. The cause often remains obscure although trauma has been implicated. Mucocele occurs most commonly in the inframandibular space (cervical) but can be located orally (ranula) or in the pharyngeal wall (pharyngeal).

14. Which breeds are typically affected with a mucocele?

Toy and miniature poodles and German shepherds 2–4 years of age.

15. How should salivary gland and duct injury be managed?

SITE OF INJURY	MANAGEMENT
Parotid gland	Duct reconstruction or ligation
Zygomatic gland	Surgical excision of gland (to prevent mucocele formation)
Mandibular gland	Rarely requires treatment
Sublingual gland	Surgical excision of gland along with the mandibular gland (to prevent mucocele formation)

16. What are the treatment alternatives for mucocele (starting with the best option)?

- Surgical excision of the implicated gland
- Periodic drainage (not recommended for pharyngeal mucocele)
- Marsupialization (mostly for ranula and pharyngeal mucocele)

17. What is marsupialization?

Exteriorization or exposure of a cystic cavity by resection of the superficial wall and suturing of cut edges to adjacent skin. (From the Latin *marsupium,* pouch.)

18. What is the most common complication of mucocele surgery?

Recurrence (5%), resulting from failure to remove the entire affected gland or damage to the opposite gland when the sublingual gland is removed.

19. What is the most common tumor affecting the salivary gland?

Adenocarcinoma; this tumor is locally invasive, and metastasis to regional lymph nodes is common.

20. Describe the treatment of choice for adenocarcinoma.
Aggressive surgical excision is usually not curative and needs to be combined with radiation therapy to provide permanent local control and long-term survival. Median survival rate for animals treated with surgery with or without radiation is 12 months.

21. What is the treatment of choice for sialoliths?
Incision of the duct over the sialolith and removal.

BIBLIOGRAPHY

1. Harvey CE: Salivary gland. In Slatter D (ed): Textbook of Small Animal Surgery, 2nd ed. Philadelphia, W.B. Saunders, 1993, pp 515–520.
2. Morrison WB: Cancers of the head and neck. In Morrison WB (ed): Cancer in Dogs and Cats, 1st ed. Philadelphia, Lippincott Williams & Wilkins, 1999, pp 511–519.
3. Spangler WL, Culbertson MR: Salivary gland disease in dogs and cats: 245 cases (1985–1988). J Am Vet Med Assoc 198:465–469, 1991.
4. Withrow SJ: Cancer of the salivary gland. In Withrow SJ, MacEwen EG (eds): Small Animal Clinical Oncology, 2nd ed. Philadelphia, W.B. Saunders, Philadelphia, 1996, pp. 240–241.

21. BRACHYCEPHALIC SYNDROME

Holly S. Mullen, D.V.M., Dip. A.C.V.S.

1. What does brachycephalic mean?
Brachycephalic animals are characterized by a short, wide face. The bones of the base of the skull have reduced length and normal width. The soft tissues of the face, nose, and nasopharynx are relatively normal but excessive for a shortened skull.

2. Name some brachycephalic breeds.
Dogs
• Bulldog
• Boston terrier
• Boxer
• Lhasa apso
• Pug
• Pekingese
• Shar-pei
Cats
• Himalayan
• Persian

3. Why are brachycephalics predisposed to upper respiratory obstructive conditions?
Their shortened skulls cause compression and distortion of the nasal passages. During inspiration, these changes, plus redundant soft tissue in the nose and nasopharynx, increase negative pressure in the airway and cause secondary anatomic changes.

4. What are congenital components of the brachycephalic syndrome?
• Stenotic nares
• Elongated soft palate
• Hypoplastic trachea

5. What are acquired components of the brachycephalic syndrome?
• Everted laryngeal saccules
• Laryngeal edema

- Laryngeal collapse
- Redundant (edematous) pharyngeal folds

6. List the clinical signs of brachycephalic syndrome.
- Exercise intolerance
- Respiratory distress
- Gagging and dysphagia
- Open mouth or stertorous breathing
- Sleep apnea
- Cyanosis
- Collapse
- Death as a result of respiratory obstruction

7. What is the best way to evaluate brachycephalic syndrome?
Thoracic radiography and **oral examination** of the dog under anesthesia (simultaneous surgical correction). Tracheoscopy and bronchoscopy may also be done.

8. What are some important anesthetic considerations in a brachycephalic patient?
Preoxygenation and rapid induction followed by prompt endotracheal entubation prevent hypoxemia and hypercapnea. Several sizes of endotracheal tubes need to be available in case the trachea is smaller than expected. A laryngoscope and spay hook can be used to move aside tissues (including an elongated soft palate) for a complete oral examination.

9. What is a hypoplastic trachea?
A congenital narrowing, **not shortening,** of the trachea.

10. List the three dog breeds, in descending order, with the highest incidence of hypoplastic trachea.
1. English bulldog (approximately 55% of dogs with hypoplastic trachea)
2. Boston terrier (approximately 15%)
3. Boxer (approximately 5%)

11. Has hypoplastic trachea been reported in the cat with brachycephalic syndrome?
No.

12. Is there a sex predilection for hypoplastic trachea?
Males are affected twice as often as females.

13. What is the clinical significance of hypoplastic trachea?
Reduced tracheal size means less respiratory volume per breath. In the absence of other respiratory or cardiac abnormalities, a hypoplastic trachea is usually fairly well tolerated. In combination with upper respiratory abnormalities, severe dyspnea can result.

14. Is there any effective treatment for hypoplastic trachea?
No. If there are underlying cardiac or respiratory conditions, correcting them may improve the situation.

15. Compare a normal and elongated soft palate.

NORMAL SOFT PALATE	ELONGATED SOFT PALATE
Extends to caudal aspect of tonsils	Extends beyond the tonsils into the larynx
Tip of palate barely touches epiglottis	Tip of palate falls into laryngeal opening, blocking air flow

16. List the surgical options for reduction of an elongated soft palate
- Traditional excision
- Carbon dioxide laser excision

17. What is the optimal patient positioning for soft palate resection (staphylectomy)?
- Sternal recumbency, head elevated, mouth open
- Patient at end of table

18. How is soft palate excision performed?
1. Grasp the tip of the elongated soft palate with an Allis tissue forceps.
2. Place a 4–0 absorbable suture at one end of the proposed incision, leaving the suture long.
3. Excise one half of the redundant tissue.
4. Close oral mucosa to nasopharyngeal mucosa with a simple continuous suture pattern.
5. Excise the remaining half of redundant palate.
6. Continue the closure using the same suture pattern.

19. What are perioperative concerns with soft palate surgery?
1. Avoid cautery or crushing tissues; both cause increased swelling.
2. Minimize swelling in the first 24 hours by administering corticosteroids.
3. Leave the endotracheal tube in as long as possible; partially deflate the cuff when extubating to help remove blood clots that may have fallen into the tracheal lumen.

20. What kind of postoperative care is needed?
1. Feed soft foods for 1 week.
2. Avoid situations that stimulate barking or heavy breathing for 1 week.

21. How soon after surgery can improvement be noted?
Immediately, unless there is a lot of postoperative swelling; improvement should continue over the next 1–2 weeks as healing occurs.

22. What are stenotic nares?
Mild-to-severe reduction of the nostril lumen resulting from excessively thickened or medially displaced nasal and alar folds.

23. What are some problems caused or enhanced by stenotic nares?
- Increased respiratory effort, leading to increased inspiratory pressure.
- Increased inspiratory pressure, leading to everted saccules.
- Increased mouth breathing, causing increased swelling and dryness of oral membranes; nasal filtration and humidification systems are bypassed by mouth breathing.

24. In what three cat breeds are most stenotic nares noted?
- **Persians** and **Himalayans**—same mechanism as dogs
- **Scottish fold**—nonbrachycephalic; nasal folds may roll into the lumen of the nares, as a result of the same cartilaginous defect affecting ears

25. What is the best treatment for stenotic nares?
Nasal fold revision by horizontal, vertical, or lateral wedge resection, or by laser ablation.

26. What are everted laryngeal saccules, and how do they occur?
The saccules are the mucosal lining of the laryngeal ventricles. With chronic upper airway obstruction, this lining everts into the lumen of the larynx.

27. What is the appearance of everted saccules?
Velvety pink, soft, round masses protruding into the ventral laryngeal lumen, just rostral to the vocal folds.

28. What is the surgical treatment for everted saccules?
Grasp one saccule with an Allis tissue forceps, exert craniomedial traction, and simply excise (no cautery) it at its base using surgical scissors. Repeat for the other side. Temporary extubation greatly facilitates removal of the saccules. Replace the endotracheal tube after bilateral sacculectomy to allow good oxygenation during recovery.

29. What is the most severe, life-threatening secondary problem seen with brachycephalic syndrome?
Laryngeal collapse.

30. What is the sequence of events leading to laryngeal collapse?
Advanced, uncorrected brachycephalic syndrome → Excess negative pressure in the airway → Pharyngeal and laryngeal edema → Greater negative airway pressure → Everted saccules → Even greater negative pressure → Cuneiform and corniculate processes of arytenoid cartilages fold during inspiration → Cartilages become chondromalacic → Arytenoid cartilages collapse into the laryngeal lumen → Complete, life-threatening obstruction.

31. What is the primary differential diagnosis for laryngeal collapse?
Laryngeal paralysis.

32. How would you differentiate the two conditions?
Oral examination.

33. What is the treatment for laryngeal collapse?
Permanent tracheostomy, a salvage procedure.

34. Are cats affected by brachycephalic syndrome?
Yes, but rarely. There are brachycephalic cat breeds, some of which have one or more component of brachycephalic syndrome.

35. What component of brachycephalic syndrome is most frequently seen in affected cats?
Stenotic nares.

BIBLIOGRAPHY

1. Coyne BE, Fingland RB: Hypoplasia of the trachea in dogs: 103 cases (1974–1990). J Am Vet Med Assoc 201:768–772, 1992.
2. Hedlund CS: Brachycephalic syndrome. In Bojrab MJ (ed): Current Techniques in Small Animal Surgery, 4th ed. Baltimore, Williams & Wilkins, 1998, pp 357–362.
3. Nelson AW: Upper respiratory system. In Slatter D (ed): Textbook of Small Animal Surgery, 2nd ed. Philadelphia, W.B. Saunders, 1993, pp 733–776.

22. LARYNGEAL PARALYSIS

Robert M. Radasch, D.V.M., M.S., Dip. A.C.V.S.

1. What is laryngeal paralysis?
The partial or, more commonly, the complete failure of the arytenoid cartilages and vocal folds to abduct during inspiration, leading to mechanical upper airway obstruction.

2. What causes laryngeal paralysis?

Interruption of the motor innervation to the intrinsic muscles of the larynx. Occasionally, it can be caused by primary laryngeal muscle dysfunction or fibrosis.

3. Which nerves supply motor innervation to the intrinsic laryngeal muscles?

The **vagus nerve** supplies all motor innervation to the intrinsic laryngeal muscles. The vagus gives rise to the cranial and caudal laryngeal nerves. The external branch of the cranial laryngeal nerve provides the sole innervation to the cricothyroideus muscle. The caudal laryngeal nerve leaves the vagus in the thorax and courses rostrally through the neck to terminate as the recurrent laryngeal nerve. The recurrent laryngeal nerve supplies motor function to all intrinsic abductor and adductor muscles except the cricothyroideus muscle.

4. What is the primary intrinsic laryngeal muscle responsible for abduction of the vocal folds and arytenoid cartilages to cause opening of the laryngeal rima glottis?

Cricoarytenoideus dorsalis muscle.

5. Name the two forms of laryngeal paralysis.
- Congenital
- Acquired

6. Which form of laryngeal paralysis is more common?

Acquired (> 80% of reported cases).

7. What is the breed predisposition for the congenital form?
- United States—Siberian Huskies and possibly Dalmatians
- Netherlands—Bouvier des Flandres
- Britain—Bulldogs

8. What is the anatomic site of the primary neurologic abnormality in dogs affected by the congenital form of laryngeal paralysis?

The nucleus ambiguus of the brain. Wallerian degeneration of the recurrent laryngeal nerves has also been observed.

9. List the causes of acquired laryngeal paralysis.
- Trauma or surgery to the cranial aspect of the thorax or cervical area, resulting in injury to the vagus or recurrent laryngeal nerves
- Intrathoracic or cervical masses that cause vagal or recurrent laryngeal nerve damage or compression
- Primary recurrent laryngeal nerve lesions
- Generalized polyneuropathy, myopathy, or myasthenia gravis
- Hypothyroidism, possibly causing distal die-back of the recurrent laryngeal nerve
- Neoplasia, either primary or metastatic, affecting the recurrent laryngeal nerve, central or peripheral portions of the vagus nerve, or larynx
- **Idiopathic,** in which no underlying cause can be found. This is the commonest form of laryngeal paralysis, usually occurring in middle-aged to older, large-breed dogs (e.g., Labrador retrievers, golden retrievers, Irish setters).

10. List characteristic clinical signs of laryngeal paralysis.

The following signs are progressive:
- Dysphonia
- Exercise intolerance
- Inspiratory stridor
- Postprandial gagging and coughing
- Respiratory distress and collapse

11. How can laryngeal paralysis be definitively diagnosed?
- Electromyography of the laryngeal muscles to confirm denervation potentials
- Histopathology of intrinsic laryngeal muscles to identify denervation atrophy
- Laryngoscopy to confirm lack of abduction of the arytenoid cartilages and vocal folds

12. Is one method of diagnosis more accurate than another?
No. One study found 100% agreement between electromyographic studies and laryngoscopy. Biopsy is impractical. Most clinicians make the diagnosis by evaluating the lack of laryngeal motion under light general anesthesia.

13. Is the plane of anesthesia important for evaluation of laryngeal paralysis?
Yes. A normal animal has no laryngeal movements when placed under a deep plane of anesthesia. The patient should be anesthetized to a point where the mouth can be opened and a swallow **laryngeal reflex** initiated if the larynx is touched.

14. What should be seen during laryngoscopy to diagnose laryngeal paralysis?
- Medial displacement of the arytenoid cartilages and vocal folds, during inspiration and expiration (absence of normal abduction during inspiration)
- Inflammation and reddening of the edges of the arytenoid mucosa
- Occasionally, fluttering or partial abduction of the arytenoid cartilages during expiration (paradoxic motions). This should not be confused with normal abduction that occurs during inspiration.

15. What other diagnostic tests should be performed before surgery if laryngeal paralysis is suspected?
Chest radiographs, cervical neck palpation, and a thorough neurologic and physical examination to rule out neoplasia and generalized polyneuropathies or myopathies. Many patients with idiopathic laryngeal paralysis exhibit mild generalized neurologic weakness. Evaluation of thyroid function should also be considered because hypothyroidism has been associated with distal axon die-back, possibly resulting in polyneuropathy (including laryngeal paralysis). If indicated, acetylcholine receptor antibody levels can be determined to rule out myasthenia gravis as a cause of polyneuropathy and laryngeal paralysis.

16. How should an animal presented with respiratory distress, resulting from laryngeal paralysis, be initially managed?
- Sedation (oxymorphone, butorphanol, acepromazine, or diazepam)
- Corticosteroids
- Cooling, if hyperthermic
- Supplemental oxygen can be considered (oxygen not helpful if the larynx is closed)

Animals failing to respond to sedation, steroids, or cooling should have an immediate temporary tube tracheostomy or definitive surgical correction of the laryngeal paralysis.

17. List surgical procedures that can be performed in patients with severe signs of respiratory distress resulting from laryngeal paralysis.
- Partial laryngectomy, combined with unilateral or bilateral ventriculocordectomy
- Modified castellated laryngofissure
- Permanent tracheostomy
- Muscle-nerve pedicle transposition to reinnervate the larynx
- Arytenoid cartilage lateralization (*tie-back* procedure)

18. What structures are removed with a partial laryngectomy?
One or both vocal folds and associated vocalis muscle; unilateral partial resection of the corniculate, cuneiform, and vocal processes of one arytenoid cartilage.

19. Name the approach used to perform a partial laryngectomy.
Oral or ventral midline laryngotomy.

20. What are the advantages and disadvantages of the oral approach for a partial laryngectomy?
- Advantages:
  Technically easy
  Short operative time
- Disadvantages: If excessive tissue is removed, glottic stenosis and aspiration of food and water can occur.

21. What are the advantages and disadvantages of ventral midline laryngotomy?
- **Advantage:** Primary closure of the mucosa can minimize excessive scar tissue formation.
- **Disadvantages:**
  Functional size of the airway cannot be evaluated during procedure
  Excessive scar tissue along the ventral laryngotomy incision
  Aspiration of food and water if excessive tissue is removed
  Demanding surgical technique

22. Discuss the possible complications associated with partial laryngectomy ventriculocordectomy.
Of dogs with bilateral **ventriculocordectomy**, 58% have aspiration pneumonia, persistent cough, increased stridor, and exercise intolerance. In one study, 38% of dogs developed severe laryngeal webbing as a result of scar tissue (requiring a second surgery). **Partial laryngectomy** has resulted in a 49% overall complication rate, including death, aspiration pneumonia, and excessive scar tissue.

23. Is there a contraindication to performing partial laryngectomy?
Yes. Dogs with laryngeal paralysis complicated by laryngeal collapse are poor surgical candidates. A 50–83% incidence of postoperative death has been reported. Laryngeal collapse complicating laryngeal paralysis has often been seen in brachycephalic breeds and should be treated by an arytenoid cartilage lateralization or permanent tracheostomy.

24. What is a castellated laryngofissure?
This procedure entails creating a stepped, or castellated, incision through the ventral surface of the thyroid cartilage. The two halves of the thyroid cartilage are then separated, staggered, and repositioned to widen the opening of the glottis. The halves of the thyroid cartilage are sutured together in this *expanded* position.

25. Why should this technique not be commonly performed?
- Technically demanding
- Associated with numerous complications
- Produces questionable results

26. Why is muscle-nerve pedicle transposition to reinnervate the intrinsic laryngeal muscles seldom used?
This procedure is technically demanding, and the reinnervation process takes 5–11 months before clinical improvement is seen. A patient in acute distress will probably die before it works, making it impractical for the management of acute respiratory distress.

27. What surgical procedure is currently recommended for an older large-breed dog with idiopathic laryngeal paralysis?
Unilateral arytenoid cartilage lateralization (laryngeal *tie-back*)

28. How effective is a laryngeal *tie-back*?
Studies have shown that the procedure results in a 70–80% increase in glottic diameter, with >90% of the patients having less respiratory distress and improved exercise tolerance.

29. What structures are *tied back*?
A nonabsorbable suture is placed through the muscular process of one arytenoid cartilage and tied back to either (1) the caudal one third of the **cricoid cartilage** near the dorsal midline or (2) the caudodorsal aspect of the **thyroid cartilage**. Sutures tied to the thyroid cartilage pull the arytenoid laterally, whereas sutures tied to the cricoid mimic the function of the cricoarytenoideus dorsalis muscle and rotate the arytenoid laterally.

30. Should arytenoid cartilage lateralization be performed bilaterally?
No, because of postoperative complications. Even though a bilateral procedure increases the glottic diameter 180%, it results in an unacceptably high rate (43%) of aspiration pneumonia.

31. List the common complications associated with arytenoid cartilage lateralization.
- Gagging and coughing after drinking water (improves with time)
- Aspiration pneumonia (incidence is less than that associated with performing a partial laryngectomy)
- Some residual inspiratory stridor, which usually does not cause any clinical problems
- Altered vocalization
- Fracture of the arytenoid cartilage resulting in recurrence of acute inspiratory stridor and respiratory distress

32. Should a permanent tracheostomy be considered as a treatment option for laryngeal paralysis?
This technique may be considered in the following situations:
1. Brachycephalic breeds presented with laryngeal paralysis complicated by laryngeal collapse
2. Extremely small patients
3. Cases in which excessive scar tissue has caused severe glottic stenosis
4. Arytenoid cartilage lateralization procedures that have failed because of fracture of the arytenoid cartilage

BIBLIOGRAPHY

1. Greenfield CL: Canine laryngeal paralysis. Comp Cont Educ Pract Vet 9:1011–1020, 1987.
2. Hedlund CS: Laryngeal paralysis. In Fossum TW (ed): Small Animal Surgery. St. Louis, Mosby, 1997, pp 628–632.
3. Nelson AW: Upper respiratory system. In Slatter D (ed): Textbook of Small Animal Surgery, 2nd ed. Philadelphia, W.B. Saunders, 1993, pp. 755–761.
4. Petersen SW, Rosin E, Bjorling DE: Surgical options for laryngeal paralysis in dogs: A consideration of partial laryngectomy. Comp Cont Educ Pract Vet 13:1531–1541, 1991.

23. TRACHEOSTOMY

D. *Michael Tillson*, D.V.M., M.S., Dip. A.C.V.S.

1. What is a tracheostomy?
An opening between the skin and tracheal lumen. It allows air to enter the respiratory tract, while bypassing the nasal cavity, nasopharynx, and upper airway. In veterinary surgery, a tracheostomy is created as an emergency or adjunct procedure.

2. What are indications for tracheostomy tube placement?
- **Life-threatening upper airway obstruction** (current or anticipated)
- Prolonged ventilatory assistance in conscious or semiconscious patients
- Removal of aspirated materials
- Maintenance of a patent airway for oxygen delivery (with or without anesthetic gases) during surgeries of the upper airway or oral cavity.

3. What changes in the respiratory tree are associated with tracheostomy tube placement?
Incision into the tracheal lumen and placement of a tracheostomy tube results in disruption of the mucociliary apparatus (retained respiratory secretions), cilia loss, epithelial ulceration, and inflammation of the submucosal layer. The disruption of the respiratory clearing mechanism predisposes the patient to bronchopneumonia or bronchi obstruction and lung atelectasis.

4. Is a temporary tracheostomy an emergency procedure?
The placement of a tracheostomy tube can be an emergency or elective procedure. Tracheostomy tube placement is rarely a **crash** procedure to prevent death from anoxia. In most cases, patients requiring tracheostomy tubes can be intubated and ventilated before and during surgery. In rare cases in which intubation is prevented because of obstructive lesions or laryngeal swelling, the insertion of a large-gauge catheter or needle into the tracheal lumen with attachment to an oxygen source is useful.

5. How is a tracheostomy tube placed?
The patient is placed in dorsal recumbency with the head extended and the neck supported or arched. The skin, subcutaneous tissues, and ventral neck muscles are incised from the larynx extending 5 to 6 rings caudally. The trachea is cleared approximately half the distance around—taking care to identify and preserve the major vessels and nerves in the area (jugular vein, carotid artery, cranial thyroid artery, recurrent laryngeal nerve, vagosympathetic trunk).
Once the proposed insertion point is identified, stay sutures are placed around a tracheal ring cranial and caudal to the proposed incision. When the site is prepared and the tube is ready, the endotracheal tube is removed, and incision is made into the tracheal lumen. While applying gentle traction to the distal stay suture, the proximal portion of the trachea is gently depressed and the tracheostomy tube is inserted. One or two simple interrupted sutures are used to close the extremes of the skin incision. A nonadherent pad is covered with a topical antibiotic and placed around the tracheostomy tube. The tube is secured around the neck with umbilical tape and a light wrap.

6. Describe three different methods for incision into the tracheal lumen.
In general, the tracheal incision is begun 3 to 5 rings below the cricoid cartilage (larynx).
1. The most common method is a **horizontal incision** (50% of circumference) between tracheal rings.
2. A second technique involves a **longitudinal (vertical) incision** across several tracheal rings.
3. The **transverse flap tracheostomy** involves the formation of a flap from the ventral wall of the trachea. This is done as either an I or **lazy U** incision.

7. What is the advantage of the transverse flap technique?
Ease in changing the tracheostomy tube: The trachea is elevated toward the skin because of relocation of the sternohyoideus muscle dorsally. No increase in stricture formation was reported when the flap method was compared with standard tracheostomy incisions.

8. List the complications associated with tracheostomy tube placement.
- **Tracheal stenosis**—tube or surgical trauma.
- **Asphyxiation**—tube kinking, occlusion, improper placement.
- **Selective bronchial intubation**—excessive tube length.

9. **What complications are associated with the maintenance of a tracheostomy tube?**
   - Occlusion of the tracheostomy tube and patient death from asphyxiation (prevented by routine removal and cleaning of the tracheostomy tube and periodic suctioning of the trachea and tracheostomy tube).
   - Respiratory tract drying (as a result of air bypassing nasal passages, oxygen supplementation, and decreased mucociliary mechanism).
   - Local wound infection.
   - Tracheal damage.
   - Subcutaneous emphysema (usually mild and self-limiting).

10. **Can tube-associated tracheal damage be minimized?**
    Yes, with use of a tube one half to two thirds of the tracheal lumen diameter, deflating the cuff.

11. **How is drying of the respiratory tract managed?**
    The best method involves humidification (nebulizer) of oxygen flowing to a patient or intermittently infusing sterile saline into the tracheostomy tube and trachea.

12. **How is suctioning of the tracheostomy tube performed?**
    The goal is to remove accumulated respiratory secretions without asphyxiating the patient. The tracheostomy tube is first cleaned to remove any accumulated material which could be dislodged into the lungs. The patient is hyperoxygenated (2–3 minutes) before suctioning. A sterile suction tube is inserted through the tracheostomy tube lumen and advanced to the level of the bronchi. Intermittent suction is applied while the tube is slowly withdrawn, gently rotating and twisting.

13. **List desirable characteristics of tracheostomy tubes.**
    - Large enough for air exchange
    - Rigid to maintain shape
    - Flexible to prevent tracheal damage

14. **What are advantages and disadvantages of a double-lumen tracheostomy tube?**
    A double-lumen tracheostomy tube allows the inner cannula to be unlocked and removed for cleaning. The outer cannula remains in place, providing a patent airway for the patient. The use of a double-lumen tube decreases the stress created by the routine removal of tracheostomy tubes for cleaning.
    The disadvantage of double-lumen tubes is the structure: A double-lumen tube provides the patient with a smaller airway compared with a single-lumen tube with the same outside diameter.

15. **When is tracheostomy tube placement an elective procedure?**
    - Upper respiratory surgeries (soft palate resections, ventriculocordectomies, laryngectomies, modified castellated laryngofissures).
    - Tracheal surgeries.
    - Surgeries involving the oral cavity when: (1) there is significant risk of postoperative airway obstruction or (2) an endotracheal tube increases the difficulty of the surgical procedure.

16. **How should a temporary tracheostomy be closed?**
    Second intention healing.

17. **What antibiotics are indicated for a patient with a temporary tracheostomy?**
    None for the tracheostomy; broad-spectrum, bactericidal agents, based on culture and sensitivity testing, for underlying disease.

18. **What is the difference between a temporary and permanent tracheostomy?**
    A **temporary tracheostomy** allows access to the respiratory system during a limited period of time. Because the objective is not to create a permanent opening, it may be more accurate to use the term **tracheotomy** (*otomy* indicating an incision into a structure).

A **permanent tracheostomy** is a definitive treatment for specific diseases. It creates a permanent opening (stoma) for the tracheal lumen on the ventral surface of the neck, bypassing the nasal and pharyngeal portions of the respiratory system.

19. What are the steps for creation of a permanent tracheostomy?
1. A portion of overlying skin is removed from the proposed stoma site.
2. The trachea is elevated by separating the sternohyoideus muscles and suturing them together dorsally to the trachea.
3. A stoma is created by removing the ventral aspect of three to four rings, including the associated annular ligaments.
4. The trachea is sutured to the subcutaneous tissues to secure it in position.
5. The tracheal mucosa is elevated and sutured to the skin edge to form a mucocutaneous junction.

20. What is most critical in creating a successful permanent stoma?
The creation of a **mucocutaneous junction.** Accurate apposition of tracheal mucosa to skin edge is vital to prevent postoperative stricture of the stoma.

21. What is the aftercare for a permanent tracheostomy?
Because the surgical procedure creates a direct communication between the environment and the tracheal lumen, care must be taken to prevent aspiration of foreign materials (grasses, excessive dust, leaves, water), hair must be trimmed, and daily wound cleansing must be performed. Obese patients need to lose weight, and, in some cases, surgical removal of excessive skin is necessary.

BIBLIOGRAPHY

1. Fingland RB: Temporary tracheostomy. In Bonagura JD (ed): Kirks' Current Veterinary Therapy XII—Small Animal Practice. Philadelphia, W.B. Saunders, 1995, pp 179–183.
2. Hedlund CS: Tracheal resection and reconstruction. Prob Vet Med 3:210–228, 1991.
3. Hedlund CS, Tangner CH: Permanent tracheostomy: Perioperative and long-term data from 34 cases. J Am Anim Hosp Assoc 24:585–591, 1988.
4. Macintire D, Henderson RA: Transverse flap tracheostomy: A technique for temporary tracheostomy of intermediate duration. J Vet Emerg Crit Care 5:25–31, 1995.

24. TRACHEAL RESECTION AND ANASTOMOSIS

D. Michael Tillson, D.V.M., M.S., Dip. A.C.V.S.

1. What is the normal anatomy of the trachea?
The trachea is a semirigid tube connecting the oral cavity to the lower respiratory tract. In the dog and cat, it is composed of 35–45 C-shaped rings formed from hyaline cartilage (providing rigid support), a dorsal tracheal membrane (the trachealis muscle), and fibrous connective tissues stretching between the cartilage rings (annular ligaments). The tracheal lumen is covered by a ciliated columnar epithelium that is part of the mucociliary system. Blood vessels in the lateral pedicles provide a segmental vascular supply to the trachea.

2. List the clinical signs in animals with a tracheal lesion requiring resection and anastomosis.
- Dyspnea with noisy inspiratory (stertor) or wheezy expiratory (stridor) sounds.
- Exercise intolerance.

- Coughing (productive or with blood).
- Subcutaneous emphysema.
- Cyanosis or syncopial episodes.
- During hot weather, heat stress or stroke.

3. **What are the indications for tracheal resection and anastomosis?**
   - Any obstructive lesion of the lumen that results in a significant compromise in air passage: neoplastic lesions, inflammatory lesions, and strictures.
   - Tracheal avulsion after trauma.

4. **List the most common neoplastic diseases of the canine or feline trachea.**

   - Tumors of cartilage (chondromas, osteochondromas, chondrosarcomas)
   - Osteomas
   - Osteosarcomas
   - Leiomyomas
   - Mast cell tumors
   - Adenocarcinomas
   - Lymphosarcomas
   - Squamous cell carcinomas
   - Chondromas
   - Epidermal cell cancers

5. **What techniques are used for lesion localization?**
   Radiographs are useful for intraluminal lesions because the air within the lumen tends to highlight intraluminal obstructions. **Tracheoscopy** is helpful for lesion localization and biopsy (neoplastic or granulomatous lesions).

6. **Describe the surgical approaches to the trachea.**
   The **cervical** trachea is approached using a ventral midline incision. The trachea is found under the sternohyoideus muscle. Care must be taken during retraction and dissection to avoid injury to the contents of the carotid sheath (vagosympathetic trunk, carotid artery, internal jugular vein, and recurrent laryngeal nerve) and the segmental blood supply to the trachea. In many cases, the midline cervical incision allows access to the trachea extending back to the second intercostal space. Incision through the manubrium and a few cranial sternebrae (limited sternotomy) may allow resection of lesions ranging from the cervical trachea into the proximal portion of the thoracic cavity.
   Lesions closer to the **tracheal bifurcation** require a lateral thoracotomy for adequate exposure. The trachea is approached through a left third or fourth intercostal incision. The third intercostal space allows better exposure to the more proximal trachea, whereas the fourth space permits better exposure to the bifurcation and distal trachea. Median sternotomy offers limited exposure to the thoracic trachea and is especially difficult in large, deep-chested animals.

7. **Name two methods of tracheal anastomosis.**
   1. **Split ring technique:** Using a sharp scalpel blade, the trachea is incised through the cartilage rings, proximal and distal to the lesion. The anastomosis is performed by placing a nonabsorbable, monofilament suture around the rings, gently apposing them. In most cases, there is minimal telescoping of the distal portion into the larger proximal portion.
   2. **Annular ligament anastomosis:** A suture is placed around the first cartilage ring on either side of the incision.

8. **Which method is preferred for tracheal resection and anastomosis?**
   Split ring technique. The annular ligament anastomosis technique created a greater amount of luminal stenosis when evaluated 2 months after surgery compared with the split ring anastomotic technique.

9. **Is there a preferred suturing technique for tracheal anastomosis?**
   A study showed that although a simple continuous suture pattern required less time to complete, tissue apposition was improved and postoperative stenosis was decreased with an **inter-**

rupted pattern. Long-lasting, monofilament, absorbable or nonabsorbable sutures can be used for tracheal surgery. Stay and tension-relieving sutures can be 2-0 or 3-0, whereas the actual anastomosis is performed with a smaller suture (4-0). After anastomosis, the stay sutures are converted into tension-relieving sutures by encircling a ring on either side of the incision.

10. How many tracheal rings can be removed?
Approximately **8–10 rings** (25%) of the trachea can be resected in the adult dog. In juvenile animals, the risk of postoperative stenosis is increased (most likely becuase of growth), and removal of fewer rings is recommended.

11. Is tracheal resection and anastomosis considered a treatment for tracheal collapse?
No.

12. What factors should be considered relative to anesthesia and airway management in dogs undergoing tracheal resection and anastomosis?
Animals in respiratory distress should be preoxygenated and closely monitored after premedication administration. Smooth, rapid induction, along with the establishment of assisted ventilation, is important. A wide selection of endotracheal tubes should be available for use because the tracheal lesions may limit the size of endotracheal tubes that can be placed. Care is taken to ensure that the endotracheal tube extends beyond the lesion or is proximal to the lesion to avoid tube obstruction.

13. How does the patient get oxygen and anesthetic gases during resection and anastomosis?
1. The distal tracheal segment is intubated by the surgeon using a sterile endotracheal tube from the surgical site.
2. The existing endotracheal tube is manipulated into the distal tracheal segment across the incision sites.
3. An endotracheal tube is placed beyond the tracheal lesion, and the trachea is resected around the tube.
4. In many cases, a combination of techniques is required for patient ventilation. Planning and good communication between the surgeon and the anesthetist are vital.

14. Discuss the postoperative complications associated with tracheal resection and anastomosis.
Most patients show minimal complications after surgery. Laryngeal, pharyngeal, or tracheal edema can result in immediate postoperative respiratory distress. Laryngeal paralysis, secondary to trauma to the recurrent laryngeal nerve, can be a major complicating factor in dogs and cats during recovery. Swelling and occlusion of the anastomotic site could cause airway obstruction. Surgery on the trachea and suture placement within the tracheal lumen can also result in mucostasis. Failure by the surgeon to clear blood and mucus from the trachea after surgery can predispose the patient to aspiration pneumonia.

Long-term complications include tracheal dehiscence as a result of vascular compromise and airway obstruction secondary to stricture or granuloma formation. Granuloma formation has been associated with the use of braided, nonabsorbable suture materials.

15. What are reasons for the postsurgical stricture formation?
1. **Tension across the anatomosis site.** Tension creates stenosis by promoting tracheal elongation as a response to increased tensile forces. As the trachea elongates, tension across the anastomotic site decreases, but the lumen diameter also decreases forming a stenotic area.
2. **Poor apposition at the resection and anastomosis site.** This is more commonly reported with the annular ring anastomosis than with the split ring anastomosis technique.

16. List techniques that can be used for reducing tension across a tracheal incision.
- Limited tracheal ring removal
- Stay or tension sutures
- Annular ligament incisions
- Flexion neck harnesses

17. What techniques are used to treat postoperative tracheal strictures?

Mild strictures are amenable to **bougienage** (dilation) and **corticosteroid therapy.** Tracheal stents can be used to help delay the reformation of strictures. The usefulness of this therapy is still debated. Severe tracheal strictures may require additional surgery (i.e., a second resection and anastomosis). Concurrent use of corticosteroids to slow the formation of fibrous tissue and re-stricture is questionable but frequently a component of stricture management.

18. What is mucostasis?

Disruption of the mucociliary transport mechanism caused by respiratory disease, mucosal trauma, or stenosis. Transport can occur across small gaps in the mucosa, but large gaps and steno-sis result in reduction of this cleansing action. Reduced mucus clearance increases the risk of res-piratory infections.

19. What clinical sign would be the most dramatic indication of a surgical dehiscence after tracheal resection and anastomosis?

The formation of severe **subcutaneous emphysema.**

In patients with a dehiscence of an intrathoracic portion of the trachea, the development of severe dyspnea is the primary clinical sign. This may indicate the development of a pneumotho-rax or possibly a life-threatening tension pneumothorax. Placement of a thoracostomy tube and continuous suction are needed to manage such a complication. Diagnostic tests, including radi-ography, tracheoscopic examination, and reoperation for direct visualization, are immediately un-dertaken to determine the cause and severity of the leakage. Immediate reoperation may be the most prudent option because chances of spontaneous healing is slight in cases with significant leakage. It is possible to see subcutaneous emphysema in cases of thoracic tracheal leakage in-stead of pneumothorax. This occurs when the pleura has healed, forcing leaking air to remain within the mediastinum. The air migrates through the thoracic inlet into the subcutaneous tissues.

BIBLIOGRAPHY

1. Dallman MJ, Bojrab MJ: Large-segment tracheal resection and interannular anastomosis with a tension-release technique in the dog. Am J Vet Res 42:217–223, 1982.
2. Fingland RB: Tracheal resection and anastomosis. In Bojrab MJ (ed): Current Techniques in Small An-imal Surgery. Baltimore, Williams & Wilkins, 1996.
3. Hardie E, Spodnick GJ: Tracheal rupture in 16 cats. J Am Vet Med Assoc 214:508–512, 1999.
4. Hedlund CS: Tracheal anastomosis in the dog: A comparison of two end-to-end techniques. Vet Surg 13:135–142, 1984.

25. PULMONARY LOBECTOMY

Robin Holtsinger, D.V.M.

1. List the indications for pulmonary lobectomy in the dog and cat.
- Primary pulmonary neoplasia
- Lung abscesses
- Pneumothorax resulting from bullae or cysts
- Severe pulmonary trauma
- Lung lobe torsion

2. What surgical approaches are commonly used for pulmonary lobectomy?
- Lateral intercostal thoracotomy
- Median sternotomy

3. What are the advantages and disadvantages of each of these approaches?
- **Lateral thoracotomy** allows access to a limited (specific) region of the thorax, whereas **median sternotomy** allows greater exposure to the entire thoracic cavity.
- Lateral thoracotomy is preferable to median sternotomy when access to the hilar or dorsal thoracic regions is required.
- Both approaches carry similar rates of postoperative morbodity and compromise to the patient's vital capacity.

4. Which intercostal space is most commonly chosen for lateral thoracotomy to perform pulmonary lobectomy?
The affected lung lobes are most commonly approached through a lateral 5th or 6th intercostal space thoracotomy; it allows the best access to the hilar region of all lung lobes. When in doubt, one should choose the more caudad space because ribs are more readily retracted cranially than caudally.

5. What two methods are most commonly used to perform pulmonary lobectomy?
1. Conventional lobectomy (isolation and transection of the airway and vasculature)
2. Use of surgical stapling equipment

6. What are pulmonary ligaments and why are they important?
Pleural reflections that attach the caudal lung lobes to the caudal mediastinum and diaphragm. Incision of these avascular ligaments facilitates mobilization of the lung lobes and exposure of the hilus.

7. How is a conventional pulmonary lobectomy performed?
The hilar region is approached and the bronchus identified by palpation and dissection. The pulmonary artery is isolated with right-angle forceps and triple-ligated, then divided between the distal two ligatures. The lung lobe is then retracted dorsally, and the pulmonary vein is isolated ventromedial to the bronchus and ligated and divided as the artery. The bronchus is then isolated and double-clamped with vascular forceps. It is transected leaving a 3–5 mm stump. Multiple overlapping interrupted horizontal mattress sutures are placed across the stump. The stump is then oversewn with a simple continuous pattern (use of a tapered needle and fine suture material decreases air leakage from needle passage sites).

8. How much lung tissue can be removed in the dog without compromising the animal?
50% of total lung mass. Because of its relatively smaller volume, the entire left lung can be removed if the right side is healthy. Conversely, acute removal of the entire right side is likely to be fatal, although staged excision of a greater volume may be possible.

9. Which of the currently available surgical stapling equipment is most useful for pulmonary lobectomy?
Most commonly used is the TA 30 linear vascular stapling device (United States Surgical Corporation), which fires a triple row of overlapping 2.8-mm staples, greatly speeding and simplifying lung lobectomy. The numeric designation refers to the length in millimeters of the staple row placed after discharge. The staples usually occlude the pulmonary vessels satisfactorily, but occasionally a residual leak from the bronchus necessitates hand suturing.

10. How is pulmonary lobectomy performed by stapling?
The tissue to be excised is placed in the jaws of the stapler, and they are closed. The approximating lever is gently closed to the desired degree of tissue compression. The safety catch is re-

leased, and the trigger is fired until it locks into the handle, sealing the tissue with staples. The edge of the stapling device is then used as a cutting guide for a blade to transect the tissue distal to the rows of staples. The jaws are released, and the instrument is removed. The stump is inspected closely for leakage. Additional sutures can be placed as needed.

11. When is partial lung lobectomy preferable to total lobectomy?
- Peripheral lobar lesions (such as pulmonary blebs or bullae)
- Tumor metastasis where complete lobectomy is not necessary

12. Name two methods of performing partial pulmonary lobectomy.
1. Surgical stapling using the TA 30 autostapler
2. Conventional partial lobectomy via a row of overlapping interrupted horizontal mattress sutures and a simple continuous oversew with fine monofilament absorbable sutures on a tapered needle

13. What are the advantages of the stapling technique in partial pulmonary lobectomy?
- Quicker
- Requires less tissue manipulation
- Results in less air leakage than hand-sewn partial lobectomy

14. After completion of either partial or complete pulmonary lobectomy, what steps are taken to ensure an uneventful postoperative course?
- The thorax is filled with warmed sterile saline and the surgical site evaluated during positive-pressure ventilation for air leakage (particularly from the bronchial stump).
- A chest tube is always placed before closure.
- Chest tubes are aspirated frequently (every 2–4 hours), and the amount of air is quantitated.
- Chest tubes are generally removed in 24–48 hours if air is not accumulating in the pleural space postoperatively.

15. When are most postoperative complications seen after pulmonary lobectomy?
Most occur within the critical 24-hour period after thoracotomy.

16. List the most common postoperative problems?
- Hypoventilation
- Hypoxemia
- Hypothermia
- Pain

17. What postoperative monitoring techniques are particularly helpful after lobectomy?
- Arterial blood gas measurement
- Respirometer to evaluate tidal volume
- Central venous pressure measurement
- Pulse oximetry
- Capnography

18. What does a PaO_2 of < 60 mm Hg suggest in a postlobectomy patient?
A serious problem; supplemental oxygen or positive end-expiratory pressure therapy may be required.

19. When is surgical reexploration necessary postlobectomy?
When there is continuous leakage of air resulting from inadequate closure of the bronchial stump or a tear in the pulmonary parenchyma (> 500 ml of air per 24 hours), or significant ongoing hemorrhage is observed. It is also important to rule out the primary incision and the chest tube as potential sources of air leakage before surgery is repeated.

20. What is the prognosis for a dog with a pulmonary abscess associated with chronic pneumonia?
Good, if the patient survives the critical perioperative period. There is a 20% perioperative

mortality rate, a 50% rate of resolution with surgery, and a 25% rate of recurrent or unresolved pneumonia.

21. What are the most common primary pulmonary neoplasms in the dog?
Pulmonary adenocarcinomas and **alveolar carcinomas** comprise 95% of primary lung tumors.

22. What is the prognosis for a dog with a primary neoplasm after pulmonary lobectomy?
In patients whose lymph nodes are free of tumor and complete excision has been performed, the median survival time is approximately 1 year. If there has already been spread of tumor to the regional nodes, a median survival time of 2–3 months may be expected.

23. What is the rationale for considering patients for pulmonary metastectomy via partial lobectomy?
That gross metastatic disease in the lungs is poorly responsive to chemotherapy and immunotherapy.

24. Which lung lobe is most frequently involved in lung lobe torsion?
The right middle lung lobe.

25. What is the treatment of choice for this condition?
Lateral thoracotomy and lobectomy *in situ* is recommended to prevent the release of sequestered endotoxin and other vasoactive substances into the systemic circulation.

26. In cases of spontaneous pneumothorax, what is the most commonly reported histopathologic finding that causes the clinical signs?
Bullous emphysema, resulting in rupture of a bleb or bulla and accumulation of air in the pleural space. Other reported associated conditions include heartworm disease (thromboembolic events), neoplasia, and pneumonia.

27. What is the prognosis for dogs with spontaneous pneumothorax?
Guarded. Recurrence rates for dogs treated conservatively (thoracocentesis or tube thoracostomy) approach $\geq 80\%$, whereas those treated surgically have a 25% recurrence rate (other areas of the lung may develop bullae that subsequently rupture).

BIBLIOGRAPHY

1. Fossum TW: Surgery of the lower respiratory system: Lungs and thoracic wall. In Fossum TW (ed): Small Animal Surgery. St. Louis, Mosby, 1997, pp 649–658, 661–667.
2. Holtsinger RH, Beale BS, Bellah JR: Spontaneous pneumothorax in the dog: A retrospective analysis of 21 cases. J Am Anim Hosp Assoc 29:195–210, 1993.
3. LaRue SM, Withrow SJ, Wykes PM: Lung resection using surgical staples in dogs and cats. Vet Surg 16:238, 1987.
4. Nelson WA: Lower respiratory system. In Slatter D (ed): Textbook of Small Animal Surgery, 2nd ed. Philadelphia, W.B. Saunders, 1993, pp 777–804.
5. Nelson AW: Surgery of the bronchi and lungs. In Bojrab MJ (ed): Current Techniques in Small Animal Surgery. Philadelphia, Lea & Febiger, 1983, pp 270–280.
6. O'Brien MG, Straw RC, Withrow SJ: Resection of pulmonary metastases in canine osteosarcoma: 36 cases (1983–1992). Vet Surg 22:105–109, 1993.
7. Waters DJ, Sweet DC: Role of surgery in the management of dogs with pathologic conditions of the thorax—Part I. Comp Cont Educ Pract Vet 13:1545–1556, 1991.

26. CHYLOTHORAX

Dianne Dunning, D.V.M., M.S., Dip. A.C.V.S.

1. What is chyle?

The lymphatic fluid arising from the intestine. It is high in fat content and typically contains >80% lymphocytes.

2. What constitutes a chylous effusion?

Chylothorax is the accumulation of chyle within the thoracic cavity.

Characteristics of Chylous Effusion

PARAMETER	FINDING
Color	White-to-pink, forms a cream layer when left to stand
Clarity	Opaque; remains clear when centrifuged
Specific gravity	1.019–1.050
Protein content	2.5–4.0 g/dl
Chylomicrons	Present
Total WBC/μl	1,650–24,420/μl
Predominant cell type	Lymphocytes or neutrophils
Triglyceride content	> Serum
Cholesterol content	Serum
Sudanophilic fat globules	Present
Ether clearance	Clears

WBC = white blood cells.

3. List common conditions associated with chylothorax.

Idiopathic	Cardiomyopathy
Thoracic duct ectasia	Neoplasia (mediastinal lymphoma)
Thoracic duct rupture	Lung lobe torsion
Cranial vena cava obstruction	Diaphragmatic hernia
Heartworm disease	Fungal pulmonary infections (blastomycosis)
Restrictive pericarditis	Long-term jugular catheter use

4. What are possible causes of chylothorax?

Lymphatic hypertension and subsequent transmural leakage of chyle have been proposed as causes of chylothorax. Experimental and clinical studies in dogs with idiopathic chylothorax have revealed lymphangiectasia (dilation) of the mediastinal and pleural lymphatics.

5. Which breeds are at risk for chylothorax?

Typical signalment includes a middle-aged to older animal of any breed. **Afghans, Sheba Inus, Siamese,** and **Himalayans** appear to have an increased risk. Sheba Inus may present early, at < 1 year of age.

6. What is the typical history for a dog or cat with chylothorax?

A vague history of coughing that is refractory to empiric medical management before the on-set of respiratory distress. The complaint of coughing is caused by the irritation of the pleural cavity by chylous effusion.

7. Describe the typical presenting signs.

The most common presentation is dyspnea. Increased bronchovesicular sounds may be auscultated dorsally, with absent heart and lung sounds present ventrally. In addition to compromised respiration, chronic chylothorax may also result in the debilitation of the animal because of the loss of large amounts of proteins, fats, fat-soluble vitamins, and lymphocytes into the thoracic cavity. Common electrolyte abnormalities include hyperkalemia and hyponatremia.

8. How is the diagnosis of chylothorax best established?

Diagnosis is suspected based on auscultation of dull respiratory sounds in a dyspneic animal and may be confirmed via **thoracocentesis** and **analysis of the fluid.** Given the multitude of diseases associated with chylothorax, further diagnostic evaluations, including radiography, ultrasonography, fluid culture and sensitivity, and echocardiography, are recommended to identify an underlying primary disease condition. If no underlying pathology is identified, the diagnosis of **idiopathic chylothorax** is made.

9. Discuss the medical therapy for idiopathic chylothorax.

The goal is to provide for the nutritional and metabolic needs of the patient until the effusion resolves spontaneously. The main components of medical management are **thoracocentesis** and **low-fat diet.**

- **Pleural drainage**—alleviates signs of respiratory distress.
- **Dietary management**
  Low-fat diets reduce the lipid content of the effusion but do not seem to decrease the volume. Decreasing lipid content of the effusion may enhance resorption by the pleura, but experimental evidence of this is unavailable.
  Medium-chain triglycerides (MCT) may be used to supplement the caloric content of the low-fat diet and are reportedly directly absorbed into the venous system. Experimental support for the complete bypass of the MCT into the venous system is lacking.
- **Total parenteral nutrition (TPN)**—decreases the flow of chyle through the thoracic duct by the complete bypass of gastrointestinal tract. TPN is rarely used for chylothorax in veterinary medicine because of the sometimes prohibitive cost of the TPN and the intensive care necessary to maintain a designated central line for the administration of the TPN.
- **Pharmaceuticals**
  Diuretics (furosemide) are not effective, may lead to dehydration, and are not recommended.
  Steroids may decrease inflammation and pleuritis, enabling more effective fluid resorption and, it is hoped, preventing fluid formation; however, no scientific evidence is available to support this assumption.

10. What is rutin?

A benzopyrone compound extracted from the fruit of the Brazilian Fava D'Anta (*Dimorphandra*) tree. In humans, it is used with mixed success in medical management of lymphedema associated with axillary lymph node extraction necessitated by metastatic breast cancer and elephantiasis caused by filarial disease. The overall conclusion within the human literature regarding the use of rutin in lymphedema is that it is safe, of variable effectiveness, but slow to work (months to years). Successful treatment of feline patients has been recently reported. Rutin is a flavone derivative and available as a nutrapharmaceutical, sometimes referred to as a **bioflavonoid.**

11. List the proposed mechanisms of action of rutin and benzopyrone compounds.

- Reduces leakage from blood vessels
- Increases protein removal by lymphatic vessels
- Increases phagocytosis via stimulation of macrophages
- Increases number of macrophages in tissues
- Increases proteolysis and removal from tissues

12. When are animals with idiopathic chylothorax considered surgical candidates?

In general, if they fail to respond to medical management after 5–10 days. Other indications for surgery include a loss of chyle > 20 ml/kg/day over a 5-day period or if the animal displays severe protein-calorie malnutrition and hypoproteinemia.

13. List the surgical options for chylothorax.
- Thoracic duct ligation
- Pleurodesis
- Active pleurovenous and pleuroperitoneal shunting
- Passive pleuroperitoneal shunting
- Omental pedicle drainage

14. What is the difference in surgical approaches between dogs and cats with chylous effusion?
Chyle is transported from the intestines to the venous system via the thoracic duct on the **right side in dogs** and on the **left side** of the thoracic cavity in **cats.** Because of the anatomic differences in location, the thoracic duct is approached through a **right thoracotomy in dogs** and a left **thoracotomy in cats,** at 10th or 11th intercostal space. An abdominal approach is also described for cats.

15. What does thoracic duct ligation involve?
Some authors advocate identification and dissection of the thoracic duct and all its branches; others recommend *en bloc* ligation of mediastinal tissues dorsal to aorta.

16. How is successful thoracic duct surgery defined?
Complete resolution of the chylous effusion.

17. What is the success rate of thoracic duct ligation?
20–60% for dogs and cats, with more recent studies quoting 59% for dogs and 53% for cats with idiopathic chylous effusion.

18. What preoperative and postoperative studies are required for thoracic duct ligation?
Preoperative and postoperative positive contrast lymphangiography.

19. How is new methylene blue used in surgery to delineate the thoracic duct and ensure complete ligation?
The dye (0.5–1.0 ml) is injected into an adjacent mesenteric lymphatic or lymph node that is then picked up by the thoracic duct. Complete ligation is confirmed when there is no lymphatic drainage into the chest via the thoracic duct or any of its tributaries.

20. What is pleurodesis?
A method of treating pleural effusion by inducing diffuse adhesions between parietal and visceral pleura.

21. How is pleurodesis performed?
1. *Chemical pleurodesis* uses agents such as tetracycline (drug of choice), quinacrine hydrochloride, bleomycin, fluorouracil, and talc.
2. *Mechanical pleurodesis* is performed by rubbing a dry gauze sponge on the parietal pleurae.

22. What is the difference between active and passive shunts?
- *Active pleurovenous and pleuroperitoneal shunts* relocate fluid via negative pressure created by a manual pump into a large abdominal vein or the peritoneal cavity, where it is absorbed. The inflow tube is placed in thorax, which is connected to a pump chamber placed subcutaneously over a rib. The outflow tube is placed in a large abdominal vein (such as the caudal vena cava or azygous) or free floating within the abdominal cavity.
- *Passive pleuroperitoneal shunts* rely on gravity to move fluid from the pleural space to the peritoneal cavity via fenestrations in the diaphragm. Silastic mesh implants are most commonly employed; however, long-term patency may be compromised because of adherence of liver or omentum.

23. When are shunts contraindicated?

- All shunting techniques are contraindicated with sepsis.
- Most shunting techniques are not effective in cats because of their small size.
- Pleuroperitoneal shunts have been shown be ineffective when there are disease processes present that impair absorption from peritoneal cavity, such as right-sided heart failure or diffuse lymphatic disease.

24. How is the omentum used to treat chylothorax?

An omental pedicle is advanced into the thoracic cavity for a physiologic drain and prevention of chyle accumulation via its adherent and granulation properties.

25. Why would anyone ever want to peel a lung?

Peeling refers to decortication of a lung lobe, a process performed when restrictive or constrictive pleuritis exists, a condition seen more commonly in cats than dogs. Decortication involves the removal of the fibrous adhesions coating the surface of the lung, restricting its expansion and limiting air exchange. This procedure is associated with severe hemorrhage, persistent pneumothorax, and a high incidence of morbidity and mortality.

26. Can one treat chylothorax with Superglue?

Isobutyl 2-cyanoacrylate (Superglue) is combined with positive contrast agent injected through a catheter in a mesenteric lymphatic. Fluoroscopic monitoring is performed during embolization to prevent excessive amounts of this embolic compound from entering vena cava. Complete obstruction of thoracic duct has been reported in the experimental and clinical setting, eliminating the need for a thoracotomy.

27. What are the complications that occur after thoracic duct ligation and embolization?

Recurrence of the original effusion or the appearance of a persistent nonchylous effusion. Recurrence of the chylous effusion is associated with the incomplete ligation of the thoracic duct or with the development of alternate pathways of lymph drainage within the thoracic and abdominal cavities. The development of a nonchylous effusion after thoracic duct ligation is a direct result of the inflammation associated with the residual pleuritis.

CONTROVERSY

28. Is surgery a reasonable treatment for animals with idiopathic chylothorax?

There is considerable debate whether any animal is a surgical candidate, given the multitude of primary disease conditions associated with chylothorax, the relatively low success rate (approximately 60%) with thoracic duct ligation, and the potential of recurrence because of the extensive arborization of the lymphatic system. Some clinicians advocate only medical management for the treatment for idiopathic chylous effusion. Given the sometimes vague history and late presentation of clinical signs, however, early surgical intervention has been proposed as a means to prevent constrictive pleuritis, to which cats seem particularly sensitive. With chronic effusion, cats develop severe constrictive pleural fibrosis that compromises pulmonary function with chronic effusion from the irritative effects of chyle.

BIBLIOGRAPHY

1. Fossum TW: Surgery of the lower respiratory system: Pleural cavity and diaphragm. In Duncan L (ed): Small Animal Surgery. St. Louis, Mosby, 1997, pp 691–693.
2. Kerpsack SJ, McLoughlin MA: Evaluation of mesenteric lymphangiograph and thoracic duct ligation in cats with chylothorax: 19 cases (1987–1992). J Am Vet Med Assoc 205:711–715, 1994.
3. Orton EC: Pleura and pleural space. In Slatter D (ed): Textbook of Small Animal Surgery. Philadelphia, W.B. Saunders, 1993, pp 381–399.
4. Orton EC: Pleural effusion and drainage. In: Small Animal Thoracic Surgery. Baltimore, Williams & Wilkins, 1995, pp 87–105.

5. Suess RP, Flanders JA: Constrictive pleuritis in cats with chylothorax: 10 Cases (1983–1991). J Am Anim Hosp Assoc 30:70–77, 1994.
6. Thompson MS, Cohn LA: Use of rutin for medical management of idiopathic chylothorax in 4 cats. J Am Vet Med Assoc 215:345–348, 1999.
7. Williams JM, Niles JD: Use of omentum as physiologic drain for treatment of chylothorax in a dog. Vet Surg 28:61–65, 1999.

27. THORACIC WALL RESECTION AND RECONSTRUCTION

D. Michael Tillson, D.V.M., M.S., Dip. A.C.V.S.

1. List the indications for thoracic wall reconstruction.
- *En bloc* resection of neoplastic diseases.
- *En bloc* resection for chronic infections (bacterial or mycotic).
- Severe chest wall trauma.
- Congenital defects.

2. What is *en bloc* resection?
Removal of large portions of tissues without regard to tissue planes, intralesional dissection, or preservation of structures. When a chest wall mass is removed *en bloc,* the mass is removed with the surrounding tissues to achieve a clean surgical margin. This includes the skin, superficial and deep muscle layers, involved ribs and a rib craniad and caudad to the mass, intercostal muscles, and the pleura. Extension of the disease into the thoracic cavity may result in adhesions or local tumor metastasis requiring débridement or removal of pulmonary tissue as well.

3. Which tumors are most commonly associated with the thoracic wall?
- Osteosarcoma
- Chondrosarcoma

4. Which of these tumors has a better prognosis?
Chondrosarcoma (10.7 months versus 3.3 months for osteosarcoma).

5. State the goals of thoracic wall reconstruction.
- Restoration of thoracic cavity stability
- Creation of an air-tight cavity

6. Why is restoration of thoracic wall stability important?
Respiration involves active expansion of the thoracic wall and diaphragm. This action enlarges the thoracic cavity and creates a lower intrathoracic pressure. This pressure differential allows air movement into the lungs and alveoli. Unstable chest wall conditions (paradoxic movement with flail chest) compromise respiration.

7. List several options for thoracic wall reconstruction.
- Primary closure with autogenous tissues
- Diaphragmatic advancement
- Reconstruction using prosthetic materials

8. Are there limits to the size of an *en bloc* resection?
Resection ≤ 6 ribs.

9. List the advantages and disadvantages using autogenous tissues for thoracic wall closure.

ADVANTAGES	DISADVANTAGES
Fewer complications	Increased surgery and anesthesia time
Low cost	Reduced margins because of fear of incomplete closure
Use of viable muscle tissues	Inadequate resection and contamination of flap tissues

10 What muscles are available for muscle flap elevation?

Although any of the thoracic wall muscles can be used for wound reconstruction, the **latissimus dorsi** muscle is preferred. The **latissimus dorsi** muscle is triangular, with the broad base originating from thoracolumbar fascia and the last ribs. Although some of the blood supply is ligated in raising the flap, the muscle can survive on the cranial vascular supply. The muscle can be released and rotated ventrally to close large defects.

11. What is diaphragmatic advancement?

The release and craniad movement of a portion of the diaphragmatic crus into the space normally considered to be the thoracic cavity. This action enlarges the abdominal cavity, decreases the thoracic cavity, and incorporates the body wall defect into a portion of the abdominal wall.

12. How does diaphragmatic advancement play a role in thoracic wall reconstruction?

It allows the surgeon to perform a technically simpler procedure than either prosthetic mesh implantation or muscle flap elevation and advancement.

13. List the advantages and the disadvantages in performing a diaphragmatic advancement for the repair of a chest wall defect.

ADVANTAGES	DISADVANTAGES
Technical ease	Decrease in thoracic cavity
Autogenous tissue	Decrease in tidal volume and lung capacity
Basic instrumentation	
Good cosmesis	

14. Can diaphragmatic advancement be used to convert any thoracic wall defect?

No. The diaphragm can be advanced only a certain distance without compromising respiratory function. A general guideline is diaphragmatic advancement can be used in resection of the caudad thoracic wall (ribs 9 to 13).

15. What synthetic materials can be used in thoracic wall reconstruction?

Polypropylene and **polyethylene,** nonreactive, nonabsorbable materials that maintain a high tensile strength, which are woven into mesh sheets. The open weave allows for ingrowth of fibrous tissue into the mesh. The inherent rigidity of the meshes and the ingrowth of fibrous tissue into the mesh weave help to restore chest wall stability. The primary disadvantages of the synthetic meshes are cost of the material and handling qualities. Closure of large wounds using combinations of mesh materials and supportive structures (plastic spinal plates, autogenous rib grafts, or molded methyl methacrylate) is reported in the veterinary literature. Other materials, including Silastic sheets, Dacron, and polytetrafluoroethylene (PTFE) patches, have been used to close thoracic wall defects. The flexible nature of these materials makes them less effective in reestablishing the rigidity of the chest wall unless combined with other materials.

16. How is the mesh used?

After the mesh is correctly sized, it is sutured in place using simple interrupted or mattress-type sutures (monofilament, nonabsorbable). In closing thoracic wall defects, mesh is secured to the dorsal and ventral ribs using circumcostal sutures cranially and caudally and mattress sutures in the intercostal spaces. Care must be taken to avoid damaging the intercostal vascular structures. Any locally available soft tissues are used to cover the mesh and allow for final wound closure. Some surgeons cover both sides of mesh with vascular tissue to decrease adhesion formation and increase the chances of viable skin coverage. The omentum is the most widely described tissue used for this purpose. Cutting polyethylene mesh with electrocautery is reported to seal the edges, allowing for suture placement closer to the mesh edge.

17. How is omentum used to cover the implanted mesh?
1. A **paracostal incision** is made, and the abdomen is entered with a flank approach. The omentum is grasped and pulled into the subcutaneous tissues. A subcutaneous tunnel is created to allow the omentum to be advanced to the thoracic wall defect. The omentum is then placed over and around the mesh and sutured in place.
2. A small **diaphragmatic incision** is created for passage of the omentum. This approach requires an abdominal incision because gentle manipulation is used to maintain omental blood supply.

In both cases, minimal closure is performed to avoid placing sutures around or through major omental vessels, and herniation is possible.

18. Are infections common after the implantation of synthetic materials?
No.

19. What routine precautions should be taken for prosthetic mesh implantation?
- Perioperative administration of a broad-spectrum antibiotic.
- Débridement of the surgical field before prosthetic implantation.
- Wound closure with elimination of dead space.
- Limited use of drains in the postoperative period.
- Reduced exposure of the mesh to the environment before implantation.

BIBLIOGRAPHY

1. Aronsohn M: Diaphragmatic advancement for reconstruction of the caudal thoracic wall. In Bojrab MJ (ed): Current Techniques in Small Animal Surgery. Baltimore, Williams & Wilkins, 1996.
2. Bowman KLT, Birchard SJ: Complications associated with the implantation of polypropylene mesh in dogs and cats: A retrospective study of 21 cases (1984–1996). J Am Anim Hosp Assoc 34:225–233, 1998.
3. Bright RM, Birchard SJ: Repair of thoracic wall defects in the dog with a omental pedicle flap. J Am Anim Hosp Assoc 18:277–282, 1982.
4. Ellison GW, Trotter GW: Reconstructive thoracoplasty using spinal fixation plates and polypropylene mesh. J Am Anim Hosp Assoc 17:613–616, 1981.
5. Matthiesen DT, Clark GN: En bloc resection of primary rib tumors in 40 dogs. Vet Surg 21:201–204, 1992.

28. PATENT DUCTUS ARTERIOSUS

Cathy L. Greenfield, D.V.M., M.S., Dip. A.C.V.S.

1. What is the ductus arteriosus?
A fetal connection between the descending aorta and the main pulmonary artery, which shunts blood away from the collapsed fetal lungs and into the systemic circulation.

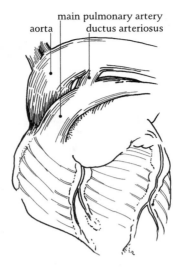

Anatomy of patent ductus arteriosus as seen through a left fourth space intercostal thoracotomy.

2. What normally happens to the ductus arteriosus after birth?
It closes; functionally at first, followed by anatomic closure.

3. What factors stimulate the ductus arteriosus to close after birth?
In the fetus, the lungs are collapsed, and pulmonary vascular resistance is high. Most of the blood flowing out of the right ventricle takes the path of least resistance and goes through the ductus arteriosus into the aorta. In the normal situation after birth, when the animal breathes air and the lungs expand, pulmonary vascular resistance decreases, allowing blood leaving the right side of the heart to flow into the lungs. Specialized smooth muscle cells in the wall of the ductus arteriosus contract and functionally close the ductus to blood flow. Anatomic closure follows.

4. When should the ductus arteriosus close?
Within the first few days of life.

5. What is a patent ductus arteriosus (PDA)?
One that is not closed, allowing blood flow to continue through it.

6. What problems does PDA cause in affected patients?
The PDA results in continued communication between the pulmonary and systemic circulations via shunting through the ductus arteriosus. In most cases, because the systemic circulation is a higher-pressure system and the inflated lungs have low vascular resistance, blood flows as a **left-to-right shunt** from the descending aorta into the main pulmonary artery. This results in volume overload of the pulmonary vascular system and the left side of the heart. Initially the left side of the heart accommodates by hypertrophy, but ultimately it also dilates. Dilation can result in stretching of the mitral annulus, secondary mitral regurgitation, and sometimes dysrhythmias.

7. What is a reverse shunting PDA?
A PDA in which the blood flows from the main pulmonary artery through the ductus arteriosus into the descending aorta, a **right-to-left shunt**.

8. Why does a reverse shunting PDA develop?

Most commonly, right-to-left shunting through a PDA develops as a long-term sequela to untreated PDA. The chronic pulmonary volume overload leads to suprasystemic pulmonary hypertension, muscular hypertrophy within the walls of the pulmonary vessels, and fibrosis. The increased pressure within the pulmonary circulation and the failing of the left side of the heart result in reversal of the blood flow through the PDA.

9. Is PDA a common abnormality in dogs and cats?

PDA is the most common congenital cardiac abnormality in dogs and occurs in approximately 1:750 live births. It is seen at a lesser frequency in cats.

10. Are reverse shunting PDAs common in dogs and cats?

No. Most dogs with untreated PDA die before the development of a reverse shunt.

11. What is the typical signalment of a dog with PDA?

- PDAs are usually seen in young puppies, within the first few months of life. Occasionally, PDAs are seen in adult dogs.
- Females are more commonly affected than males (4:1 ratio)
- PDA is commonest in purebred dogs:
- Miniature and toy poodles
- Shetland sheepdogs
- Cocker spaniels
- Pomeranians
- Yorkshire terriers
- Irish setters
- German shepherd dogs
- Collies
- English springer spaniels
- Bichon frisés
- Keeshonden

12. Describe the typical history of a patient with PDA.

Most patients with PDA are asymptomatic or have mild exercise intolerance with shortness of breath and coughing, if pulmonary edema is present. The characteristic heart murmur is usually detected on physical examination when a puppy or kitten presents for vaccination.

13. List the diagnostic tests most useful in the diagnosis of PDA.

- Physical examination
- Thoracic radiographs
- Echocardiography

14. What abnormalities are found on physical examination?

- Characteristic continuous or **machinery** murmur over the left heart base
- A palpable **thrill**
- Bounding or **water hammer** pulses—due to a large gradient between normal or high systolic followed by low diastolic pressures
- Dysrhythmias possible in severely compromised patients

15. What abnormalities are found on thoracic radiographs?

- Left atrial and ventricular enlargement
- Pulmonary overcirculation
- Dilation of the descending aorta as a result of the ductus diverticulum on the dorsoventral view
- Pulmonary edema, in some affected animals

16. What abnormalities may be found with echocardiography?

- Left atrial enlargement
- Left ventricular dilatation
- PDA may be visualized
- Dilatation of the main pulmonary artery

- Increased aortic ejection velocity
- Reverse turbulent flow in the pulmonary artery with Doppler echocardiography
- Enlargement of the mitral annulus with mitral regurgitation in about 50% of cases
- Aortic or pulmonic insufficiency possible
- Decreased fractional shortening possible

17. Name the treatment options available for PDA.
- Surgical ligation
- Surgical division
- Transcatheter coil embolization (transarterial ductal occlusion)

18. What happens if the PDA is left untreated?
Progressive left-sided heart failure and pulmonary edema develop. Most animals die at less than 1 year of age if they are not treated.

19. Should surgical ligation be performed as treatment for reverse shunting PDAs?
No. If a reverse shunting PDA is surgically ligated, the dog will die from acute right-sided heart pressure overload and subsequent ventricular failure.

20. Is there an effective treatment for reverse shunting PDA?
No.

21. What surgical approach is used for ligation of the PDA?
Left fourth (most commonly) or fifth intercostal thoracotomy. The left cranial lung lobe is retracted and packed off with saline-moistened laparotomy sponges to provide exposure to the base of the heart and the PDA.

22. Describe the anatomy and location of the PDA.
In the dog, the PDA is usually wide (around 1 cm in diameter) and short in length (<1 cm long). It is located between the descending aorta and main pulmonary artery (ventral to the aorta and dorsal to the pulmonary artery) beneath (medial) where the vagus nerve crosses between these vessels. The left recurrent nerve wraps around the ductus and can be seen in some dogs.

23. Name the two surgical techniques used for ligation of a PDA.
1. Standard ligation technique
2. Jackson/Henderson modified ligation technique

24. Describe the standard ligation technique.
The vagus nerve is identified and retracted. The pericardium is opened dorsal and parallel to the phrenic nerve, and the PDA is isolated by dissecting in front and behind it with right-angle forceps (some surgeons do not open the pericardium when using this technique). During the entire dissection, the tip of the right-angle forceps is under the thick-walled aorta, rather than under the friable ductus. Suture material (0–2 silk) is placed in the tip of the right-angle forceps and passed from cranial to caudal under the ductus. The PDA is double ligated with the aortic side tied first.

25. Describe the modified ligation technique of Jackson and Henderson.
No dissection is done around the medial (right) aspect of the PDA. The mediastinal pleura dorsal to the aorta and ventral to the thoracic duct is sharply incised, and this opening is deepened by digital dissection around the medial aspect (right side) of the aorta and aortic arch. The ventral border of the incised mediastinal pleura is elevated with forceps, and the dissection is continued to expose the lateral side of the aorta, ductus, and left pulmonary artery. A blunt, curved instrument is passed from ventral to dorsal under the medial side of the aorta in front of the duc-

tus. A doubled strand of appropriate suture material is placed in the instrument, and the instrument is withdrawn, pulling the suture to the lateral side of the aorta. Forceps are passed a second time medial to the aorta and caudal to the ductus. The free ends of the doubled suture material are placed in the jaw of the instrument, and the instrument is withdrawn, pulling the suture ends to the lateral side of the aorta. Gentle ventral traction is placed on the suture material to pull it under the ductus between the aorta and the pulmonary artery. The suture is divided to make two ligatures. The PDA is double ligated with the aortic side tied first.

26. Is there an advantage of using the Jackson and Henderson ligation technique over the standard ligation technique?

Possibly. Because dissection is not done on the medial (right) side of the ductus, there may be less of a chance for intraoperative hemorrhage (which could be fatal). In a large retrospective study of PDAs, however, a significant difference was not found in the incidence of hemorrhage between the two techniques.

27. Name the reflex that causes the heart rate to slow secondary to the increase in arterial blood pressure that occurs with PDA ligation.

The Branham reflex.

28. When should surgery be performed in the patient with PDA?

As soon as the diagnosis is made. Size of the animal should not be a factor in deciding when to do surgery because PDA surgery has been successfully performed in patients weighing < 1 lb. The longer the surgery is postponed, the greater the chance that the patient will develop heart failure. Pulmonary edema and dysrhythmias, if present, should be treated preoperatively.

29. List the most common complications that occur during or after PDA ligation.

- Hemorrhage, minor or major (**most common**)
- Pulmonary edema
- Ventricular fibrillation
- Cardiac arrest
- Iatrogenic lung damage

30. What is the success rate of surgical ligation of PDAs?

> 90%

31. What is the prognosis for patients with successful ligation of the PDA?

If the patient survives the surgical and postoperative period, chances for long-term survival are good. Secondary mitral regurgitation and associated problems often resolve after successful PDA ligation. Approximately 1–2% of patients with surgical ligation of a PDA have recanalization of the ductus requiring further surgery.

32. When should surgical division of a PDA be considered the most appropriate treatment?

Because of the anatomy (short and wide) of the PDA in the dog, it is difficult to divide the ductus and have enough room to suture the ends. Consequently, division is recommended only if an attempt to surgically ligate the PDA has failed and recanalization has occurred or if the ductus tears and severe intraoperative hemorrhage cannot be resolved by more conservative methods.

33. How is division of a PDA performed?

An identical pair of patent ductus forceps are placed across the ductus with the tips pointing cranially. The forceps are placed to leave as much tissue between them as possible (usually only a few millimeters). The PDA is divided, and the forceps are turned laterally to allow visualization and suturing of the cut ends of the vessel. The ductus is sutured closed with 4–0 to 6–0 monofilament suture material with a swaged on cardiovascular needle with a continuous mattress pattern oversewn with a simple continuous pattern or just a simple continuous pattern if there is not enough room for two rows of sutures.

34. How is transcatheter coil embolization of a PDA performed?
A catheter is passed from the femoral artery through the descending aorta to the PDA. Ductal anatomy is studied using angiography. Embolization coils are passed to the level of the ductus in a catheter, and embolization coils are released into the ductus. Angiography is used to determine if flow through the PDA is completely occluded. If significant flow remains, additional embolization coils are deployed as necessary.

35. Has transcatheter coil embolization been successfully performed in dogs?
- Yes. Occlusion with Gianturco coils was successful in 86% (37 of 43) of dogs. Of 37 dogs, 22 had complete occlusion based on angiography performed after coil deployment, and 15 of 37 had minor residual flow.

36. Is transcatheter coil embolization likely to become more common in veterinary medicine?
Yes, especially by interventional cardiologists in private referral or university practices.

BIBLIOGRAPHY

1. Birchard SJ, Bonagura JD, Fingland RB: Results of ligation of patent ductus arteriosus in dogs: 201 cases (1969–1988). J Am Vet Med Assoc 196:2011–2013, 1990.
2. Eyster GW: Basic cardiac surgical procedures. In Slatter D (ed): Textbook of Small Animal Surgery, 2nd ed. Philadelphia, W.B. Saunders, 1993, pp 897–900.
3. Fossum TW: Patent ductus arteriosus. In Fossum TW (ed): Small Animal Surgery. St. Louis, Mosby, 1997.
4. Goodwin JK, Lombard CW: Patent ductus arteriosus in adult dogs: Clinical features of 14 cases. J Am Anim Hosp Assoc 28:349–354, 1992.
5. Henderson RA, Jackson WF: Modified double ligation and division of patent ductus arteriosus. In Bojrab MJ (ed): Current Techniques in Small Animal Surgery, 4th ed. Baltimore, Williams & Wilkins, 1998, pp 652–659.
6. Miller MW, Meurs KM, Gordon SG, et al: Transarterial ductal occlusion using Gianturco vascular occlusion coils: 43 cases, 1994–1998. Proceedings of the 17th Annual Veterinary Medical Forum of the American College of Veterinary Internal Medicine, Chicago, IL, 1999, p 713.
7. Snaps FR, McEntee K, Saunders JH, et al: Treatment of patent ductus arteriosus by placement of intravascular coils in a pup. J Am Vet Med Assoc 207:724–725, 1995.

29. CARDIAC VALVULAR SURGERIES

Dianne Dunning, D.V.M., M.S., Dip. A.C.V.S.

1. What causes mitral valve insufficiency?
Mucoid valvular degeneration and myxomatous transformation of the left atrioventricular valve, a process known as **endocardiosis,** characterize mitral valve insufficiency. The cause is unknown.

2. What is the incidence of mitral valve insufficiency?
Mitral valve insufficiency is one of the most common acquired heart diseases in the dog. It is seen more often in the small-breed dog, such as the poodle, and has a documented familial predisposition in the King Charles Cavalier spaniel. Prevalence increases with age, affecting 5% of the canine population < 1 year and > 75% of population by 16 years of age.

3. Discuss the pathophysiology of mitral insufficiency.

With mitral valve insufficiency, part of the blood flow normally ejected out of the aortic valve regurgitates back through the mitral valve, increasing the blood volume in the left atrium. With this increase in blood volume the left atrium and annulus begin to dilate. With chronic dilation, the left atrium begins to press on the trachea, causing the characteristic cough of mitral insufficiency. Late in the disease course, this chronic increase of left ventricular preload leads to left ventricular dilation and contractile dysfunction.

4. How is mitral insufficiency diagnosed?

The predominant physical examination finding is a **holosystolic murmur,** best auscultated at the left heart base. Diagnosis may be confirmed by **echocardiography.**

5. Discuss the indications for mitral valvular surgery.

Recommendations for surgery are based on the animal's clinical signs and echocardiographic findings. In humans, surgery is generally recommended for patients in New York Heart Association (NYHA) classification I–II with accompanying echocardiographic signs of severe mitral regurgitation, left ventricular dysfunction, atrial fibrillation, pulmonary hypertension, and a history of thromboembolic events. In the dog, indications for repair have not yet been outlined, but surgery is usually reserved for the patient in end-stage congestive heart failure refractory to medical management.

6. Why is mitral valve surgery generally delayed in the dog?

1. Most dogs are not diagnosed with congestive heart failure resulting from mitral valve disease until much later during the disease course when compared with people.

2. The canine patient tolerates medical management reasonably well.

Delaying surgery until this late in the disease probably results in higher patient morbidity and mortality.

7. What procedures are available for mitral valve disease?

- Mitral valve repair
- Mitral valve replacement

8. What surgical procedures constitute mitral valve repair?

- **Annuloplasty:** repair of the valve's dilated ring annulus with imbrications, sutures, or a ring prothesis
- **Valvuloplasty:** repair of the valve leaflets

9. What are the two basic types of valves available for mitral valve replacement?

- Mechanical valves
- Bioprosthetic/tissue valves (usually porcine in origin)

10. What are the benefits and drawbacks of replacement versus repair?

	BENEFITS	DRAWBACKS
Replacement	Long lifespan of the prothesis	Anticoagulation required because of the risk of thromboembolic disease
	Can be used at any stage of the disease	Failure of valves is a catastrophic event, usually resulting in the death of the patient
	Guaranteed to be competent	
Repair	Reduced risk of sepsis	Advanced stage of disease may make repair difficult
	Valve prosthesis not required	Sharp learning curve of surgery, leading to a high initial mortality rate
	Long-term anticoagulation not required	Unclear if human techniques are applicable in the dog

11. What is the incidence of pulmonic stenosis?
- Common in dogs and uncommon in cats.
- Estimated to occur in 1 in every 1,000 live births in dogs

12. Which canine breeds are at risk for pulmonic stenosis?
- English bulldogs
- Beagles
- Cocker spaniels
- Chihuahua
- German shepherds
- Miniature schnauzers
- Samoyeds
- Mastiffs
- Terrier breeds

13. What is the commonest anatomic anomaly in pulmonic stenosis?
Pulmonic stenosis is a congenital narrowing of the pulmonic valve, pulmonary artery, or right ventricular outflow tract. In dogs, the stenosis is usually **valvular,** although supravalvular stenosis and subvalvular stenosis have also been reported. Valvular stenosis may be simple or dysplastic:
- **Simple** valvular stenosis consists of an incomplete separation of the bicuspid leaflets.
- **Dysplastic** valvular stenosis is characterized by a hypoplastic valvular annulus and thickened immobile valve leaflets. Of dogs with pulmonic valvular stenosis, 78% are dysplastic.

14. Are there any other concurrent anomalies commonly associated with pulmonic stenosis?
English bulldogs and boxers have a high concurrent incidence of an **aberrant left coronary artery,** which crosses directly over the stenotic valve. This artery is important to identify before attempting medical dilation or primary surgical enlargement of the pulmonary outflow tract because laceration or rupture of this vessel results in the death of the animal. These animals require a valved or nonvalved conduit placed between the right ventricle and pulmonary artery.

15. What is a typical history suggesting pulmonic stenosis?
Young animals are often asymptomatic. Older animals present with signs of exercise intolerance, syncope, or right-sided heart failure.

16. What physical examination findings suggest pulmonic stenosis?
The predominant physical examination finding is a **systolic ejection murmur,** loudest at the left heart base. Electrocardiogram findings are consistent with a right axis shift resulting from right heart enlargement or hypertrophy.

17. How is the diagnosis of pulmonic stenosis confirmed?
Echocardiography. Cardiac catheterization (the diagnostic gold standard in human medicine) is usually not necessary unless one suspects an aberrant left coronary artery.

18. What are the indications to treat pulmonic stenosis?
- Presence or development of clinical signs
- Progression of right ventricular enlargement
- Systolic pressure gradients obtained from echocardiography:

SYSTOLIC PRESSURE GRADIENT	GRADE OF PULMONIC STENOSIS	TREATMENT
< 50 mm Hg	Mild	Medical management
50–75 mm Hg	Moderate	Medical management, ± balloon dilation
> 75 mm Hg	Severe	Patch graft valvuloplasty or valved/nonvalved conduit

19. What is the medical management of pulmonic stenosis?
- Symptomatic treatment of congestive heart failure
- Percutaneous balloon valvuloplasty (used mostly for moderate grades of pulmonic stenosis)
- Balloon dilation for simple valvular stenosis (should be used with caution in dogs with aberrant left coronary arteries)

20. What surgical treatments are available for pulmonic stenosis?
- **Transventricular valve dilation:** used mostly in animals with moderate pressure gradients, simple valvular stenosis, and moderate right ventricular hypertrophy
- **Patch graft valvuloplasty:** reserved for animals with severe pressure gradients, dysplastic valvular stenosis, and severe right ventricular hypertrophy

21. Describe the technical details of transventricular valve dilation.
Surgery is performed via a left fourth intercostal thoracotomy. The pericardium is opened over the right outflow tract. A buttressed mattress suture is placed in the right ventricular outflow tract, ventral to the stenosis. A stab incision is made through the ventricle, and a dilating instrument, such as a Hegar or Cooley valve dilator, is passed through the incision into the right ventricular outflow tract and across the pulmonic valve. After dilation, the instrument should be removed, and the ventricular incision should be closed with the preplaced mattress suture.

22. Describe the technical details of patch graft valvuloplasty.
Open patch graft correction may be performed under mild hypothermia and inflow occlusion or full cardiopulmonary bypass. Surgery is performed via a left fourth intercostal thoracotomy. The pulmonary outflow tract is opened, and a patch graft is sutured with a simple continuous suture pattern, reinforced with the pledget-buttressed (stented) mattress sutures.

23. What are the advantages and disadvantages of full-bypass patch graft valvuloplasty?
- **Advantages:** It provides ample time for full evaluation of the right ventricular outflow tract, ensuring correct patch size and positioning and a reduced operative mortality when compared with inflow occlusion.
- **Disadvantages:** It requires a bypass unit and surgical team, and animal weight must be >15 kg.

24. If an aberrant left coronary artery is present, what surgical procedure can be used to treat a dog with pulmonic stenosis?
A valved or nonvalve conduit may be placed between the right ventricle and the pulmonary artery. This vascular conduit allows blood to bypass the stenosis, alleviating the right ventricular pressure overload.

25. List common complications associated with the patch graft technique.
- Failure to relieve stenosis and recurrence of stenosis
- Patch failure and leakage
- Coronary artery damage from an inappropriately positioned patch graft
- Hemorrhage
- Cardiac arrhythmias
- Complications associated with inflow occlusion or cardiopulmonary bypass

26. What is the incidence of aortic stenosis?
- Second or third most common congenital heart defect in the dog
- Uncommon in the cat

27. Which canine breeds are at risk for aortic stenosis?
- Newfoundland (genetic basis)
- Golden retriever
- Rottweiler
- German shepherd
- Boxers
- Samoyeds

28. Describe the most common anatomic anomaly in aortic stenosis.
A congenital narrowing of the aortic valve, aorta, or left ventricular outflow tract. In >90% of dogs, the stenosis is **subvalvular;** the severity and morphology of the lesion can vary greatly. The typical lesion is a discrete fibrotic ring located beneath the valve annulus and is associated with mild aortic insufficiency and left ventricular septal hypertrophy. In severe cases of aortic stenosis, mitral insufficiency is commonly present because of the reflection of the fibrous ring lesion onto the adjacent mitral valve leaflets.

29. What is a typical history suggesting aortic stenosis?
Ranging from asymptomatic to exhibiting exercise intolerance, collapse, syncope, or sudden death.

30. Describe physical examinations findings suggestive of aortic stenosis?
The predominant finding is a **systolic ejection murmur,** loudest at the left heart base but radiating to the right side of the thorax and thoracic inlet. Femoral pulses are weak and hypokinetic. Electrocardiogram findings are consistent with a left axis shift resulting from left heart enlargement or hypertrophy.

31. What is the most common cause of death in dogs with aortic stenosis?
Sudden death due to cardiac arrhythmias.

32. How is the diagnosis of aortic stenosis confirmed?
Systolic pressure gradients may be calculated from the peak aortic velocity.

33. What are the indications to treat aortic stenosis?
- Presence or development of clinical signs
- Progression of left ventricular hypertrophy
- Systolic pressure gradients obtained from echocardiography:

SYSTOLIC PRESSURE GRADIENT	GRADE OF AORTIC STENOSIS	TREATMENT
25–50 mm Hg	Mild	Medical management
50–75 mm Hg	Moderate	Medical management, ± balloon dilation
> 75 mm Hg	Severe	Valve dilation or open fibrotic ring resection under cardiopulmonary bypass

34. What is the medical management of aortic stenosis?
- Symptomatic treatment of congestive heart failure
- β-adrenergic blocker therapy
- Balloon dilation for moderate aortic stenosis

35. What surgical treatments are available for aortic stenosis?
- **Transventricular valve dilation:** Acute relief of stenosis is achieved, but pressure gradients usually recur within 3 months. This technique is not recommended.
- **Open fibrotic ring resection:** Reserved for animals with severe pressure gradients and significant left ventricular hypertrophy. Cardiopulmonary bypass allows for direct visualization of the fibrotic ring. Operative mortality rates are 10–12%, and surgery is not protective against sudden death.

36. Describe the technical details of fibrotic ring resection.
Surgery is accomplished via the right fourth intercostal thoracotomy under cardiopulmonary bypass. A curvilinear incision is made on the aortic outflow tract, and the aortic valve leaves are gently retracted. The subvalvular ring is sharply resected, taking care not to damage the adjacent mitral valve or the conduction tissues along the septal wall. The aortotomy is closed with a continuous horizontal mattress suture pattern with the pledgets (stents), which is then oversewn with a simple continuous suture pattern.

37. List common complications associated with open fibrotic ring resection.
- Hemorrhage
- Rupture of the aorta
- Cardiac arrhythmias
- Restenosis
- Complications associated with cardiopulmonary bypass

38. Is there any surgical treatment for tricuspid valve dysplasia?
Medical management is more commonly employed; surgery is considered when medical management of right-sided congested heart failure is unsatisfactory but before end-stage right-sided heart failure. The valve may be repaired or replaced. If replacement is undertaken, a bio-prosthetic valve is preferred because it reduces the risk of thromboembolic disease.

BIBLIOGRAPHY

1. Boggs, LS, Dewan SJ: Mitral valve reconstruction in a toy-breed dog. J Am Vet Med Assoc 209:1872–1876, 1996.
2. Caywood DD: Cardiovascular surgery. In: Complications in Small Animal Surgery. Baltimore, Williams & Wilkins, 1996, pp 265–286.
3. Kanemoto I, Shibata S: Successful mitral valvuloplasty for mitral regurgitation in a dog. Jpn J Vet Sci 52:411–414, 1990.
4. Komtebedde J, Ilkiw JE: Resection of subvalvular aortic stenosis: Surgical and perioperative in seven dogs. Vet Surg 22:419–430, 1993.
5. Linn K, Orton EC: Closed transventricular dilation of discrete subvalvular aortic stenosis in dogs. Vet Surg 21:441–445, 1992.
6. Monnet E, Orton EC: Open resection for subvalvular aortic stenosis. J Am Vet Med Assoc 209:1255–1261, 1996.
7. Orton EC: Small Animal Thoracic Surgery. Baltimore, Williams & Wilkins, 1995.
8. Orton EC: Surgery of the cardiovascular system. In Fossum TW (ed): Small Animal Surgery. St Louis, Mosby, 1997, pp 575–608.

30. PERSISTENT RIGHT AORTIC ARCH

Cathy L. Greenfield, D.V.M., M.S.

1. What are the aortic arches?
Paired vessels that connect the paired dorsal and ventral aortas to each other in the normally developing fetus.

2. What is a vascular ring anomaly?
A congenital malformation of the great vessels and their branches that arises from abnormal development of the embryologic aortic arches.

3. Which aortic arches are involved in vascular ring anomalies?

The third, fourth, and sixth, because these are the ones that are maintained and form the great vessels. Abnormalities of the third arch alone do not cause clinical signs because a complete ring encircling the esophagus and trachea does not exist.

4. Which vascular ring anomalies have been reported in dogs and cats?

- **Dogs**
  Persistent right aortic arch (PRAA)
  Double aortic arches
  Persistent right ligamentum arteriosum
  Aberrant left subclavian artery
  Aberrant right subclavian artery
- **Cats**
  PRAA

5. Which vascular ring anomaly is most common in dogs and cats?

PRAA.

6. What percentage of vascular ring anomalies are PRAA in the dog?

95%.

7. Between what structures does the esophagus become entrapped in PRAA?

The ligamentum arteriosum on the left; the heart base and main pulmonary artery ventrally; the aortic arch on the right.

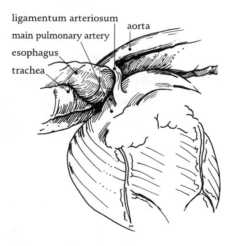

Pertinent anatomy of persistent right aortic arch as seen through a left fourth space intercostal thoracotomy.

8. Name four other anomalies that may be seen in conjunction with PRAA.

1. Persistent left cranial vena cava (40% of cases with PRAA)
2. Patent ductus arteriosus (a murmur is rarely heard, and the diagnosis is made at surgery)
3. Prominent left hemiazygos vein
4. Aberrant left subclavian artery

9. Of what clinical significance are these other anomalies?

None are of any hemodynamic significance. The left cranial vena cava is retracted to allow adequate exposure of the constricting band of tissue. Because no murmur is heard even if a patent ductus arteriosus is present rather than a ligamentum arteriosum, it is best to double-ligate the ligamentum and ductus before dividing it in all cases of PRAA. If a prominent left hemiazygos vein is obstructing exposure of the esophageal constriction, the vessel should be ligated and divided. An aberrant left subclavian artery can also be ligated and divided if it is contributing to the esophageal constriction.

10. What clinical problems do vascular ring anomalies cause in the dog and cat?

The abnormal location of the great vessels results in entrapment of the esophagus and trachea between these vessels and the base of the heart. Clinical signs are due to esophageal obstruction and sometimes tracheal compression (only with double aortic arches).

The main clinical sign is postprandial **regurgitation,** which usually begins at the time of weaning. Aspiration pneumonia may be present.

11. What is the typical signalment with PRAA?

- Young puppies and kittens, < 6 months of age. There are also reports of older dogs (10 years of age).
- There is no sex predisposition.
- German shepherd dogs, Irish setters, and Boston terriers are predisposed, although it is also seen in other breeds and mixed-breed dogs.
- Siamese and Persian cats may be predisposed.
- More than one animal in a litter may be affected.

12. What is the typical history of dogs with PRAA?

Regurgitation starting around the time of weaning with the introduction of solid foods. The affected animal is often smaller than its littermates and may be emaciated and dehydrated.

13. What is the recommended treatment for PRAA?

Surgical ligation and division of the band of tissue responsible for constricting the esophagus.

14. When should surgery be performed?

As soon as possible after the diagnosis is made. In most cases, the longer PRAA goes without definitive treatment, the greater the damage to the esophageal muscles and nerves. Although some of the esophageal dilation present preoperatively may resolve after surgery, the esophagus rarely returns completely to normal.

15. What preoperative workup is indicated in cases of suspected PRAA?

- **Thoracic radiography:** esophageal dilation cranial to the heart base with or without aspiration pneumonia. Occasionally, esophageal dilation caudal to the base of the heart.
- **Esophagram:** esophageal constriction at the base of the heart and esophageal dilation cranially
- **Fluoroscopy:** to evaluate esophageal motility
- **Complete blood count:** if there is evidence of aspiration pneumonia
- **Angiography:** is not commonly performed or necessary

16. What therapy should be instituted before surgery is performed in a patient with PRAA?

- Aspiration pneumonia should be treated with appropriate **antibiotics.**
- The dog should be fed a gruel from an elevated site to allow gravity to assist getting the food into the stomach.
- **Nutritional support** through a gastrostomy tube may be helpful in severely debilitated patients.
- **Fluid therapy** is indicated preoperatively in dehydrated patients.

17. Name the surgical approach that should be used to treat PRAA.

Left fourth intercostal thoracotomy. Occasionally a left fifth intercostal thoracotomy is used in cats.

18. Describe the surgical procedure that is performed to treat PRAA.

The ligamentum arteriosum is located at the caudal end of the dilated esophagus, over the heart base. The ligamentum arteriosum is bluntly dissected off of the underlying esophagus with right-angle forceps and double-ligated (0 or 2–0 silk) before it is divided. A Foley or other balloon-type catheter is passed down the esophagus and dilated in the area under the ligamentum arteriosum. Remaining bands of fibrous tissue are carefully transected.

19. What is the postoperative care for PRAA?
- Routine postoperative care for a thoracotomy is performed.
- Elevated oral alimentation may be resumed, or feeding through a gastrostomy tube is continued until adequate food consumption per os is maintained.
- Antibiotics should be continued if the patient has aspiration pneumonia.

20. List the main postoperative complications seen in surgically treated PRAA patients.
- Continued **regurgitation**
- Unresolved neuromuscular damage from the megaesophagus, leaving poor esophageal function in some animals
- Aspiration pneumonia

21. What management steps should be recommended when the patient is released from the hospital?

The animal should be fed gruel in an upright position for the first weeks after surgery and maintained in an upright position for approximately 20 minutes after it is fed. After the first few weeks, different kinds and consistencies of food should be tried to determine what the animal tolerates best. The goal is to get the animal back to eating normally.

22. Is PRAA believed to be heritable, and should affected animals be taken out of the gene pool (i.e., neutered)?

Yes, and yes.

23. What is the short-term prognosis for dogs with surgically treated PRAA?

Fair; 11–40% of patients surgically treated for PRAA die within 3 weeks of surgery or are euthanized because of continued related problems.

CONTROVERSY

24. What is the long-term prognosis for dogs with surgically treated PRAA?

Unknown. In one study, 92% of dogs followed for >6 months after surgery did not regurgitate after eating, and 8% regurgitated less than once per week. In another study, of the 60% of PRAA cases that survived long-term, only 9% had excellent results with return to normal function, 67% had good results with occasional related problems, and 24% had poor results with continued frequent problems.

BIBLIOGRAPHY

1. Ellison GW: Surgical correction of persistent right aortic arch. In Bojrab MJ (ed): Current Techniques in Small Animal Surgery, 4th ed. Baltimore, Williams & Wilkins, 1998, pp 659–662.
2. Fingeroth JM: Surgical diseases of the esophagus. In Slatter D (ed): Textbook of Small Animal Surgery, 2nd ed. Philadelphia, W.B. Saunders, 1993, pp 538–557.
3. Fingeroth JM, Fossum TW: Late-onset regurgitation associated with persistent right aortic arch in two dogs. J Am Vet Med Assoc 191:981–983, 1987.
4. Fossum TW: Vascular ring anomalies. In Fossum TW (ed): Small Animal Surgery. St. Louis, Mosby, 1997.
5. Helphry M: Vascular ring anomalies. In Bojrab MJ (ed): Disease Mechanisms in Small Animal Surgery, 2nd ed. Philadelphia, Lea & Febiger, 1993, pp 350–354.
6. Muldoon MM, Birchard SJ, Ellison GW: Long-term results of surgical correction of persistent right aortic arch in dogs: 25 cases (1980–1995). J Am Vet Med Assoc 210:1761–1763, 1997.
7. Shires PK: Persistent right aortic arch in dogs: A long-term follow-up after surgical correction. J Am Anim Hosp Assoc 17:773–776, 1981.

31. PERICARDIECTOMY

Cathy L. Greenfield, D.V.M., M.S.

1. What is the pericardium?

A saclike structure surrounding the heart and base of the great vessels. It is composed of an outer fibrous layer and an inner serous layer. The inner serous layer covers the surface of the heart (visceral layer = epicardium) and lines the inside of the fibrous pericardium (parietal layer).

2. List the functions of the pericardium.
- Maintains the heart in its normal anatomic position within the thoracic cavity
- Protects the heart during thoracic trauma
- Prevents great vessel kinking
- Provides a smooth gliding surface for heart motion
- Prevents spread of disease from the pleural space to the heart
- Prevents overdilation of the heart

3. In most pericardial diseases, what causes the clinical signs in the patient?

Pericardial effusion resulting in pericardial tamponade.

4. What are the general causes of pericardial effusion seen in small animal patients?

Neoplasia or **idiopathic** hemorrhagic pericardial effusion. Infectious pericarditis also occurs but is seen less frequently. Pericardial disease of all types is rare in cats. Infectious pericardial effusion has been seen in cats with feline infectious peritonitis, toxoplasmosis, and bacterial infections.

5. What is pericardial tamponade?

A condition caused by a rise in intrapericardial fluid pressure that interferes with cardiac function (filling and contraction of the ventricles) by compression of the heart.

6. What clinical signs are seen in animals with pericardial tamponade?

Because the right ventricle is thin walled, clinical signs are primarily attributed to **right-sided heart failure** and include weakness, exercise intolerance, lethargy, abdominal distention, dyspnea, weight loss, and anorexia.

On physical examination, muffled heart sounds, dyspnea or tachypnea, tachycardia, weak arterial pulses, pale mucous membranes, abdominal splinting, and shock may be present.

7. What is the typical signalment of a dog that presents with pericardial effusion?

Middle age or older large and giant-breed dogs. Male dogs are affected more frequently with nonmalignant effusion than females. German shepherd dogs and golden retrievers are predisposed to cardiac hemangiosarcoma, and brachycephalic breeds are predisposed to aortic body tumors.

8. Discuss the diagnostic tests that are most useful in diagnosing pericardial effusion.

Echocardiography is the most useful test and demonstrates fluid between the fibrous pericardium and the epicardium. Other useful diagnostic tests include **thoracic radiography** (globoid enlargement of the heart, with or without pulmonary edema, with or without pleural effusion) and **electrocardiography,** which may have electrical alternans (beat-to-beat voltage variations in the QRS complexes), diminished QRS voltages, and ST segment depression.

9. What should the initial treatment be for a patient presenting with pericardial effusion?

If the patient has signs of pericardial tamponade, **pericardiocentesis** should be performed.

10. In addition to removing a portion of the pericardial fluid to relieve the pericardial tamponade, what diagnostic tests should be performed on the fluid obtained?
- **Cytology**—to determine the type of fluid (i.e., transudate, exudate, or sanguineous effusion) and cells (possibly neoplastic) if present.
- **Culture and susceptibility testing**—to identify any infectious causes (bacterial and fungal).

11. What types of tumors commonly cause pericardial effusion in dogs?
- Hemangiosarcoma
- Mesothelioma
- Chemodectoma
- Ectopic thyroid carcinoma located at the heart base
- Metastatic neoplasia to the heart

12. What types of tumors cause pericardial effusion in cats?
Primarily **lymphosarcoma,** although other types are occasionally diagnosed.

13. When should surgery be considered for treatment in cases with pericardial effusion?
In 50% of cases, effusion recurs frequently and/or rapidly after pericardiocentesis, and surgery should be performed. Surgery should also be recommended for suspected neoplastic masses (diagnosis, mass resection) or when the underlying cause of the effusion cannot be determined without a biopsy specimen of the pericardium.

14. What surgical procedure is recommended to treat pericardial effusion?
Pericardiectomy—removal of all or part of the fibrous pericardium.

15. Why does pericardiectomy help in cases of pericardial effusion?
Pericardiectomy is used to remove the tissue producing the effusion and allows remaining fluid to drain into the thoracic cavity, where a large pleural surface is available for resorption of fluid.

16. List the two surgical approaches that can be used for pericardiectomy.
- Median sternotomy
- Lateral thoracotomy

17. What are the advantages and disadvantages of median sternotomy and lateral thoracotomy?

	ADVANTAGES	DISADVANTAGES
Median sternotomy	Increased exposure to both sides of the pericardium	More painful surgical approach
Lateral thoracotomy	Less painful surgical approach Easier access to the base of the heart for resection of masses in this area	Poor exposure to the contralateral side of the thoracic cavity

18. What is the difference between total and subtotal pericardiectomy?
In **total pericardiectomy,** the entire pericardium is removed.
In **subtotal pericardiectomy,** less than the total pericardium is removed.

19. What is the most common type of subtotal pericardiectomy performed in the dog?
Subphrenic pericardiectomy.

20. Has the surgical approach or procedure been shown to be related to survival time or complication rate?
No.

21. How is a pericardiectomy performed?

In most cases, a **subtotal (subphrenic) pericardiectomy** is performed. A t-shaped incision is made through the pericardium with one arm of the t ventral and parallel to the phrenic nerve and the other arm of the t extending from the first incision to the apex of the heart. Both incisions are extended to the contralateral side of the heart. The pericardiophrenic ligament is divided, allowing the incised pericardium to be removed. The pericardium can be incised with an electrosurgical device to help control hemorrhage from the thickened, granulomatous pericardium. Culture and biopsy samples of the pericardium should be obtained, and a sternal lymph node biopsy specimen should be obtained, if possible. A thoracostomy tube should be obtained, if possible. A thoracostomy tube should be placed before closure of the thoracic cavity and used postoperatively.

22. What other, less invasive, type of surgery can be used to perform a pericardiectomy?

Partial pericardiectomy can be performed using **thoracoscopy** to create a pericardial window (less pericardium is removed than in the open thoracic cavity surgical procedures).

23. What is the most common complication of pericardiectomy?

Postoperative pleural effusion.

24. List positive and negative prognostic indicators that have been shown to aid in predicting outcome in dogs with pericardial effusion.

- Positive
  Presence of ascites preoperatively
- Negative
  Echocardiographic evidence of a right atrial mass
  Radiographic evidence of pulmonary metastasis
  Development of pleural effusion > 30 days after pericardiectomy

25. What is the prognosis for dogs with idiopathic hemorrhagic pericardial effusion after pericardiectomy?

Good. Median survival time after pericardiectomy varies between 460 and 792 days (15.3–26.4 months). Prolonged survival can be expected compared with neoplastic disease.

26. What is the prognosis for dogs with heart or heart base tumors treated by pericardiectomy?

Poor. Reported median survival times after pericardiectomy include 52 days (for all neoplastic diseases combined), 16 days for dogs with hemangiosarcoma, and 13.6 months for dogs with mesothelioma. Dogs with chemodectoma that can be partially or completely excised, along with pericardiectomy, may have prolonged survival. Performing a pericardiectomy does not extend the disease-free interval or median survival time of dogs with right atrial hemangiosarcoma or mesothelioma.

BIBLIOGRAPHY

1. Aronson LR, Gregory CR: Infectious pericardial effusion in five dogs. Vet Surg 24:402–407, 1995.
2. Berg RJ: Surgical treatment of pericardial diseases and cardiac neoplasms. In Bojrab MJ (ed): Current Techniques in Small Animal Surgery, 4th ed. Baltimore, Williams & Wilkins, 1998, pp 671–676.
3. Bouvy BM, Bjorling DE: Pericardial effusion in dogs and cats. Comp Cont Educ Pract Vet 13:417–424, 633–641, 1991.
4. Dunning D, Monnet E, Orton CE, et al: Analysis of prognostic indicators for dogs with pericardial effusion: 46 cases (1985–1996). J Am Vet Med Assoc 212:1276–1280, 1998.
5. Eyster GE: Basic cardiac surgical procedures. In Slatter D (ed): Textbook of Small Animal Surgery, 2nd ed. Philadelphia, W.B. Saunders, 1993, pp 912–913.
6. Eyster GE, Gaber CE, Probst M: Cardiac disorders. In Slatter D (ed): Textbook of Small Animal Surgery, 2nd ed. Philadelphia, W.B. Saunders, 1993, pp 886–887.
7. Fossum TW: Pericardial effusion and pericardial constriction. In Fossum TW (ed): Small Animal Surgery. St. Louis, Mosby-Year Book, 1997, pp 596–601.
8. Kerstetter KK, Krahwinkel DJ, Millis DL, et al: Pericardiectomy in dogs: 22 cases (1978–1994). J Am Vet Med Assoc 211:736–740, 1997.
9. Rush JE, Keene BW, Fox PR: Pericardial disease in the cat. A retrospective evaluation of 66 cases. J Am Anim Hosp Assoc 26:39–46, 1990.

32. ESOPHAGEAL FOREIGN BODIES

Douglas M. MacCoy, D.V.M., Dip. A.C.V.S.

1. List the clinical signs of a patient with an esophageal foreign body.
- Difficulty in swallowing
- Excessive salivation
- Regurgitation
- Fever, malaise
- Cervical swelling or drainage
- Pleuritis, pneumothorax, or pyothorax
- Inappetence (cats)

2. How does the shape of the foreign body affect clinical signs?
1. Hollow bones may permit passage of fluids or semisolids.
2. Balls may completely obstruct the esophageal lumen.
3. Hooks and needles cause perforation and infection.

3. What are common foreign bodies?
Anything that can be ingested (i.e., needles, hooks, bones, metal fragments, plastic, wood, rubber balls, tennis balls, corncobs, socks, underwear, carving knives).

4. Where do things get stuck?
Hooks or sharp objects lodge anywhere the point engages the esophageal mucosa.
Other objects lodge at the proximal esophagus, thoracic inlet, base of the heart, or the diaphragmatic hiatus.

5. How is the diagnosis made?
- Suspicion based on clinical signs and history
- Survey or contrast radiography (obstruction, air or dye leakage)
- Endoscopy (direct visualization)

6. How are objects removed nonsurgically?
- Endoscopic retrieval
- Balloon inflation to dislodge embedded objects
- Gentle aboral dislodgment into the stomach
Success rates may be nearly 90%.

7. List some postretrieval protocols.
- Endoscopic evaluation of the esophageal lumen.
- Radiographs looking for free gas in tissues or body spaces.
- Broad-spectrum, bactericidal antibiotics to protect against infection.
- Prokinetic (metoclopramide, cisapride) drugs to increase gastric motility and increase lower esophageal sphincter pressure (decreasing risk of esophageal reflux).
- Corticosteroids to reduce stricture formation.
- Soft or slurried foods for 24 hours after procedure.
- Mucosal protectants (carafate slurry).
- Histamine H_2-receptor blockers (cimetidine, ranitidine, famotidine) or proton pump inhibitors (omeprazole) to limit acid reflux.
- Monitor (clinical signs or endoscopically) for stricture formation.

8. What are indications for surgical removal of a foreign object?
- Embedded objects
- Suspected perforations greater than 3 mm
- Prolonged unsuccessful endoscopy

9. What are the surgical approaches to the esophagus?
Ventral cervical or lateral thoracotomy.

10. What are some protocols for surgery?
- Longitudinal incision over healthy tissue.
- If possible, horizontal closure of a longitudinal incision to enlarge the esophagus and limit stricture formation.
- Closure in two layers:
1. Mucosa/submucosa and muscularis/adventitia in simple interrupted pattern using monofilament absorbable (polydioxanone) or nonabsorbable (polypropylene) material with swaged-on, taper needle.
2. External patching with a section of cervical strap muscles or lung to aid healing.
3. A feeding tube gastrostomy tube to place the esophagus at rest during healing.

11. Which is the holding layer of the esophagus?
Tunic submucosa.

12. What is the postoperative care?
- Nothing by mouth for 24 hours.
- Antibiotics for 7 days.
- Feeding through gastrostomy tube for 7 days.
- Soft foods for 7 days if feeding gastrostomy is not used.
- H_2-receptor blockers (cimetidine, ranitidine) for 7 days.
- Protectants (carafate slurry) for 7 days.

13. What are causes of dehiscence after esophageal surgery?
- Lack of serosal (omental) coverage for devitalized lesions
- Inadequate segmental blood supply or disruption of intramural vascular elements
- Excessive tension or motion (ingesta)
- Patient debilitation

14. What is a relatively safe amount of esophagus that can be resected in cases of severe circumferential necrosis?
All necrotic tissue to a length equal to three vertebrae. If a significant amount of esophagus is resected, tension-relieving techniques, such as advancing the cardia of the stomach into the chest, tension sutures on the esophagus, and a harness to flex the neck, are needed. Suture materials and patterns as well as aftercare are similar to protocols of esophagotomy.

15. What is a partial circumferential myotomy?
Incision of the longitudinal (not inner circular) muscle layer and preservation of the blood supply to the submucosa performed 2 to 3 cm proximal and distal to the surgery site. Experimentally, it has been shown to decrease significantly (by ⅔) suture line tension after extensive (30%–50%) esophageal resection.

CONTROVERSY

16. What type of contrast media can be used?
Iodinated liquids are relatively safe (less tissue irritation) if they escape through a perforation but provide poor contrast, especially if diluted by esophageal fluids.

Liquid barium suspensions provide excellent contrast but are irritating to tissues if there is a perforation. The risk from barium irritation is less than the danger of not recognizing a perforation; barium may be removed during surgery.

BIBLIOGRAPHY

1. Dallman MJ: Functional suture-holding layer of the canine esophagus. J Am Vet Med Assoc 192:638–640, 1988.
2. Fingeroth JM: Surgical techniques for the esophagus. In Slatter D (ed): Textbook of Small Animal Surgery, Philadelphia, W.B. Saunders, 1993, pp 549–561.
3. Hedlund CS: Surgery of esophagus. In Fossum TW (ed): Small Animal Surgery. St. Louis, Mosby, 1997, pp 243–245.
4. Lemarie RJ, Hosgood G: Esophagotomy and esophageal anastomosis. In Bojrab MJ (ed): Current Techniques in Small Animal Surgery, 4th ed. Baltimore, Williams & Wilkins, 1998, pp 193–197.
5. Muangsombut J: Circular myotomy to facilitate resection and anastomosis of the esophagus. J Thorac Cardiothorac Surg 78:522–530, 1974.
6. Oakes MG, Hosgood G: Esophagotomy closure in the dog. Vet Surg 22:451–456, 1993.
7. Spielman BL, Shaker EH, Garvey MS: Esophageal foreign body in dogs: A retrospective study of 23 cases. J Am Anim Hosp Assoc 28:570–574, 1992.

33. DIAPHRAGMATIC HERNIA

D. Michael Tillson, D.V.M., M.S., Dip. A.C.V.S.

1. What is a diaphragmatic hernia?

A disruption in the diaphragm resulting in the abnormal positioning of abdominal viscera within the thoracic cavity. Diaphragmatic hernias involve a tear in the diaphragm allowing abdominal viscera to enter into the pleural cavity (**pleuroperitoneal**) or a failure of the diaphragm to fuse separately from the pericardial sac (**pericardioperitoneal**). Acquired diaphragmatic hernias are seen most frequently in young male dogs and are associated with traumatic events. The formation of an iatrogenic hernia by improper surgical closure of the diaphragm or incisional dehiscence is also possible.

2. What is the proposed cause of traumatic diaphragmatic hernias?

Diaphragmatic hernias are tears in the diaphragm resulting from the creation of an excessive pressure differential between the abdominal and thoracic cavity when the glottis is open. The abdomen is compressed, increasing the intraabdominal pressure. This pressure is transmitted across the diaphragm to the thoracic cavity. If the glottis is closed, the pressure is equalized across the diaphragm. An open glottis allows air within the lungs to escape, leaving the thoracic cavity less full than the abdomen. The higher abdominal pressure tears the diaphragm, creating the hernia.

3. Should trauma patients have thoracic radiography performed before surgery?

Yes. The high correlation between traumatic accidents (automobiles) and diaphragmatic hernias means that every dog with a history of such trauma should receive thoracic radiographs to rule out the presence of a diaphragmatic hernia and other life-threatening cardiopulmonary injuries.

4. Will a diaphragmatic hernia heal on its own?

No. **Surgical repair** is appropriate as soon as the patient has been stabilized.

5. What are the clinical signs associated with traumatic diaphragmatic hernias?

Some dogs have no clinical signs, with the diaphragmatic hernia being an incidental finding on thoracic films, whereas other dogs are in acute respiratory distress and shock, with cardiac dysrhythmias (12%).

6. List useful diagnostic tests.
- Radiography (disruption in diaphragmatic outline or detail, increased soft tissues with gas loops in the thorax, effusion).
- Ultrasonography (as above).
- Peritoneography (air or contrast).

7. What are the types of tears in the diaphragm?
A **radial** tear begins in the central, muscular portion of the diaphragm and radiates outward. A **circumferential** tear denotes an avulsion of the diaphragm away from the abdominal wall. Commonly, both are present.

8. What is the difference in prognosis between acute versus chronic diaphragmatic hernias?
- **Acute** hernia deaths are related to complications associated with performing anesthesia and surgery on an unstable patient (e.g., hypovolemic, cardiac arrhythmias, or respiratory or cardiovascular complications associated with the hernia itself).
- **Chronic** diaphragmatic hernia deaths are related to chronic organ compromise, adhesions between abdominal and thoracic structures, and postoperative complications (reperfusion injuries).

9. Discuss reperfusion injuries.
Reperfusion injury refers to a cascade of events occurring at the cellular level in response to the sudden reintroduction of highly oxygenated blood into an anaerobic environment. As the oxygen returns, there is generation of a large number of **free oxygen** radicals and other highly reactive compounds. These compounds have a short half-life and are unstable. They are generated and interact immediately with cells. This interaction can severely damage cellular integrity and generate more free radical molecules. Only by reacting with a **free radical scavenger** is the cycle interrupted.

This situation is important in chronic diaphragmatic hernia management because reexpansion of chronically atelectic lungs and restoring blood flow to chronically compromised portions of liver or gastrointestinal tract results in generation of free radicals. Conditions such as **reexpansion pulmonary edema** and **liver shock,** reported as complications of chronic diaphragmatic hernia repair, may be blunted by careful consideration of the potential for reperfusion injury. No single method is effective in preventing or managing reperfusion events in patients. Medications, such as steroids or free radical scavengers, and management practices, such as lobectomy for severely compromised liver lobes and slow gradual reinflation of compromised lung tissue over several days, may decrease the severity of reperfusion injury.

10. If acute diaphragmatic hernias have a high mortality rate, when should a diaphragmatic hernia be considered an emergency procedure?
- Entrapment of a distending hollow organ (stomach) in the thoracic cavity.
- Visceral (spleen, liver, intestines) and vascular compromise.
- The inability to stabilize the trauma patient.

11. What are anesthetic guidelines for surgical patients?
- IV catheter.
- Supplemental oxygenation.
- Premedications to reduce anxiety.
- Rapid induction.
- ECG and pulse oximetry.
- Controlled ventilation.
- Avoid nitrous oxide.

12. Why shouldn't nitrous oxide be used in animals anesthetized for diaphragmatic hernia repair?

Postoperatively, nitrous oxide exacerbates the pneumothorax by diffusing into the chest cavity, reexpanding the gas space, and inhibiting lung expansion.

13. What is the surgical management for diaphragmatic hernia?
- Generous surgical site clipping
- Ventral midline celiotomy
- Gentle return of abdominal contents
- Débridement and closure of hernia
- Gentle breakdown of adhesions
- Restoration of negative thoracic pressure

14. List intraoperative complications of diaphragmatic hernia surgery.
- Reexpansion and reperfusion injury of lungs.
- Hemorrhage.
- Chronic adhesions, strictures, or tears.
- Loss of diaphragmatic tissue for repair.

15. Describe the best way to close a diaphragmatic hernia.
- Dorsal closure working proximally toward the surgeon.
- Use of monofilament synthetic absorbable or nonabsorbable sutures in continuous, interrupted, or interlocking patterns.
- Closure of radial tears first.
- Use of long stay sutures.

16. What is done if the diaphragmatic tear cannot be closed by reapposing the natural tissues?

A number of options are available to fill in gaps left in the diaphragm:
- Muscle flaps
- Prosthetic mesh
- Silastic sheeting
- Omental flaps
- Advancement of diaphragm

17. How can negative intrathoracic pressure be reestablished?

By placing a thoracostomy tube or percutaneous or transdiaphragmatic thoracocentesis. **Transdiaphragmatic thoracocentesis** is ideal because it allows the surgeon to see the restoration of negative thoracic pressure as the diaphragm resumes its normally curved shape. Failure to reestablish or maintain the transdiaphragmatic pressure differential (restoring normal shape and curvature) alerts the surgeon to the presence of significant leaks and helps identify other diaphragmatic lesions.

18. Which parameters should be most closely monitored in the postoperative period?
- Respiratory rate and quality (tachypnea and cyanosis indicate problems).
- Analgesics.
- Continued intravascular fluid support.
- Cardiac rate and rhythm.

19. Are antibiotics required after repair of a diaphragmatic hernia?

In the absence of a long surgical procedure (>2 hours), use of a prosthetic mesh, or organ compromise, prophylactic antibiotic administration is not required. Otherwise, administration of a first-generation cephalosporin or aminopenicillin is appropriate. The most commonly compromised organ is the liver, and the antibiotic chosen should be effective against *Clostridium* organisms.

20. What is empty abdomen syndrome?

Adaptation of abdominal musculature in chronic cases to having less viscera in the abdomen. After returning the misplaced organs to the abdominal cavity, room is at a premium, and closure is tight. Care must be taken to avoid incorporating the viscera in the abdominal closure or creating excessive pressure within the abdominal cavity and compromising vascular supply. Although the abdominal cavity may be tight, it accommodates the viscera in a short time.

CONTROVERSY

21. Is a thoracostomy tube required after repair of a diaphragmatic hernia?
Not routinely. When continued accumulation of fluid or air is expected during the initial post-surgical period, a thoracostomy should be placed. A thoracostomy tube can be used for intrapleural administration of bupivacaine for analgesia. One advantage of **not** placing a thoracostomy tube is that patients with compromised (atelectic) lungs are less likely to suffer reexpansion pulmonary edema secondary to excessive efforts to restore negative intrapleural pressure. Tubes require diligent maintenance to avoid iatrogenic problems.

BIBLIOGRAPHY

1. Boudrieau RJ, Muir WW: Pathophysiology of traumatic diaphragmatic hernia in dogs. Comp Cont Educ Pract Vet 9:379–385, 1987.
2. Hosgood G: Diagnosis and management of diaphragmatic diseases. Waltham Focus 6:2–9, 1996.

34. HEPATIC LOBECTOMY

Sheldon Padgett, D.V.M., M.S., Dip. A.C.V.S.

1. What are indications for partial or total hepatic lobectomy?
• Mass lesion (neoplasia, abscess, cyst)
• Fracture or damage to lobe with severe hemorrhage
• Hepatic arteriovenous fistula

2. What is a maximum amount of canine liver that can be removed, assuming normal function of the remaining liver?
70%–80%; regeneration via hyperplasia and hypertrophy of the remaining portion occurs within 6 weeks.

3. During lobectomy, which afferent vessels to the liver need to be identified and preserved to avoid fatal iatrogenic hemorrhage?
• Hepatic arteries (the number varies between 2 and 5)
• Portal vein

4. If bleeding from the liver is uncontrolled and a source not readily identified, what potential life-saving measure can be performed by the surgeon at the time of laparotomy?
The **Pringle maneuver** acutely obstructs afferent sources of blood to the liver parenchyma. This obstruction is accomplished by occluding the structures (hepatic artery and portal vein) in the hepatoduodenal ligament between the thumb and forefinger at the level of the epiploic foramen.

5. List some local methods for controlling mild hepatic lobular hemorrhage secondary to trauma.
• Ligature of vessels
• Cautery
• Clips

- Fibrin glue
- Pressure by packing the area or reapposing the capsule with large mattress sutures
- Removal of affected lobe

6. What is the effect of ligating a hepatic artery supplying a liver lobe that is to remain in place?
No effect; collateral circulation supplies the affected lobe.

7. What is the effect of ligating a hepatic duct draining a lobe that is to remain in place?
Either lobar atrophy or biliary diversion to an adjacent lobe.

8. What is the effect of ligating a portal vein?
Acute, persistent ligation results in portal hypertension and death.

9. Does surgical stapling have a place in hepatic lobectomies?
Although both blunt dissection with ligation and surgical stapling are associated with minimal morbidity when performed correctly, stapling (Autosuture, TA 90, 55, or 30) is quicker and more complete.

BIBLIOGRAPHY

1. Bjorling DE: Surgical management of hepatic and biliary disease in cats. Comp Cont Educ Pract Vet 13:1419–1425, 1991.
2. Fossum TW: Surgery of the liver. In Fossum TW (ed): Small Animal Surgery. St. Louis, Mosby-Year Book, 1997, pp 367–388.
3. Lewis DD, Bellanger CR, Lewis DT, et al: Hepatic lobectomy in the dog: A comparison of stapling and ligation techniques. Vet Surg 19:221–225, 1990.
4. Tobias KS: Hepatobiliary system. In Harara J (ed): Small Animal Surgery. Media, PA, Williams & Wilkins, 1996, pp 143–155.

35. PORTOSYSTEMIC SHUNTS

Sheldon Padgett, D.V.M., M.S., Dip. A.C.V.S.

1. What are the two major anatomic categories of portosystemic shunts (PSS)?
- Extrahepatic
- Intrahepatic

2. How are most extrahepatic PSS characterized?
Single (60%–80%) congenital shunts in small dogs.

3. Which persistent fetal vessel commonly creates a single intrahepatic PSS?
The ductus venosus.

4. What side of the liver usually contains a persistent (patent) ductus venosus?
The left.

5. In single extrahepatic shunts, what are the common vessels of origin for the shunt?
- Portal vein
- Left gastric vein
- Splenic vein
- Cranial or caudal mesenteric vein
- Gastroduodenal vein

6. What physiologic abnormality leads to the development of multiple (extrahepatic) portosystemic shunts?
Portal hypertension.

7. List common physical examination findings in patients with a PSS.
- Small body size
- Other congenital abnormalities, such as a heart murmur or cryptorchidism
- Ascites (acquired shunt)

8. What physical examination finding is common in cats with PSS?
Ptyalism, and cats with copper-colored eyes.

9. List the commonest clinical signs associated with PSS.
- Neurologic signs (disorientation, seizures, coma) referable to hepatoencephalopathy (increased ammonia, aromatic amino acids)
- Polyphagia
- Vomiting or diarrhea
- Polyuria and polydypsia
- Prolonged anesthetic recovery

10. List common laboratory findings associated with PSS.
- Increased liver enzymes
- Decreased blood urea nitrogen
- Decreased albumin
- Increased fasting ammonia
- Elevated bile acids
- Ammonium biurate crystalluria

11. Why do many animals with PSS have urinary calculi?
One of the functions of the liver is to conjugate nitrogen-containing proteins into urea. With inadequate hepatic function, the high concentration of ammonium in the urine leads to calculi containing ammonium biurate.

12. Are ammonium biurate urinary calculi pathognomonic for PSS?
No, only for liver disease and Dalmatians.

13. A young dog presented with clinical signs of hepatoencephalopathy and blood work to support the diagnosis of a PSS (elevated serum bile acids, low albumin, and low blood urea nitrogen). At the time of exploratory surgery, no extrahepatic shunt is found. An intraoperative portogram is performed, and there is no evidence of a vascular anomaly. How do you explain the laboratory and clinical abnormalities?
The syndrome of **hepatic microvascular dysplasia** is most likely occurring. This condition consists of normal gross vascular anatomy, but shunting at the level of the hepatic sinusoids. Gross appearance and portography are normal. The diagnosis is confirmed on histologic examination of the liver tissue.

14. What is transcolonic scintigraphy?
Use of sodium pertechnetate (technetium 99m) applied colonically; in animals with PSS, blood is shunted away from the liver into systemic circulation, and nuclear activity is detected in the heart and lungs before the liver.

15. What other diagnostic test may be useful in diagnosing a PSS?
Ultrasonography.

16. What are the basic items used in medical therapy of a PSS and how are they beneficial?
- **Lactulose**—decreases colonic pH, decreasing the amount of ammonia absorbed.

- **Oral antibiotics**—decrease the number of urease-producing bacteria in the colon, decreasing the amount of toxins absorbed.
- **Protein restriction**—decreases the substrate for production of ammonia.

17. What are anesthetic concerns for patients with PSS?
- **Hepatic dysfunction** or **insufficiency**—increased and unpredictable effect of drugs (diazepam, isoflurane are recommended).
- **Pressure changes**—hypotension resulting from hypoalbuminemia and surgical manipulations; decrease in central venous pressure after ligation of shunt (increase in portal pressures).
- **Hypothermia** and **hypoglycemia** in young, small patients.

18. In what three intraabdominal areas should one look for a PSS?
- Right mesenteric root
- Epiploic foramen
- Left mesenteric root (traversing the diaphragm, as in a portoazygous shunt)

19. Once a shunt is found at surgery, what is done next?
Complete occlusion is the eventual goal; this can be done acutely via ligation or gradually with an ameroid constrictor or other gradual occlusion technique (such as cellophane banding).

20. What is the primary morbidity associated with acute occlusion of the anomalous vessel?
Severe portal hypertension (which can be fatal).

21. What is done to avoid acute portal hypertension during ligation?
Portal pressures are measured, via a manometer and portal vessel (mesenteric) catheter during slow ligation of the shunt. Portal pressures are maintained less than 10 cm H_2O over preligation pressures. If full ligation of the shunt is not possible, partial ligation is performed.

22. What other *objective* parameter can be measured during ligation to signal hypertension?
Central venous pressure can be measured via a jugular catheter; there should be less than a 1-cm drop in preligation pressures.

23. What are some *subjective* intraoperative methods to detect acute portal hypertension?
- Pulsating of splanchnic vasculature
- Congestion, or cyanosis, or both of the small intestine
- Hypermotility of the small intestine

24. How does an ameroid constrictor decrease morbidity?
The constrictor, when placed around the anomalous vessel, slowly (over weeks) decreases the lumen of the vessel. This allows the hepatic parenchyma to accommodate the increased blood flow gradually, decreasing the chance of portal hypertension.

25. What is an ameroid constrictor?
Casein in the ring expands because of its hygroscopic properties. The metal jacket around the constrictor forces inward expansion and, when placed around a shunt, leads to obliteration of the lumen.

26. Are there any treatments for multiple extrahepatic PSS?
Medical therapy is recommended. Banding of the posthepatic vena cava can be done to increase the caval pressure. Consequentially, this decreases the amount of blood that *runs off* into the cava, increasing portal flow. Although patients can tolerate caval banding with some morbidity, this procedure has not been shown to change long-term survival or quality of life.

27. What are the commonest postoperative complications associated with ligation of a PSS?
- **Ascites:** prognosis good if mild.
- **Portal hypertension:** prognosis poor to grave if not treated by relieving portal hypertension.
- **Generalized motor seizures:** prognosis guarded to poor if not suppressed.

28. Are any animals more likely to seizure after ligation of a PSS?
Older animals (>1.5 years).

29. There has been a lot of discussion about partial versus complete ligation of portosystemic shunts; does it really matter?
Yes, partial ligation patients have a much higher incidence (50%) of long-term problems because of their shunt (persistent hepatoencephalopathy, gastrointestinal signs, or urinary calculi).

30. How can you avoid these late complications?
By using an ameroid constrictor or by repeating a laparotomy 1–4 months after the initial partial ligation and attempting full ligation at that time.

31. Are there any predictors for full shunt ligation?
Animals that are not encephalopathic have a greater chance (approaching 100%) of recovery from full ligation versus those with encephalopathy (60% chance that full ligation can be performed without causing fatal portal hypertension).

32. How can successful recovery from PSS surgery be documented?
- Absence of clinical signs and patient growth
- Minimal dietary requirements
- Repeat nuclear scintigraphy or portography

BIBLIOGRAPHY

1. Allen L, Stobie D: Clinicopathologic features of dogs with microvascular dysplasia. J Am Vet Med Assoc 214:218–220, 1999.
2. Boothe HW, How LM, Edwards JF, et al: Multiple extrahepatic portosystemic shunts in dogs: 30 cases (1981–1993). J Am Vet Med Assoc 208:1849–1854, 1996.
3. Hottinger HA, Walshaw R, Hauptman J: Long-term results of complete and partial ligation of congenital portosystemic shunts in dogs. Vet Surg 24:331–336, 1995.
4. Komtebedde J, Koblik PD, Breznock EM: Long-term clinical outcome after partial ligation of single extrahepatic vascular anomalies in 20 dogs. Vet Surg 24:379–383, 1995.
5. Vogt JC, Krahwinke DJ, Bright RM: Gradual occlusion of extrahepatic portosystemic shunts in dogs and cats using the ameroid constrictor. Vet Surg 25:495–502, 1996.
6. Youmans KR, Hunt GB: Experimental evaluation of four methods for progressive venous attenuation in dogs. Vet Surg 28:38–47, 1999.

36. BILIARY SURGERY

Sheldon Padgett, D.V.M., M.S., Dip. A.C.V.S.

1. What are the most important functions of the biliary tree?
Accumulation, concentration, storage, and delivery of bile.

2. Where is the gallbladder located?
Between the quadrate and right medial hepatic lobes.

3. Describe the anatomy of the extrahepatic biliary system.

Each liver lobe is drained by its own hepatic duct. The cystic duct supplies and empties the gallbladder. The cystic duct and the hepatic ducts converge to form the common bile duct (CBD). The CBD is located in the lesser omentum (hepatoduodenal ligament) and drains into the proximal duodenum (in dogs, at the major duodenal papilla with the ventral pancreatic duct).

4. What is the composition of canine choleliths?

Choleliths in the dog are usually formed from calcium salts of biliary pigment.

5. Are choleliths the commonest cause of extrahepatic biliary obstruction?

In humans, yes; in dogs, no. Most cases of cholelithiasis are clinically silent.

6. What is the commonest cause of extrahepatic biliary obstruction in dogs?

Obstruction (usually because of inflammation) of the CBD as it passes through the pancreatic area and empties into the duodenum.

7. List other possible causes of extrahepatic biliary obstruction in small animals.
- Inflammation of the biliary tract (cholangitis, cholecystitis)
- Biliary stasis
- Neoplasia (either of the biliary tree or extraluminal neoplasia leading to lumen compromise)
- Diaphragmatic hernias
- Parasitic infestation of the liver
- Congenital dysplasia

8. Should a coagulation profile be performed on a patient with chronic posthepatic biliary obstruction?

Yes. Fat absorption may be impaired with biliary obstruction; fat-soluble vitamin K is not well absorbed. Coagulation factors VII, IX, and X are vitamin K dependent and may not be produced in quantities sufficient for normal coagulation. Treatment with vitamin K_1 for 24–48 hours before surgery restores adequate vitamin K factors.

9. What is the commonest type of biliary neoplasia?

Bile duct carcinoma is the second commonest type of hepatic tumor and the commonest type of tumor in the biliary tree.

10. What is cholecystitis?

Inflammation and infection of the gallbladder.

11. What are the commonest pathogenic organisms of cholecystitis?

Escherichia coli and *Klebsiella*.

12. When a physician client asks you if Charcot's triad is seen in canine cholecystitis, what is your response?

Although biliary colic (pain) and fever is present, as it is in humans, jaundice is not seen as often as vomiting in dogs.

13. What pathologies can cause biliary tract rupture and consequentially bile peritonitis?
- Trauma
- Necrotizing cholecystitis
- Cholelithiasis

14. What portion of the biliary tree most commonly ruptures?

CBD.

15. What are causes of biliary ruptures?
- **Trauma** causes about 6% of gallbladder and 98% of bile duct ruptures.
- **Cholecystitis** causes approximately 30% of gallbladder ruptures.
- **Cholelithiasis** causes only 2% of bile duct ruptures and nearly 70% of gallbladder ruptures.

16. Discuss the preferred method of repair for biliary trauma.
Primary repair alone is usually not possible except in cases of avulsion of the CBD from its duodenal insertion. If trauma to the length of the CBD is minimal, primary closure with stenting via an intraluminal stent may be possible. If the CBD is severely traumatized, biliary diversion, as in cholecystenterotomy, should be performed. Trauma to the hepatic ducts is usually treated by ligation of the duct, and auxiliary routes drain bile from the affected lobe.

17. Discuss the preferred surgical treatment for cholecystitis.
Cholecystectomy is indicated to remove the infected tissue. This procedure involves dissection of the gallbladder from the hepatic fossa, freeing the cystic duct and accompanying vessels, and ligation at the junction with the CBD.

18. What are the indications for a cholecystotomy?
To remove contents from the gallbladder or CBD that cannot be removed by a less invasive method, such as aspiration. When performing a cholecystotomy for cholelith removal, one should consider performing a cholecystectomy because the survival rate is higher with the latter procedure for the treatment of choleliths.

19. When creating a stoma in the gallbladder and intestine for a cholecystenterotomy, what are guidelines for the dimensions of the opening?
Over time, the orifice strictures to approximately half of the original length. The stoma should be either the entire length of the gallbladder, from the apex to the infundibulum, or 4 cm in length, whichever is less.

20. What is the sequela of creating a stoma that is not large enough?
Chronic, recurrent ascending cholangiohepatitis.

21. What is the difference between cholecystoduodenostomy versus cholecystojejunostomy?
Location of the anastomosis of the gallbladder within the intestinal tract (duodenum [more physiologic] or jejunum).

22. What are treatment options for bile peritonitis?
Culture of the peritoneal cavity is indicated, and perioperative and postoperative antibiotics (enrofloxacin, amikacin, trimethoprim/sulfadiazine, second- or third-generation cephalosporin) should be given. The source of the biliary effusion should be identified and treated. High-volume lavage should be performed at the time of surgery. Open abdominal management of severe peritonitis is indicated, with all the attending management concerns (hypoproteinemia, sepsis, nutritional support).

23. What are some prognostic factors of bile peritonitis?
Sterile biliary effusions have a much higher survival rate than those with septic effusions. **Average neutrophil count** in animals that survive biliary rupture is significantly lower than those who do not survive.

BIBLIOGRAPHY

1. Bjorling DE: Surgical management of hepatic and biliary disease in cats. Comp Cont Educ Pract Vet 13:1419–1425, 1991.
2. Kirpensteijn J, Fingland RB, Ulrich T, et al: Cholelithiasis in dogs: 29 cases (1980–1990). J Am Vet Med Assoc 202:1137–1142, 1993.

3. Ludwig LL, McLoughlin MA, Grafes TK, et al: Surgical treatment of bile peritonitis in 24 dogs and 2 cats: A retrospective study (1987–1994). Vet Surg 26:90–98, 1997.
4. Parchman MB, Flanders JA: Extrahepatic biliary tract rupture: Evaluation of the relationship between the site of rupture and the cause of rupture in 15 dogs. Cornell Vet 80:267–272, 1990.
5. Tobias KS: Hepatobiliary system. In Harari J (ed): Small Animal Surgery. Media, PA, Williams & Wilkins, 1996, pp 143–155.

37. GASTRIC DILATATION–VOLVULUS

Bradley R. Coolman, D.V.M., M.S.

1. What is gastric dilatation–volvulus (GDV)?

An acute, life-threatening, medical and surgical emergency affecting primarily large and giant breeds of dogs. The stomach of affected dogs becomes distended with gas and malpositioned, leading to shock and rapid deterioration of the patient if not properly treated.

2. What causes GDV?

The exact cause of GDV is not known; however, several risk factors have been identified.

3. What are some specific risk factors that have been associated with GDV in dogs?

- **Age**—middle-aged and old dogs are at an increased risk.
- **Body weight**—breeds with a higher average adult body weight are at increased risk for GDV. Obesity is not a risk factor.
- **Body conformation**—dogs with deep, narrow thoracic conformation have an increased risk for GDV.
- **Diet**—dogs that eat few meals each day or ingest meals rapidly have increased susceptibility to GDV.
- **Genetics**—Purebred dogs have a higher risk of GDV than mixed-breed dogs.
- **History**—dogs with a family history of GDV have an increased risk of developing the syndrome.

4. List the clinical signs for a dog with acute GDV.

- Restlessness and pain.
- Increased respiratory rates.
- Nervous pacing.
- Abdominal distention (bloat).
- Repeated vomiting (often nonproductive)
- Hypersalivation (ptyalism)

5. What comes first, dilation or volvulus?

This is the proverbial *chicken or the egg* question of the GDV syndrome. Most investigators believe that gastric dilation precedes rotation of the stomach. Analysis of the stomach gas from dogs with GDV shows that the gas filling the bloated stomach is essentially room air, and aerophagia is likely the cause of gastric dilation. Chronic partial gastric volvulus without dilation is also reported to occur.

6. In which direction does the stomach normally rotate during GDV?

Usually in a clockwise direction (to 270°) as viewed ventrodorsally into the abdomen (i.e., the position of the patient prepared for a ventral midline laparotomy).

7a–c. Discuss the pathophysiology of GDV.

   a. Cardiovascular: Dogs with GDV present in shock. Dilation of the stomach causes compression of the caudal vena cava and portal vein, resulting in sequestration of blood in the caudal half of the body and markedly decreased venous return to the heart (**hypovolemic shock**). Decreased cardiac output and decreased arterial blood pressure result, which, in turn, lead to cellular hypoxia and a shift to anaerobic metabolism. Myocardial ischemia can lead to decreased contractility and arrhythmias, which contribute to cardiac dysfunction (**cardiogenic shock**). Stasis of the portal circulation decreases the ability of the hepatic monocyte-macrophage defense system to clear bacteria and endotoxins from the circulation, and consequently **distributive or vasogenic shock** may also ensue. Vascular stasis, hypoxia, acidosis, and circulating endotoxin can predispose to the development of **disseminated intravascular coagulation**.

  b. **Respiratory:** The grossly distended stomach pushes on the diaphragm and results in decreased pulmonary compliance. The respiratory impairment leads to a **ventilation-perfusion mismatch,** which further decreases blood oxygenation and exacerbates tissue hypoxia.

  c. **Gastric:** Increased luminal pressure and twisting of the stomach on its mesenteric axis causes compression of the thin-walled gastric veins, resulting in vascular stasis and edema of the gastric wall. Avulsion of the short gastric vessels along the greater curvature of the stomach often occurs secondary to volvulus and can contribute to **gastric wall ischemia.** Ultimately, partial-thickness or full-thickness necrosis of the gastric wall may occur, most commonly along the left side of the greater curvature and fundus.

8. How is GDV diagnosed?

Usually based on **signalment, clinical signs,** and **physical examination.** Radiographs may be necessary in some cases.

9. Which radiographic view is recommended?

The right lateral recumbent view is considered the view of choice for confirming a diagnosis of GDV. Dogs with gastric volvulus have a distinct compartmentalization line between the gas-filled fundus and pylorus (**double bubble** or **pillar** sign).

10. Is it important to distinguish between simple gastric dilation and GDV?

No. Dogs with acute gastric dilation should be treated identically to dogs with GDV.

11. List some differential diagnoses for GDV in dogs.

- Mesenteric volvulus
- Splenic torsion
- Ascites
- Hemoabdomen
- Abdominal neoplasia

12. What are the emergency treatments for a dog that presents with acute GDV?

- Aggressive shock treatment (see Chapter 3).
- Gastric decompression with an orogastric tube or via percutaneous trocarization.

13. List the goals of surgery for GDV.

- Gastric decompression and repositioning
- Assessment of abdominal organ viability
- Permanent gastropexy of the stomach to the body wall

14. List methods for intraoperative gastric decompression.

- Orogastric tube passed by an assistant and guided through the gastroesophageal junction by the surgeon.
- Trocarization with a large-bore needle (14–18 gauge) attached to the surgical suction hose.
- Temporary gastrostomy tube.

15. Is gastrotomy useful for intraoperative gastric decompression?

Gastrotomy should be avoided if possible and used only if a gastric foreign body or desiccated, packed gastric contents are present.

16. What is the first structure seen during an emergency celiotomy for GDV?

The omentum covering the distended stomach.

17. How is the stomach repositioned in a dog with a 180° clockwise rotation?

Carefully, to avoid organ trauma. With the surgeon standing on the dog's right side, the right hand reaches up toward the dog's left dorsal body wall and grabs the pylorus. The left hand pushes down on the stomach as the right hand gently lifts up and back on the pylorus. The stomach should flip back into a normal position. Complete derotation is confirmed by visualizing the esophagus, pylorus, omentum, and spleen in their normal positions.

18. What percentage of dogs with GDV have gastric necrosis?

Approximately 10%.

19. What criteria are used to determine gastric and splenic viability?

Evidence of **gastric** necrosis includes gastric contents in the peritoneal cavity, discoloration and thinning of the stomach wall, and lack of active bleeding after gastric incision.

Splenic necrosis, avulsion of splenic mesenteric vessels, and thrombosis of the splenic vessels are indications for splenectomy. An engorged spleen may return to normal size and color several minutes after repositioning.

20. Is intravenous fluorescein dye injection valuable for assessment of gastric viability?

No; it has no advantage over subjective assessment.

21. Which clinical laboratory assay has been described as useful in identifying gastric necrosis in dogs with GDV?

Preoperative plasma lactate concentration greater than 6 mmol/L.

22. Does splenectomy decrease the recurrence rate of GDV in dogs?

No.

23. List methods for partial gastrectomy.

- Surgical resection and two-layer inverting, hand-sewn closure.
- Resection and closure with automated surgical stapling equipment (i.e., TA 90 or GIA 55 staplers, United States Surgical Corporation).
- Invaginating the necrotic portion into the gastric lumen and oversewing of the gastric wall.
- For all gastrectomy techniques, an orogastric tube should be placed first to maintain patency of the esophageal-gastric opening.

24. What techniques are commonly used for permanent gastropexy?

- Tube gastropexy
- Circumcostal gastropexy
- Belt-loop gastropexy
- Incisional gastropexy
- Ventral midline gastropexy

25. Which gastropexy method creates the strongest adhesion in experimental cases?

Circumcostal gastropexy.

26. Is the increased strength of the circumcostal gastropexy clinically important?

No. All of the methods listed are associated with a low rate of recurrence (< 10%). Surgeons should select a familiar and consistently successful method.

27. Should pyloromyotomy or pyloroplasty be routinely performed on dogs that have GDV?

No. These procedures do not increase gastric emptying rates or prevent future episodes of gastric dilation; they do increase the postoperative complication rates.

28. What is the case fatality rate of dogs with acute GDV?

15%–33%.

29. What factors are associated with an increased risk of perioperative mortality?

- Poor physical condition on hospital admission (i.e., depressed or comatose dogs)
- Gastric necrosis or gastric rupture
- Splenectomy or partial gastrectomy
- Preoperative cardiac dysrhythmias
- Disseminated intravascular coagulation

30. List the primary immediate postoperative complications encountered in dogs with GDV.

- Shock
- Ventricular dysrhythmias
- Vomiting and gastritis
- Hypokalemia
- Hypoproteinemia
- Anemia
- Gastric atony
- Gastric necrosis
- Peritonitis
- Disseminated intravascular coagulation
- Death

CONTROVERSY

31. What is the optimal timing of surgery for a GDV patient?

Most surgeons believe that the dog should be taken to surgery as soon as possible immediately after initiating shock therapy; others argue that the dog should be subjected to surgery only after a more extensive period of medical stabilization (12–24 hours). The timing of surgery ultimately depends on the condition of the patient, the response to shock treatment, the judgment of the attending clinician, and the availability of a surgeon.

BIBLIOGRAPHY

1. Brockman DJ, Washabau RJ, Drobatz KJ: Canine gastric dilatation/volvulus syndrome in a veterinary critical care unit: 295 cases (1986–1992). J Am Vet Med Assoc 207:460–464, 1995.
2. Brourman JD, Schertel ER, Allen DA, et al: Factors associated with perioperative mortality in dogs with surgically managed gastric dilatation-volvulus: 137 cases (1988–1993). J Am Vet Med Assoc 208:1855–1858, 1996.
3. de Papp E, Drobatz KJ: Plasma lactate concentration as a predictor of gastric necrosis and survival in dogs with GDV. J Am Vet Med Assoc 215:49–53, 1999.
4. Glickman LT, Glickman NW, Schellenberg DB, et al: Multiple risk factors for the gastric dilatation-volvulus syndrome in dogs: A practitioner/owner case-control study. J Am Anim Hosp Assoc 33:197–204, 1997.
5. Glickman LT, Lantz GW, Schellenberg DB, et al: A prospective study of survival and recurrence following the acute gastric dilatation-volvulus syndrome in 136 dogs. J Am Anim Hosp Assoc 34:253–259, 1998.
6. Lantz GC: Treatment of gastric dilatation-volvulus. In Bojrab MJ (ed): Current Techniques in Small Animal Surgery, 4th ed. Baltimore, Williams & Wilkins, 1998, pp 223–231.
7. Meyer-Lindenberg A, Harder A, Fehr M, et al: Treatment of gastric dilatation-volvulus and a rapid method for prevention of relapse in dogs: 134 cases (1988–1991). J Am Vet Med Assoc 203:1303–1307, 1993.
8. Matthiesen DT: Gastric dilatation-volvulus syndrome. In Slatter D (ed): Textbook of Small Animal Surgery, 2nd ed. Philadelphia, W.B. Saunders, 1993, pp 580–593.

38. GASTRIC OUTFLOW OBSTRUCTION

Cathy L. Greenfield, D.V.M., M.S.

1. List the commonest causes of gastric outflow obstruction in dogs and cats.
- Foreign bodies
- Pyloric stenosis
- Chronic hypertrophic pyloric gastropathy
- Infiltrative fungal diseases
- Gastric neoplasia
- Lesions near the stomach that compress the outflow tract (pancreatic or hepatic abscesses or neoplasia)

2. What is pyloric stenosis?
A congenital lesion characterized by a benign thickening of the circular smooth muscle of the pylorus.

3. What is the typical signalment of animals affected with pyloric stenosis?
Young animals that start to show clinical signs after weaning. Brachycephalic dogs are most commonly affected, especially bulldogs, Boston terriers, and boxers. Siamese cats have also been diagnosed with this condition.

4. What is chronic hypertrophic pyloric gastropathy?
An acquired, benign condition involving hypertrophy of the pylorus. This name may refer to only mucosal hypertrophy or to mucosal and muscular hypertrophy.

5. List other names used synonymously with chronic hypertrophic pyloric gastropathy.
- Chronic antral mucosal hypertrophy
- Antral pyloric hypertrophy
- Chronic hypertrophic gastritis
- Acquired pyloric stenosis
- Multiple gastric polyps

6. What is the typical signalment of a patient presenting with chronic hypertrophic pyloric gastropathy?
Middle-aged to older, small-breed dogs weighing less than 10 kg are most commonly affected.

7. Is there a sex predisposition in chronic hypertropic pyloric gastropathy?
Male dogs are affected approximately twice as often as female dogs.

8. What type of infiltrative fungal disease may cause gastric outflow obstruction?
Pythiosis, caused by *Pithium insidiosum*. Ingested spores penetrate the gastric mucosa, enter lymphatics, and result in the development of granulomas within the submucosa and muscularis. The granulomas may cause gastric outflow obstruction. It may affect all portions of the gastrointestinal tract.

9. What is the typical signalment of dogs affected with pythiosis?
Young, large-breed, male dogs living in the Gulf Coast areas of the southeastern United States.

10. What types of gastric neoplasia are seen in dogs and cats?
- **Gastric adenocarcinoma**—the commonest type of gastric neoplasia in dogs.

- **Leiomyomas and leiomyosarcomas**—smooth muscle tumors. Leiomyomas are the most common benign gastric tumor in the dog.
- Lymphoma—the commonest type of gastric neoplasia in the cat; also seen in dogs.

11. **Which portions of the stomach are usually affected with gastric neoplasia?**
   - **Adenocarcinomas**—pyloric antral region or along the lesser curvature
   - **Leiomyomas**—the cardia
   - **Lymphoma**—discrete masses of the gastric wall or a diffusely infiltrative disease
   The intestinal tract may also be involved.

12. **What is the typical signalment of a patient presenting with gastric neoplasia?**
   Older dogs (8–9 years of age for **adenocarcinoma**). There is a breed predisposition in Belgian shepherd dogs, and male dogs of this breed are more frequently affected than females.
   There is a breed predisposition for **leiomyomas** in beagles, with very old dogs (17–18 years) affected most commonly.
   Lymphoma affects primarily middle-aged to older dogs (average 6 years).

13. **Describe the common clinical signs seen in patients with gastric outflow obstruction.**
   Chronic intermittent vomiting which may be projectile. Cats, especially, may regurgitate and have esophagitis. Some animals may be dehydrated and have electrolyte and acid-base imbalances, depending on the chronicity and severity of the obstruction.

14. **What diagnostic tests are useful when working up a patient with gastric outflow obstruction?**
   - Complete blood count, chemistry profile, and urinalysis.
   - Abdominal radiographs—usually unrewarding, but may reveal an enlarged stomach.
   - Contrast radiographs—filling defects, irregular mucosal surfaces, gastric wall thickening, or delayed gastric emptying.
   - Thoracic radiographs—to evaluate for metastatic disease.
   - Abdominal ultrasound examination—to evaluate for metastatic disease.
   - **Gastroscopy**—the best diagnostic test, to identify and biopsy the lesion.

15. **What is the definitive treatment for gastric outflow obstruction?**
   Surgery.

16. **What medical management should be provided before performing surgery?**
   The patients should be stabilized before any anesthetic episode by rehydrating affected patients and correcting electrolyte and acid-base abnormalities. If esophagitis is present, H_2-receptor blockers or a protein-pump inhibitor should be administered. Perioperative antibiotics may be started preoperatively.

17. **List the surgical procedures that can be used for treatment of gastric outflow obstruction.**
   - Fredet-Ramstedt pyloromyotomy
   - Heineke-Mikulicz pyloroplasty
   - Y-U pyloroplasty
   - Billroth I gastroenterostomy
   - Billroth II gastroenterostomy

18. **What type of suture material should be used when closing gastric incisions?**
   Synthetic, monofilament, absorbable suture material, usually in 3–0 or 4–0 sizes for most small animal patients. Chromic gut suture material should not be used because it is rapidly removed when exposed to digestive enzymes and does not reliably retain its holding strength for an adequate period to allow for sufficient wound healing.

19. What is a Fredet-Ramstedt pyloromyotomy?

An incision through the serosa and muscularis over the pylorus, without penetrating the submucosa or mucosa. It is the least aggressive of the pyloric surgeries and used to be recommended for minor pyloric outflow obstructions (congenital pyloric stenosis). Because of rapid healing and fibrosis of the pyloromyotomy incision, long-term efficacy of this procedure is questioned, and many surgeons no longer recommend it.

20. Who were Fredet and Ramstedt?

Wilhelm Ramstedt (1867–1963) was a German surgeon who described pyloromyotomy. At the same time, Pierre Fredet (1870–1946), a French surgeon, reported a similar procedure.

21. What is a pyloroplasty?

One or more full-thickness incisions through the pylorus with subsequent suturing of the pyloric incisions together in a different direction, widening the gastric outflow tract. Pyloroplasty is indicated with mild pyloric outflow obstruction, when full-thickness excision of the gastric wall is not necessary to relieve the obstruction.

22. What is the Heineke-Mikulicz pyloroplasty?

A full-thickness, longitudinal incision centered over the pylorus on the ventral surface of the pylorus. The incision extends equal distances into the pyloric antrum and proximal duodenum and is closed transversely using a simple interrupted suture pattern.

23. Who were Heineke and Mikulicz?

Walter Hermann Heineke (1834–1901) was a German surgeon. Little information regarding his career is available from surgery history textbooks. Johann von Mikulicz-Radecki (1850–1905) began his career as an assistant to Billroth in Vienna. He was an active contributor to the surgical literature and is credited with being the first surgeon to require facemask usage during operations.

24. Describe the Y-U pyloroplasty.

An advance flap pyloroplasty procedure in which a full-thickness Y-shaped incision is made over the duodenum, pylorus, and pyloric antrum. The incision is then closed in a U shape.

25. What are the advantages of the Y-U pyloroplasty over the Heineke-Mikulicz pyloroplasty?

Adequate exposure is afforded to allow excessive pyloric mucosa to be resected. The longitudinal direction of the incisions results in less alteration of pyloric function.

26. What is a Billroth I gastroenterostomy?

A pylorectomy with a gastroduodenostomy. It is indicated when full-thickness resection of the stomach wall is required to relieve the obstruction and when the disease is localized to the pylorus and distal pyloric antral region.

27. What is a Billroth II gastroenterostomy?

A distal gastrectomy with gastrojejunostomy. It is indicated when extensive, full-thickness resection of the distal portion of the stomach, pylorus, and proximal duodenum is necessary and when the extent of the resection precludes the surgeon from performing an end-to-end anastomosis between the remaining stomach and duodenum.

28. Who was Billroth?

Theodor Billroth (1829–1894) was Germany's most celebrated surgeon. He was an outstanding surgical technician able to bring his experimental successes to the practical side of clinical surgery. He established one of the earliest surgical training programs at the University of Vienna, authored several texts, and pioneered numerous gastrointestinal surgical procedures.

29. What adjacent anatomic structures must be carefully protected during a gastroenterostomy?

The common bile duct and pancreatic ducts.

30. What treatment is appropriate if either of these structures becomes damaged during the gastroenterostomy or if the disease process involves these structures?

A cholecystoenterostomy may be necessary to reestablish biliary outflow from the gallbladder. If the pancreatic ducts are damaged, the patient may develop pancreatic exocrine insufficiency and needs to be treated with enzymes to allow for food digestion.

31. What complications may be seen in association with pyloromyotomy?

Inadequate long-term relief from the clinical signs associated with most types of gastric outflow obstruction. Consequently, it is recommended only for use in mild cases of congenital pyloric stenosis.

32. What complications may be seen in association with pyloroplasty?

- Suture line dehiscence or leakage and peritonitis
- Inadequate resection of tissues resulting in inadequate relief of clinical signs
- Duodenal-gastric reflux (is not as much of a problem with the Y-U pyloroplasty).

33. What complications may be seen in association with gastroenterostomy?

- Suture line dehiscence or leakage and peritonitis
- Inadequate resection of tissues resulting in inadequate relief of clinical signs
- Recurrence of neoplastic disease at the surgical site
- Metastasis of malignant neoplasms

34. What is the prognosis for a patient with surgically treated pyloric stenosis?

Excellent, if the condition is treated properly.

35. What is the prognosis for a patient with surgically treated chronic hypertrophic pyloric gastropathy?

Excellent. Surgery should be curative for this disease, assuming all abnormal tissue was resected.

36. Discuss the prognosis for a patient with gastric neoplasia that has been surgically treated.

If the tumor is benign (i.e., leiomyoma), surgery should be curative. Most gastric tumors are malignant, however, and are usually relatively refractory to adjunct chemotherapy. Consequently a guarded to poor prognosis for long-term survival must be given in these cases. The exception is lymphoma, which may respond to chemotherapy.

BIBLIOGRAPHY

1. Fossum TW: Surgery of the stomach. In Fossum TW (ed): Small Animal Surgery. St. Louis, Mosby-Year Book, 1997, pp 266–270, 283–286, 289–292.
2. Kapatkin AS, Mullen HS, Matthiesen DT, et al: Leiomyosarcoma in dogs: 44 cases (1983–1988). J Am Vet Med Assoc 201:1077–1079, 1992.
3. Matthiesen DT, Walter MC: Surgical treatment of chronic hypertrophic pyloric gastropathy in 45 dogs. J Am Anim Hosp Assoc 22:241–247, 1986.
4. Matthiesen DT: Chronic gastric outflow obstruction. In Slatter D (ed): Textbook of Small Animal Surgery, 2nd ed. Philadelphia, W.B. Saunders, 1993, pp 561–568.
5. Sikes RI, Birchard S, Patnaik A, et al: Chronic hypertrophic pyloric gastropathy: A review of 16 cases. J Am Anim Hosp Assoc 22:99–104, 1986.
6. Stanton MLE: Gastric surgery. In Bojrab MJ (ed): Disease Mechanisms in Small Animal Surgery, 2nd ed. Philadelphia, Lea & Febiger, 1993, pp 232–236.
7. Walter MC, Matthiesen DT, Stone EA: Pylorectomy and gastroduodenostomy in the dog: Technique and clinical results in 28 cases. J Am Vet Med Assoc 187:909–914, 1985.

39. GASTROINTESTINAL FOREIGN BODIES

Bradley R. Coolman, D.V.M., M.S.

1. Why are gastrointestinal foreign bodies a common problem in small animals?

Small animals (especially juveniles) have a high orolingual curiosity. The oropharyngeal entrance to the gastrointestinal tract has a larger diameter than any other portion of the digestive system.

2. What clinical signs are associated with foreign bodies in the stomach and intestine?
- Vomiting
- Dehydration
- Anorexia
- Depression
- Fever
- Abdominal pain

3. List the characteristic radiographic findings in an animal with mechanical obstruction of the intestine.
- Multiple loops of gas-filled or fluid-filled, dilated small intestine
- Radiopaque foreign material in the gastrointestinal tract
- Delayed passage (or retention) of gastrointestinal contrast material

4. Can gastric and intestinal foreign bodies be successfully removed with an endoscope?

Yes, for **gastric** foreign bodies.

No, for foreign bodies from the **small intestine.**

5. How long should an internist attempt endoscopic removal of a gastric foreign body before the patient is taken to surgery?

A time limit should be set at the start of the procedure (e.g., 30 minutes) to prevent excessive anesthesia time and patient trauma. The efficiency of removing the foreign body or the ability to decide that surgical retrieval is necessary often increases if the surgeon is present during the endoscopy.

6. Is conservative management (supportive care only) successful for gastric or intestinal foreign bodies?

Limited information is published concerning conservative management of gastrointestinal foreign bodies in small animals. In human patients (mainly pediatrics), 80%–90% of ingested foreign bodies will pass without intervention and cause no adverse effects. In one report, 9 of 19 cats with linear foreign bodies responded successfully to conservative management after freeing the sublingually lodged string.

7. What are linear foreign bodies?

String, fabric, thread, or other objects that become fixed proximally in the gastrointestinal tract, extend distally, and cause partial gastrointestinal obstruction.

8. Describe the pathophysiology of a linear foreign body.

After the linear foreign body becomes fixed proximally, the intestine becomes plicated on the string because of repeated peristaltic activity. The linear foreign body becomes taut at the mesenteric border of the intestine and eventually begins to cut into the mucosa. If the string is not removed or released, the foreign body eventually cuts through the bowel. The end result is localized or generalized peritonitis, with extensive adhesions at the mesenteric border.

9. What radiographic findings are characteristic of linear foreign bodies?
- Plication of the intestine with sharp turns and irregular gas bubbles

- Loss of serosal detail or free gas in the abdominal cavity, which indicate bowel perforation and peritonitis

10. Where do linear foreign bodies typically lodge?
- **Cats**—around the base of the tongue
- **Dogs**—at the pylorus

11. Where do nonlinear gastric and intestinal foreign bodies typically become lodged?
- Pylorus
- Transverse portion of the duodenum
- Ileocecocolic valve

12. List the indications for surgical removal of a gastric or intestinal foreign body.
- Complete gastrointestinal obstruction
- Increased vomiting or abdominal pain
- Fever, lethargy, or deterioration of patient status
- Failure of a foreign body to move (based on radiographs) for more than 8 hours
- Failure to pass a foreign body per rectum in 36 hours

13. What is the surgical treatment for a gastric foreign body?
Gastrotomy. The gastrotomy incision should be made in an avascular region of the body of the stomach and closed in one or two layers using either an appositional or an inverting pattern. Excessive inversion of the stomach should be avoided.

14. What are the surgical treatments for an intestinal foreign body?
Enterotomy made just distal to the foreign body (in healthy bowel) and closed in a single-layer appositional pattern. Linear foreign bodies typically require a **gastrotomy** and one or more enterotomies for complete removal.

15. When should intestinal resection and anastomosis be performed?
- If the foreign body obstruction has caused necrosis of the bowel
- If perforation and localized peritonitis are present (i.e., linear foreign body)
- If the viability of the intestine is in question

16. Should a biopsy specimen of the bowel be obtained when removing a foreign body?
Yes, if the bowel is thickened or stenotic at the level of the obstruction.

17. Why should a biopsy be performed in this situation?
Patients can develop a foreign body obstruction secondary to neoplastic impingement into the bowel lumen. Neoplasia must always be considered in middle-aged and older patients.

18. What is the incidence of intestinal dehiscence in dogs and cats?
7%–15.7%.

19. What risk factors have been associated with increased rates of intestinal dehiscence in small animals?
- Traumatic intestinal injuries
- Intestinal foreign body
- Peritonitis present at the initial surgery

20. What is the average length of time elapsed between intestinal surgery and the identification of gastrointestinal wound dehiscence?
4 days—this corresponds to the end of the lag phase of intestinal healing.

21. What is the mortality rate for patients that experience intestinal dehiscence?
73%-80%.

BIBLIOGRAPHY

1. Basher AWP, Fowler JD: Conservative versus surgical management of gastrointestinal linear foreign bodies in the cat. Vet Surg 16:135–138, 1987.
2. Evans KL, Smeak DD, Biller DS: Gastrointestinal linear foreign bodies in 32 dogs: A retrospective evaluation and feline comparison. J Am Anim Hosp Assoc 30:445–450, 1994.
3. Hedlund CS, Fossum TW: Surgery of the digestive system. In Fossum TW (ed): Small Animal Surgery. St. Louis, Mosby, 1997, pp 200–306.
4. Michels GM, Jones BD, Huss BT, et al: Endoscopic and surgical retrieval of fishhooks from the stomach and esophagus in dogs and cats: 75 cases (1977–1993). J Am Vet Med Assoc 207:1194–1197, 1995.
5. Orsher RJ, Rosin E: Small intestine. In Slatter D (ed): Textbook of Small Animal Surgery, 2nd ed. Philadelphia, W.B. Saunders, 1993, pp 593–612.
6. Van Sluys FJ: Gastric foreign bodies. In Slatter D (ed): Textbook of Small Animal Surgery, second edition. Philadelphia, WB Saunders, 1993, pp 568–571.
7. Wylie KB, Hosgood G: Mortality and morbidity of small and large intestinal surgery in dogs and cats: 74 cases (1980–1992). J Am Anim Hosp Assoc 30:469–474, 1994.

40. INTUSSUSCEPTION

Douglas M. MacCoy, D.V.M.

1. Define intussusception.
An **intussusception** is the prolapse of one part of the intestine into the lumen of an immediately adjoining part. The portion entering the adjoining part is called the **intussuscipiens**. The part receiving the bowel is called the **intussusceptum**. Jejunum and ileum are most commonly involved; however, ileum into colon and stomach into esophagus also occur. The intussusception may be sliding (first forming, then self-reducing) and produce resolving clinical signs. Intussusceptions are usually a strangulating obstruction of the bowel.

2. What are the types of intussusception?
- **Colic**—involving segments of the large intestine
- **Enteric**—involving only the small intestine
- **Ileocolic**—ileum prolapses through the ileocecal valve into the colon
- **Cecocolic**—cecum prolapses into colon

3. What causes intussusception?
The exact cause is unknown. It is considered a sign of an underlying disorder, such as:
- Parvovirus infection
- Severe intestinal parasitism
- Intestinal obstruction
    Foreign body
    Mass (neoplastic, fungal, or
      granulomatous)

4. List the clinical signs of a patient with an intussusception.
- Vomiting (severity depends on location)
- Abdominal pain
- Melena or hematochezia
- Palpable abdominal mass

5. What is the differential diagnosis for intussusception?
- Intestinal foreign body
- Intestinal mass (neoplastic, fungal, granulomatous)
- Abdominal abscess
- Intestinal volvulus
- Inflammatory bowel disease
- Peritonitis

6. How is the diagnosis made?
 1. Recognition of classic clinical signs.
 2. Palpation of a bowel loop leading into an abdominal mass or a sausagelike mass associated with the intestines.
 3. Survey radiography indicating bowel obstruction—gas-dilated or fluid-dilated loops of intestine proximal to the intussusception and a tissue density mass in the abdomen.
 4. Contrast radiography:
     a. Upper gastrointstinal view shows obstructive pattern sometimes with constriction of the dye column.
     b. Barium enema may outline the intussuscipiens.
 5. Ultrasonography.

7. What is the initial medical management?
 Correction of electrolyte, acid-base, and fluid imbalances with intravenous crystalloids, corticosteroids, antibiotics, and glucose.

8. When should surgery be performed?
 After hemodynamic resuscitation or if worsening clinical status despite medical treatments.

9. Discuss the surgical options.
 Manual reduction
 • The bowel proximal to the intussusception is gently supported, while the intussuscipiens is squeezed out of the intussusceptum.
 • There is no correlation between the duration of signs and ability to reduce the intussusception manually.
 • The degree of damage is related to the degree of vascular compromise.
 • Small serosal tears may occur and do not necessarily compromise the bowel wall (think of pyloromyotomy incisions).
 Resection and anastomosis:
 • Assess bowel viability to decide if resection is necessary.
   Color
   Peristalsis
   Arterial pulsations
   Pulse oximetry
   Intravenous fluorescein dye injection—lack of fluorescence under ultraviolet light
 • Consider for an irreducible lesion, questionable viability, or tearing through the muscularis layer.

10. How is intestinal resection and anastomosis performed?
 Isolate affected bowel and ligate mesenteric vascular supply. Gently *milk* intestinal contents away from lesion and apply noncrushing (Doyen) forceps to remaining intestine. Angling the clamps and incision permits luminal parity between segments. Anastomosis is via a single-layer, simple interrupted or continuous approximating pattern. To reduce mucosa eversion, excess tissue can be resected before anastomosis or intramural sutures are placed to avoid the lumen. Synthetic absorbable monofilament or nonabsorbable monofilament sutures are used.

11. Can skin staplers be used for intestinal anastomosis?
 Yes; simple, safe, and rapid end-to-end anastomoses can be performed.

12. How can leakage from anastomotic sites be minimized?
 • Good operative technique
 • Wrapping of the site with omentum
 • Serosal patching via attachment of adjoining bowel loops

13. What is short-bowel syndrome?
Intractable diarrhea associated with malabsorption and bacterial overgrowth secondary to extensive (70%–80%) bowel resection (with or without ileocecal valve function).

14. What is the postoperative care?
- Nothing by mouth for 24 hours.
- Antibiotics for 7 days if there is serosal tearing.
- Start feeding with mild foods when consistent borborygmus are heard.
- Continue to correct electrolyte and fluid deficits as required.
- Monitor for signs of intestinal breakdown and leakage.

15. What are the commonest postoperative complications after reduction of an intussusception?
- Recurrence of intussusception
- Breakdown of anastomosis
- Peritonitis

CONTROVERSY

16. Should enteropexy be performed after reduction or resection?

For

30% of patients that do not receive an enteropexy have another intussusception in the postoperative period. Enteropexy is a simple technique of suturing the antimesenteric borders of the bowel side-by-side in a series of gentle loops using an absorbable suture. It has been recommended that three loops of plicated bowel be used proximal and distal to the anastomosis or reduced intussusception.

Against

70% of patients do not suffer another intussusception after surgery. and the technique may increase operating time in a patient who is compromised. There is also a potential for complications directly related to the procedure.

BIBLIOGRAPHY

1. Bellenger CR, Beck JA: Intussusception in 12 cats. J Sm Anim Pract 35:295–298, 1994.
2. Coolman BR, Ehrhart N: Evaluation of a disposable skin stapler for jejunal anastomosis in the dog. Vet Surg 28:389, 1999 (abstract).
3. Ellison GW: Intestinal resection and anastomosis. In Bojrab MJ (ed): Current Techniques in Small Animal Surgery, 4th ed. Baltimore, Williams & Wilkins, 1998, pp 248–254.
4. Kyles AE, Schneider TA, Clare A: Foreign body intestinal perforation and intra-abdominal abscess formation as a complication of enteroplication in a dog. Vet Rec 143:112–113, 1998.
5. Lamb CR, Mantis P: Ultrasonographic features of intestinal intussusception in 10 dogs. J Sm Anim Pract 39:437–441, 1998.
6. Oakes MG: Enteroplication to prevent recurrent intestinal intussusception. In Bojrab MJ (ed): Current Techniques in Small Animal Surgery, 4th ed. Baltimore, Williams & Wilkins, 1998, p 254.

41. INTESTINAL VOLVULUS

Joseph Harari, M.S., D.V.M., Dip. A.C.V.S.

1. What is intestinal volvulus?
Abnormal twisting of the bowel on its mesenteric axis. It can include **intestinal torsion,** which is a rotation of the bowel along its long axis.

2. What are the patient data for this condition?

Infrequently identified in veterinary patients, intestinal volvulus occurs in young, medium to large dogs presented with peracute abdominal discomfort and pain, vomiting, bloody diarrhea, shock, and unexpected death. German shepherd dogs were most often reported as affected patients. Associated events before hospital admission include athletic activity, trauma, gastrointestinal disease, and dietary indiscretion.

3. What diagnostic parameters are useful in identifying the condition antemortem?
- Peracute, highly morbid clinical signs.
- Radiographic evidence of severe bowel distention.
- Abdominocentesis yielding a modified transudate.
- Blood work variable.
- Ultrasonography and laparoscopy may help determine diagnosis.
- **Surgery** or **necropsy** provides conclusive evidence.

4. What treatments should be instituted?
- Immediate fluid resuscitation for shock, including acid-base restoration
- Corticosteroid and antibiotic medications
- Exploratory celiotomy

5. List other conditions that should be considered in the differential diagnosis.
- Cecocolic volvulus
- Intestinal entrapment
- Gastric dilation or volvulus
- Splenic torsion
- Intestinal obstruction or intussusception
- Pancreatitis
- Hemorrhagic gastroenteritis
- Viral enteritis

6. What gross anatomic changes or pathology have been found at surgery or necropsy with this condition?
- Dilated, discolored, and ischemic bowel loops rotated clockwise around the mesenteric axis
- Thrombosis of the mesenteric vasculature

7. Which surgical procedures are recommended?
- Derotation and repositioning of the bowel and mesentery
- Intestinal resection and anastomosis
- Abdominal lavage and drainage
- Intraoperative euthanasia when the severity of the condition warrants

8. What conditions are the pathologic basis for the high degree of morbidity (or mortality) associated with intestinal volvulus?
- Intestinal obstruction and hypoxia
- Vascular compromise
- Endotoxemia
- Circulating shock
- Cardiovascular failure
- Postresuscitation injury

9. What is meant by *postresuscitation injury*?

After restoration of blood pressure, continued ischemia and progressive tissue injury may occur because of persistent hypoperfusion (no reflow phenomenon), reperfusion injury, and oxygen debt.

10. What is meant by *reperfusion injury*?
Toxic metabolites accumulating during ischemia are washed out during reflow and delivered to distant organs. These oxygen radicals react with cell membrane lipids (peroxidation) to produce a chain reaction of toxin generation and cell injury.

11. What is the prognosis for this disease?
Grave; mortality is nearly 100%.

BIBLIOGRAPHY

1. Cairo J, Font J: Intestinal volvulus in dogs: A study of four clinical cases. J Sm Anim Pract 40:136–140, 1999.
2. Carberry C, Flanders JA: Cecal-colic volvulus in two dogs. Vet Surg 22:225–228, 1993.
3. Carberry C, Harvey HJ: Small intestinal volvulus in a dog. Comp Cont Educ Pract Vet 11:1322–1325, 1989.
4. Marino PL: The ICU Book, 1st ed. Media, PA, Williams & Wilkins, 1991, pp 135–137.
5. Shealy PM, Henderson RA: Canine intestinal volvulus. Vet Surg 21:15–19, 1992.

42. OPEN PERITONEAL DRAINAGE

Cathy L. Greenfield, D.V.M., M.S.

1. What is the peritoneum?
A semipermeable membrane of mesodermal origin that lines the abdominal cavity and covers the visceral surface of the abdominal organs.

2. What is the peritoneal cavity?
The cavity is the cavity lined by peritoneum that includes the abdominal cavity, portions of the pelvic cavity and the vaginal processes in the dog and cat.

3. What are the functions of the peritoneum?
- **Peritoneal fluid production**—produces a small amount of fluid for lubrication between viscera.
- **Protection of the peritoneal cavity**—removes excessive fluid and small particulate matter, deposits fibrin for formation of adhesions.

4. What are the most common causes of aseptic peritonitis in small animal patients?
Urine or bile leakage.

5. What are the most common causes of septic peritonitis in small animal patients?
Rupture of **gastrointestinal organs** (resulting from spontaneous diseases, such as gastric dilation–volvulus syndrome, intussusception, neoplasia, or perforating foreign bodies, or surgical incision dehiscence), **uterus** (pyometra), or **prostatic** or **pancreatic abscesses**.

6. List some clinical signs of a patient that presents with peritonitis.
- Depression
- Vomiting
- Anorexia
- Diarrhea
- Pyrexia
- Abdominal distention
- Abdominal pain
- Shock (tachycardia, dehydration, prolonged capillary refill time, injected mucus membranes)
- Presence of free fluid in the abdominal cavity

7. What diagnostic tests should be performed in a patient suspected to have generalized peritonitis?

A complete blood count and chemistry profile and the changes present reflect the cause and duration of the peritonitis. Abdominal radiographs may show the presence of free fluid or air in the peritoneal cavity, a radiopaque foreign body, or an abdominal mass. If the animal had recent trauma and urinary tract rupture is suspected, an excretory urogram with or without contrast cystogram helps determine the sites of urinary tract rupture. Ultrasonography may be helpful in locating the cause of the peritonitis. The most definitive test to diagnose peritonitis is **abdominocentesis**. Fluid obtained should be evaluated cytologically and cultured.

8. What are the characteristics of peritoneal fluid from an animal with aseptic peritonitis?
Urine peritonitis
- Yellowish to serosanguineous fluid
- Neutrophils—may be degenerate
- Creatinine of peritoneal fluid higher than that of peripheral blood

Bile peritonitis
- Greenish brown fluid
- Large numbers of red blood cells, neutrophils, and bile pigment in fluid

9. What are the cytologic characteristics of peritoneal fluid from an animal with septic peritonitis?
- Cloudy fluid with some color (yellow, yellowish red, greenish brown)
- Large (> 500/μL) numbers of degenerative neutrophils, some with intracellular bacteria
- Plant material, ingesta, and debris

10. How many neutrophils with intracellular bacteria are necessary to confirm a diagnosis of septic peritonitis?
One.

11. What are the cytologic characteristics of a postoperative peritoneal tap?

Regardless of the surgeon's training, inflammation (and peritonitis) is created when surgery is performed. A postoperative peritoneal tap has 7,000–9,000 leukocytes/μL with mild-to-moderate peritonitis and more than 9,000 leukocytes/μL with severe peritonitis. Intracellular bacteria should *not* be present.

12. What is the definitive therapy for generalized peritonitis?

Exploratory celiotomy to identify and correct the underlying problem; to remove peritoneal exudates; and, in cases of septic peritonitis, to establish a method for continued drainage of peritoneal exudates during the postoperative period.

13. Should the patient with generalized peritonitis be taken to surgery immediately after the diagnosis is made? Why or why not?

In most cases, no. Patients with generalized peritonitis are in critical condition and should be stabilized with good medical management before anesthesia and surgery. Most are moderately to severely dehydrated and require intravenous fluid therapy. Electrolyte imbalances should be corrected. A regimen of antibiotics that covers aerobic and anaerobic organisms should be started in patients with septic peritonitis.

14. Which antibiotics should be given to the patient with septic peritonitis?
- Intravenous administration of ampicillin plus enrofloxacin
- Amikacin plus clindamycin or metronidazole

- Cefoxitin for anaerobic organisms plus one of the aforementioned agents for aerobic organism coverage

15. If the underlying problem causing peritonitis is corrected and the peritoneal cavity is thoroughly lavaged, why is it necessary to provide a method for continued drainage of peritoneal exudates?

Even with thorough lavaging, bacteria are usually still present at the completion of the surgical procedure (growth of bacteria is usually present on cultures taken just before completion of the surgical procedure in septic peritonitis cases). If a method for continued drainage of peritoneal exudates is not provided, the closed peritoneal cavity essentially becomes an abscess cavity, and infection continues or is exacerbated.

16. What methods are available for continued drainage of peritoneal exudates?
- Gravity-dependent drains, such as sump-Penrose drains
- Continuous or intermittent peritoneal lavage
- Open peritoneal drainage

17. What is the problem with using passive drainage systems, such as sump-Penrose drains?

These drains become walled off from the peritoneal cavity within hours. Although some drainage can continue for 48 hours after the drains are placed, successful drainage for longer periods of time in patients with severe peritonitis has not been demonstrated.

18. What is open peritoneal drainage?

A surgical technique in which the abdominal incision is left open to allow peritoneal exudates to drain postoperatively out of the cavity and into a sterile bandage.

19. When is open peritoneal drainage indicated?

For generalized septic peritonitis to allow for continued drainage of exudates after the underlying problem has been surgically corrected and the peritoneal cavity is extensively lavaged. It is not usually necessary to perform open peritoneal drainage in cases of aseptic peritonitis caused by chemical irritants, such as urine or bile.

20. How is open peritoneal drainage performed?

After correcting the underlying cause of the peritonitis and thorough lavage of the peritoneal cavity, a culture of the peritoneal surface is taken to determine which bacteria are still present and what their susceptibility patterns are. The linea alba is loosely closed with two strands of monofilament, nonabsorbable suture material placed in a simple continuous pattern. One strand of suture material is started at each end of the incision, and suturing is done toward the middle of the incision. Each suture pass should be placed close to the adjacent suture to provide a meshwork of suture material to prevent herniation of abdominal contents during the postoperative drainage period. The two strands of suture material are tied to each other in the middle of the incision. A gap of 1 to 4 cm is left between the edges of the linea alba along the entire incision to allow drainage in the postoperative period (see figure). The subcutaneous layer and skin are left completely open and are not sutured at this time.

A urinary catheter is placed in all male dogs and is left in place until the abdominal incision is closed. Sterile bandaging material is placed over the open incision to collect drainage and protect the abdominal viscera. The bandaging material closest to the incision should be a nonadherent wound dressing (petrolatum impregnated gauze works well). Outside of this layer, various layers of sterile absorbent bandaging material are placed. The type and amount of materials used depend on the size of the patient, the expected volume of drainage, and materials that are available. The bandage is secured to the dog by wrapping stretchable gauze and stretchable adhesive-backed or nonadhesive tape circumferentially around the dog's torso.

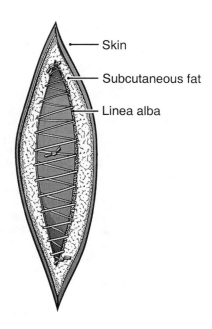

Simple continuous suture pattern used to close the linea alba loosely during open peritoneal drainage.

21. Discuss postoperative care for the patient with open peritoneal drainage.

The patient should be placed in an **intensive care unit** with constant monitoring for complications associated with the underlying disease and the surgical procedure performed. Large volumes of fluid as well as some red cells and protein are lost through the open peritoneal incision and patients need to have these parameters closely monitored. The patient must be prevented from destroying the bandage.

22. How often should the bandage be changed?

Any time it is wet or soiled or a minimum of once every 24 hours.

23. Describe the bandage changing procedure.

All bandage changes should be done using strict aseptic technique. Materials should be sterilized before use. Bandages can be preassembled, sterilized, then used, or individual components can be sterilized and the bandage can be assembled using aseptic technique at the time that it is applied to the patient.

24. When is it time to close the open peritoneal drainage incision?

When the infection has been controlled as evidenced by:
- Improved to normal appetite and mentation
- Maintenance of normal body temperature
- Decreased fluid production so once-daily bandage changes are adequate, and only small amounts of fluid are present in the bandage
- Cytology of the peritoneal fluid reveals no evidence of intracellular bacteria
- When the patient is difficult to control in the intensive care unit

25. How is closure of the incision done?

The animal is anesthetized. The bandage is removed and the surgical field is aseptically prepared. Sterile, dry, laparotomy sponges are placed in the open incision to prevent scrub soap from

entering the abdomen during patient preparation. The central knot holding the two strands of suture material together is cut. Before closing the abdominal incision, a culture of the peritoneal surface is obtained. The two strands of suture material are tightened until the edges of the linea alba are apposed. The subcutaneous tissue and skin are débrided if necessary, followed by routine closure.

26. Should reexploration of the abdominal cavity be done before closure?
Not unless the patient has not responded properly to treatment and there are possible problems that need to be surgically addressed. Some authors do recommend routine reexploration of the peritoneal cavity during the period of open peritoneal drainage or before closure.

27. What should be done if bacteria grow from the closure culture?
Positive bacterial growth on cultures taken at the time of abdominal closure is not unusual. When different organisms are present than those cultured at the first surgery, the infection is often considered to be **nosocomial**. The significance of these nosocomial infections is questionable. Treatment for 1–2 weeks with an appropriate antibiotic is recommended. If the same organism is cultured at the time of abdominal closure as was originally cultured, it may mean that there is a continued source of contamination, which may warrant further surgical exploration. In either case, if the patient is doing well, close monitoring and antibiotic therapy may be all that is indicated.

28. When can the patient be released from the hospital?
1–2 days after closure of the abdominal incision *and* after the closure culture results are available to ensure that the correct antibiotic is prescribed to go home with the animal, if necessary.

29. What is the prognosis for patients with generalized septic peritonitis?
Guarded. Septic peritonitis is an acute, life-threatening disease with a mortality rate of up to 67%. With open peritoneal drainage, probably the most effective method of treating this disease, mortality rates in two case series of patients with naturally occurring septic peritonitis have been 33%–48%.

BIBLIOGRAPHY

1. Greenfield CL: Open peritoneal drainage for peritonitis. In Bojrab ME (ed): Current Techniques in Small Animal Surgery, 4th ed. Baltimore, Williams & Wilkins, 1998, pp 330–335.
2. Greenfield CL, Walshaw R: Open peritoneal drainage for treatment of contaminated peritoneal cavity and septic peritonitis in dogs and cats: 24 cases (1980–1986). J Am Vet Med Assoc 191:100–105, 1987.
3. Hardie EM: Life-threatening bacterial infection. Compend Contin Educ Pract Vet 17:763–777, 1995.
4. Hosgood G: Drainage of the peritoneal cavity. Comp Cont Educ Pract Vet 15:1605–1616, 1993.
5. Hosgood G, Salisbury SK: Generalized peritonitis in dogs: 50 cases (1975–1986). J Am Vet Med Assoc 193:1448–1450, 1988.
6. Woolfson JM, Dulisch ML: Open abdominal drainage in the treatment of generalized peritonitis in 25 dogs and cats. Vet Surg 15:27–32, 1986.

43. MEGACOLON

Giselle Hosgood, B.V.Sc., M.S., F.A.C.V.Sc., Dip. A.C.V.S.

1. What is megacolon?
Overdistention of the colon, often associated with obstipation (**megacolon** = "big" colon).

2. How is megacolon associated with obstipation?
Megacolon is the physical increase in size of the colon associated with obstipation. **Obstipation** is intractable constipation and is an acquired condition in dogs and cats. Impaction from

material within the colon constitutes primary obstipation. External compression or obstruction of the colon or conditions that cause pain during defecation and subsequently prohibit defecation cause secondary obstipation.

3. List common causes of obstipation in dogs and cats.

Dog
- Perineal hernias
- Perianal fistulas
- Anal sac disease
- Previous pelvic fractures
- Rectal strictures secondary to neoplasia

Cat
- Idiopathic megacolon
- Rectal neoplasia

4. Differentiate between idiopathic megacolon in cats and Hirschsprung's disease in humans.

Hirschsprung's disease is a congenital disease of humans characterized by absence of ganglionic cells in the colonic wall. The aganglionic segment of the colon is spastic, and the colon proximal to this segment dilates.

Idiopathic megacolon has no obvious cause and no histologic changes in the colonic wall. Segmental agangliosis has been documented in the colon of two cats, and myenteric ganglia were absent from the distal end of the resected colonic segment in two other cats.

5. Describe the clinical features of obstipation and megacolon.

Clinical signs include weight loss, anorexia, apparent abdominal pain, scant or thin feces, and fresh blood in the feces. Animals may vomit, sometimes, what appears to be fecal material. A firm, tubular mass (feces in colon) may be palpated in the abdomen. Hematologic abnormalities can reflect chronic disease and include anemia and acid-base and electrolyte imbalances.

6. How is a diagnosis of megacolon made?
- Abdominal palpation
- Rectal examination
- Abdominal radiographs

7. Is megacolon considered a disease by itself?

Megacolon is only a feature of and not, by itself, a disease. The inciting cause of the obstipation must be determined. Only in the cat, when no other causes are determined, is **idiopathic megacolon** considered a disease.

8. What is the treatment of choice?

In the case of idiopathic megacolon in **cats,** subtotal colectomy can be performed and is the treatment of choice from a surgeon's perspective. Minimal complications are reported, and the clinical results are good.

In the case of megacolon in **dogs,** the approach is to treat the underlying cause. Should the megacolon be retractable, subtotal colectomy can be performed in dogs, but the loss of colonic function in dogs generally results in diarrhea, electrolyte imbalances, and bacterial overgrowth of the small intestine. Subtotal colectomy may not be a viable option.

9. Is there an alternate to treatment besides surgery?

Not from a surgeon's perspective for the treatment of feline **idiopathic megacolon.** Cisapride has been used but appears to have limited success and only delays the inevitable subtotal colectomy.

For the **dog,** prokinetic drugs, such as cisapride, should be used before performing subtotal colectomy but only after the inciting cause has been addressed. In view of the morbidity of subtotal colectomy in the dog, the merit of performing surgery should be questioned.

10. If colectomy is performed, is it imperative to preserve the ileocolic valve?

In the **cat,** because bacterial overgrowth of the small intestine is not a problem, preservation of the ileocolic valve is unnecessary. Removing the colon at the level of the ileum facilitates the procedure and the preservation of the vascular supply to the ileum by reducing tension on the ileocolic anastomosis. Attempts should be made to preserve as much ileum as possible. In the **dog,** because bacterial overgrowth is a problem, **preservation** of the ileocolic valve should be attempted.

11. How much of the descending colon should be removed?

As much as possible without entering the pelvic canal. If a large segment of descending colon is left, recurring problems are likely.

12. How does one anastomose a small ileal segment to the large colonic remnant?

Never make the big end smaller; always make the small end bigger. The discrepancy in the intestinal segments can be corrected by *fish mouthing* the ileal segment by making a longitudinal antimesenteric incision (avoiding the antimesenteric vessels of the ileum) until the cut surface of the ileum matches that of the colonic segment.

13. What are perioperative considerations?

Perioperative antibiotics (second-generation and third-generation cephalosporins) with bactericidal activity against gram-negative and anaerobic bacteria are indicated. The colon is not evacuated of feces before surgery. Enemas and laxatives are not effective and liquefy intestinal contents at the time of surgery. A preoperative morphine epidural provides intraoperative and immediate postoperative analgesia and facilitates recovery. Tenesmus may be present in the immediate postoperative period, and a preemptive epidural may have some benefit in these animals. Antibiotics are not indicated beyond the perioperative period. Hydration in the first few days after surgery should be monitored closely because the animals have loose stools.

14. What is the prognosis for surgical patients?

For subtotal colectomy (idiopathic megacolon) in cats, excellent. Surgical complications (dehiscence, stricture, necrosis) are rare. Generally the stool is pastelike and becomes firm over several weeks. The frequency of defecation may be increased, but the cats are continent.

15. Will enteric function be normal?

Yes. Evaluation of the enteric function in four cats undergoing subtotal colectomy was similar to normal cats.

BIBLIOGRAPHY

1. Bertoy RW, MacCoy DM, Wheaton LG, et al: Total colectomy with ileorectal anastomosis in the cat. Vet Surg 18:204–210, 1989.
2. Bright RM, Burrows CF, Goring R, et al: Subtotal colectomy for treatment of acquired megacolon in the dog and cat. J Am Vet Med Assoc 188:1412–1416, 1986.
3. Dvorak J, Willard MD, Floyd E: Panfibrinonecrotic colitis in a dog treated by subtotal colectomy. J Am Vet Med Assoc 198:264–266, 1991.
4. Gregory CR, Guilford WG, Berry CR, et al: Enteric function in cats after subtotal colectomy for treatment of megacolon. Vet Surg 19:216–220, 1990.
5. Hasler AH, Washabau RJ: Cisapride stimulates contraction of idiopathic megacolonic smooth muscle in cats. J Vet Intern Med 11(6) 313–318, 1997.
6. Holt D, Johnston DE: Idiopathic megacolon in cats. Comp Cont Educ Pract Vet 13:1411–1417, 1991.
7. Kudisch M, Pavletic MM: Subtotal colectomy with surgical stapling instruments via a trans-cecal approach for treatment of acquired megacolon in cats. Vet Surg 22:457–463, 1993.
8. Matthiesen DT, Scavelli TD, Whitney WO: Subtotal colectomy for the treatment of obstipation secondary to pelvic fracture malunion in cats. Vet Surg 20:113–117, 1991.

44. RECTAL TUMORS

Giselle Hosgood, B.V.Sc., M.S., F.A.C.V.Sc., Dip. A.C.V.S.

1. How common are rectal tumors?

Primary tumors of the colon and rectum are common; the rectum is more frequently affected than the colon. Tumors of the colon and rectum represent 36%–60% of all canine intestinal neoplasia and 15% of all feline intestinal neoplasia. In the **dog,** twice as many tumors are malignant as opposed to benign. In the **cat,** tumors are almost always malignant.

2. What sort of tumors occur?

Most primary tumors exist as a solitary mass. In the dog, benign adenomas (polyps) are most frequent; adenocarcinomas (annular intraluminal and pedunculated forms) are second most common. Malignant transformation of adenomas, lymphosarcoma, leiomyosarcoma, and leiomyoma are also reported in the dog. In the cat, leiomyosarcoma, adenocarcinoma, and lymphosarcoma are the most frequent types of tumors diagnosed.

3. Where in the rectum are tumors most common?

Distal in the rectum; very distal tumors may even prolapse during defecation. Note however, that mid-rectal tumors also occur and a negative rectal exam does not rule out a tumor (even if one has a long finger).

4. List common clinical findings.
- Hematochezia
- Tenesmus
- Rectal prolapse
- Rectal bleeding
- Palpable rectal mass
- Palpable rectal constriction

5. What is the best way to confirm disease?
Colonoscopy:
- Determines location of the tumor
- Permits biopsy
- Rules out multiple tumors (uncommon)

6. Discuss the value of a biopsy.

A biopsy is extremely helpful, yet not always definitive. Biopsy specimens should always be taken before treatment is performed. The biopsy diagnosis may not always be in agreement with the final histologic diagnosis of the excised tumor (e.g., adenoma on biopsy may turn out to be adenocarcinoma on excised tumor). Several biopsy specimens should be taken. In the case of lymphosarcoma, the tumor area is often surrounded by marked lymphocytic-plasmacytic infiltrates, which may be misleading. An excisional biopsy of pedunculated tumors can be performed using a submucosal resection. As large of a margin should be taken as possible because this may be a curative treatment if the tumor is benign. Diagnosis of a malignant tumor necessitates reoperation.

7. What is a possible complication of rectal wall biopsy?

Rectal perforation after biopsy of an intramural lesion.

8. How rare is metastasis?

Metastasis occurs readily for malignant disease, and the disease must be staged (evaluation of the sublumbar lymph nodes, abdominal radiographs, ultrasound, and fine-needle aspirate of enlarged lymph nodes) before treatment. **Pulmonary metastasis** is rare, and thoracic radiographs are only indicated if multicentric lymphoma is suspected.

9. Is surgical resection the treatment of choice?

Depends on the diagnosis, stage of the disease, and location of the tumor. **Surgery** is the treatment of choice for adenoma, polypoid adenocarcinoma, and other solitary tumors. **Chemotherapy** is indicated for lymphosarcoma. **Radiation therapy** may be indicated for nonresectable tumors.

10. How much tissue should be excised?

A submucosal resection may be curative for adenomas; however, a **full-thickness rectal resection** is required for malignant tumors.

11. What are some surgical approaches to the rectum?

The **dorsal** or **ventral** approach, which requires removal of the pubis, both offer limited access and do not always allow direct visualization of the tumor. The best method is a **rectal pull-through** procedure. This is a difficult procedure and despite grossly clear margins, local recurrence of malignant tumors often develop within two to three months.

12. What is the Swenson pull-through procedure?

An abdominal-anal pull-through procedure for terminal colonic or proximal rectal tumors. This procedure involves colorectal resection through a celiotomy with eversion of the colonic and rectal stumps through the anus by means of stay sutures. Considerable tension on the left colic artery may develop. Caution is required to avoid devascularization of the remaining colonic segment when a large section of colon or rectum is removed.

13. How much of the rectum can be removed without compromising function?

The rectum contributes to fecal continence by acting as a functional reservoir. Resection of a large portion of the rectum affects continence. Resection of **4 cm of rectum** allows normal rectal function in the dog, but resection of 6 cm results in fecal incontinence.

14. What is the prognosis for rectal tumors?

For **malignant tumors,** poor because of recurrence. A **benign tumor** can also recur if not adequately resected. This is particularly applicable to benign tumors that are "lopped" off for a diagnosis and follow-up resection is not performed. Malignant transformation of benign tumors can occur. Rechecks at 90-day intervals are indicated to closely monitor animals that have had tumors resected, even if the diagnosis was benign.

15. Has colostomy been performed in dogs?

Yes. Diverting flank colostomies have been described in dogs with pelvic and rectal tumors. Minimal complications (skin excoriation) were noted, and long-term home management was readily accomplished by owners.

BIBLIOGRAPHY

 1. Anson LW, Betts CW, Stone EA: A retrospective evaluation of the rectal pull-through technique: Procedure and postoperative complications. Vet Surg 17:141–146, 1988.
 2. Fucci V, Newton JC, Hedlund CS: Rectal surgery in the cat: Comparison of suture versus staple technique through a dorsal approach. J Am Anim Hosp Assoc 28:519–526, 1992.
 3. Hardie EM, Gilson SD: Use of colostomy to manage rectal disease in dogs. Vet Surg 26:270–274, 1997.
 4. Holt D, Johnston DE, Orsher R: Clinical use of a dorsal surgical approach to the rectum. Comp Cont Educ Pract Vet 13:1519–1529, 1991.
 5. Slawienski MJ, Mauldin GE: Malignant colonic neoplasia in cats: 46 cases (1990–1996). J Am Vet Med Assoc 211:878–881, 1997.
 6. Valerius KD, Powers BE, McPherron MA, et al: Adenomatous polyps and carcinoma in situ of the canine colon and rectum: 34 cases (1982–1994). J Am Anim Hosp Assoc 33:156–160, 1997.
 7. Williams FA Jr, Bright RM, Daniel GB, et al: The use of colonic irrigation to control fecal incontinence in dogs with colostomies. Vet Surg 28:348–354, 1999.

45. PERIANAL FISTULAE

Giselle Hosgood, B.V.Sc., M.S., F.A.C.V.Sc., Dip. A.C.V.S.

1. Are perianal fistulae a disease specific to German shepherd dogs?

No. They appear to afflict German shepherd dogs most frequently, although they are reported in other breeds, including Irish setters, spaniels, and mixed-breed dogs.

2. Are perianal fistulae a disease primarily of the anal sacs?

No. The disease appears to begin in the perineal epithelium with extension into the adnexal structures characterized by superficial necrosis and ulceration. Progressive involvement results in deep inflammation and creation of subcutaneous sinus tracts. The anal sacs become secondarily involved.

3. What is the cause of perianal fistulae?

Unknown. Historically, theories have cited hypothyroidism and bacterial pyodermatitis combined with anatomic predisposition, such as increased density of apocrine sweat glands in the zona cutanea of the perianal region, and conformational characteristics, such as a low tail head position. An immune-mediated cause has also been proposed. The occurrence of perineal fistula has also been linked to concurrent inflammatory bowel disease and colitis.

4. Are these true fistulae?

No. By definition, a fistula is a communication between one epithelial surface and another. Unless they communicate between the skin and the rectum or the skin and the anal sac, the tracts, by definition, are **sinuses** (extend from a nonepithelial surface to an epithelial surface).

5. When are most clinical cases presented for treatment?

In a fairly advanced stage because early lesions are difficult to visualize.

6. What is the clinical presentation of early lesions?

Early lesions are characteristically pinpoint **holes** in the perianal surface and may go undetected unless the owner is prompted to look closely at the perineum of the dog after noticing bleeding from the area, excessive licking of the perianal region by the dog, or the dog straining to defecate (**tenesmus**). The dog may also show anorexia and weight loss. Fecal incontinence can occur and surface tissue loss may be present.

7. Should perianal fistulae be differentiated from neoplasia before treatment is instituted?

Yes. Although perianal fistulae do not require histologic examination to confirm a diagnosis made on clinical findings, it is prudent to rule out neoplastic disease as a cause of the clinical findings. Perianal adenocarcinoma can present as a diffuse, ulcerated, dissecting lesion and should be on the differential list for a dog with perianal lesions. Histologic features of perianal fistulae are compatible with hidradenitis and necrotizing pyogranulomatous inflammation.

8. What is deroofing?

Excision of intact skin and, sometimes, granulation and necrotic tissue from the top of each tract to create a saucer-shaped wound.

9. What is fulguration?

Passage of a spark across a gap greater than 1 mm into tissues to create destruction (from Latin, *fulgur*—lightning).

10. Is medical management a treatment option?

The only medical management that has shown promise is administering **oral cyclosporine.** The cost of oral cyclosporine may be prohibitive, although it is similar to the cost for surgical treatment. Concurrent administration of a cytochrome p-450 inhibitor such as ketoconazole may reduce the dosing requirements and cost of cyclosporine but may cause side effects. Anecdotal reports of successful treatment using local installation of cyclosporine (eye ointment) at a reduced cost over oral cyclosporine treatment have been reported.

Other medical management is the administration of oral prednisone, metronidazole, or sulfasalazine for the treatment of concurrent inflammatory bowel disease.

11. Are stool softeners indicated or contraindicated for this disease?

Indicated. Usually, stool softeners that increase the bulk but decrease the consistency of the stool are preferred (i.e., psyllium). Diet management, in conjunction with treatment for inflammatory bowel disease, may achieve the same result.

12. What is the best approach to take when presented with a dog with perianal fistulae?

1. Be aggressive with therapy, do not give false hope to the owners, and closely monitor the dog—lesions can get out of hand in 3 weeks.

2. Offer surgical and medical management and the pros and cons of each.

3. Cyclosporine therapy is emerging as the treatment of choice because of the low morbidity and encouraging results.

4. Inform the owners of the necessity for close monitoring and daily cleansing (garden hose) of the perianal region that will be required of them.

5. Rechecks every 2–3 weeks regardless of how the owner perceives the dog to be doing are highly recommended.

CONTROVERSY

13. Is surgery the treatment of choice for perianal fistulae?

Not necessarily. Many surgical approaches have been described, including cryosurgery, chemical cauterization (iodine, silver nitrate), en bloc resection and rectal pull-through, neodymium-yttrium-aluminum-garnet (Nd. YAG) laser débridement, and surgical débridement (deroofing) and fulguration. All have disadvantages, including failure to control disease, postoperative rectal and anal stricture, tissue sloughing, and fecal incontinence. Of the surgical treatments, deroofing and fulguration (preferably in conjunction with tail amputation) is preferred by the author. The key to surgical success is thorough débridement, with close follow-up and timely reoperation, if necessary.

14. Is tail amputation necessary for success of surgical treatment?

No, but it may help in the postoperative management of the perianal region. The only report evaluating tail amputation cited a 50% success rate of tail amputation alone (at the level of the second or third coccygeal vertebrae) in the treatment of perianal fistulae. Tail amputation may facilitate the postoperative management of the disease by allowing easy cleansing and aeration of the area and easy visualization of the lesions as they regress or progress.

15. Should the anal sacs be removed regardless of whether or not they are affected?

There is no literature to support either option. If surgical débridement is being performed, both anal sacs could be removed, regardless of their degree of involvement. Never remove just one. If medical management is being pursued, judgment is reserved based on disease regression or progression.

BIBLIOGRAPHY

1. Ellison GW: Treatment of perianal fistulas in dogs. J Am Vet Med Assoc 206:1680–1682, 1995.
2. Ellison GW, Bellah JR, Stubbs WP, et al: Treatment of perianal fistulas with ND:YAG laser—results in twenty cases. Vet Surg 24:140–147, 1995.
3. Goring RL, Bright RM, Stancil ML: Perianal fistulas in the dog: Retrospective evaluation of surgical treatment by deroofing and fulguration. Vet Surg 15:392–398, 1986.
4. Harkin KR, Walshaw R, Mullaney TP: Association of perianal fistula and colitis in the German Shepherd dog: Response to high-dose prednisone and dietary therapy. J Am Anim Hosp Assoc 32:515–520, 1996.
5. Mathews KA, Ayres SA, Tano CA, et al: Cyclosporin treatment of perianal fistulas in dogs. Can Vet J 38:39–41, 1997.

46. PERINEAL HERNIA

John T. Silbernagel, D.V.M.

1. What is the pelvic diaphragm?

The pelvic diaphragm is the major component of the perineum. It consists of the levator ani and coccygeal muscles, along with their fascial coverings. It is attached to the caudal vertebrae dorsally and pelvis ventrally, affording a stable closure to the pelvic outlet.

2. What are the major neurovascular structures pertinent to perineal hernia surgery?

Pudendal nerve—	Dorsolateral to the internal obturator, coccygeus, and levator ani muscles
Sciatic nerve—	Craniolateral to the sacrotuberous ligament
Caudal rectal nerve—	Caudal border of the levator ani muscle
Caudal gluteal artery and vein—	Lateral to the internal obturator muscle
Internal pudendal artery and vein—	Dorsolateral to the internal obturator, coccygeus, and levator ani muscles
Caudal rectal artery and vein—	Caudal borders of the levator ani muscles

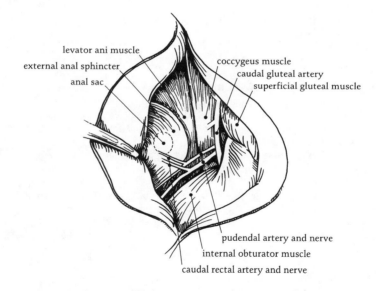

Important surgical landmarks for perineal herniorrhaphy.

3. List the typical clinical signs seen with perineal hernia.

- Perineal swelling
- Tenesmus
- Constipation
- Dyschezia
- Hematochezia
- Diarrhea
- Fecal incontinence
- Flatus

4. What is the prevalence of perineal hernia?

- 0.1%–0.4% in dogs.
- Rare in cats.

5. What is the typical signalment of perineal hernia?

Most dogs are intact males, 7–9 years old or older. Reports in females are rare. Boston terrier, boxer, collie, Kelpie, Old English sheepdog, and Pekingese are overrepresented breeds.

6. Is medical management an option for animals with perineal hernia?

Yes, but not a good one. **Medical** and **dietary treatments** including high-fiber and high-moisture diets, bulk-forming laxatives, docusates, and hormone therapy, are better **adjuncts** to surgical management than sole treatments.

7. What surgical options are available for repair of perineal hernia?
- Standard herniorrhaphy
- Internal obturator muscle transposition
- Transposition of the superficial gluteal muscle
- Semitendinosus muscle flap

8. List the advantages of internal obturator transposition over other surgical techniques.
- Less tension is placed on the repair.
- Less lateral deviation of the external anal sphincter.
- Procedure aids in closure of the ventral aspect of the hernia, typically the region most difficult to close.

9. What are the most commonly found hernial contents?
- Rectal sacculation or flexure
- Prostate gland
- Fluid
- Omentum
- Fat
- Urinary bladder

10. What secondary rectal abnormalities can be seen in conjunction with perineal hernias?
- **Rectal deviation:** Sigmoid curvature of the rectum.
- **Rectal diverticulation:** Mucosal protrusion within the pelvic canal resulting from separation of the muscular coat.
- **Rectal sacculation:** Unidirectional outpouching of the rectal wall usually toward the side of the hernia with all layers intact (**most common**).

11. What are the major postoperative complications of perineal hernia repair?
- Surgical site infection and abscess formation
- Rectal prolapse
- Hernia recurrence
- Fecal incontinence
- Hemorrhage
- Sciatic nerve entrapped in a suture
- Suture placed in the rectal lumen or anal sac
- Urethral damage

12. Which factors contribute to the recurrence of a hernia?
- Relative size of the defect when compared with the remaining levator ani, coccygeal, and external anal sphincter muscles
- Surgeon's inexperience
- Previous perineal surgery
- Males remaining sexually intact

BIBLIOGRAPHY

1. Bellenger CR, Canfield RB: Perineal hernia. In Slatter D (ed): Textbook of Small Animal Surgery, 2nd ed. Philadelphia: W.B. Saunders, 1993, pp 471–482.
2. Hosgood G: Perineal herniorrhaphy: Perioperative data from 100 dogs. J Am Anim Hosp Assoc 31:331–342, 1995.
3. Krahwinkel DJ Jr: Rectal diseases and their role in perineal hernia. Vet Surg 12:160–165, 1983.

4. Marretta SM, Matthiesen DT: Problems associated with the surgical treatment of diseases involving the perineal region. Prob Vet Med April 1:215–242, 1989.
5. Matthiesen DT: Diagnosis and management of complications occurring after perineal herniorrhaphy in dogs. Comp Cont Educ Pract Vet 11:797–822, 1989.
6. Welches CD, et al: Perineal hernia in the cat: A retrospective study of 40 cases. J Am Anim Hosp Assoc 28:431–438, 1992.

47. ANAL SAC DISEASE

John T. Silbernagel, D.V.M.

1. What are the anal sacs (versus anal glands)?

The **anal sacs** are paired cutaneous diverticula located at approximately 4 and 8 o'clock with respect to the anus in all carnivores. They are situated between the internal and external anal sphincter muscles, each connecting to the skin surface by a duct that opens at the level of the anocutaneous junction.

Anal glands or anal apocrine glands are located in the submucosa around the anus at the anocutaneous junction.

2. What are the functions of the anal sacs?

The exact function is unknown, although their putrid contents may play a role in social communications, sexual attraction, and delineation of territory by releasing **pheromones.** They also play a role in defense in skunks and stripe-necked mongooses.

3. What are the three classifications of nonneoplastic anal sac disease?

1. Impaction   2. Sacculitis   3. Abscessation

4. Describe the pathophysiology of nonneoplastic anal sac disease and predisposing factors.

Although the specific cause of anal sac disease is unknown, prolonged retention of secretions (i.e., impaction) in the sacs may be the initiating factor. Secondary bacterial infection leads to sacculitis and abscessation in many cases. Contributing factors include diarrhea, glandular hypersecretion, and poor muscle tone of the anal sphincter in small and obese dogs.

5. List common clinical signs of anal sac disease.

- Tenesmus
- Discomfort when sitting
- Licking or biting the anal area
- Scooting
- Tail chasing
- Perianal discharge

6. What are the differential diagnoses for animals with anal sac disease?

Vaginitis, proctitis, ectoparasites, endoparasites, flea allergy, perianal fistulae, and perianal tumor.

7. What is the most common tumor of anal sacs?

Adenocarcinoma of the apocrine glands. These tumors tend to be highly malignant, invade surrounding soft tissue, and frequently metastasize to regional lymph nodes.

8. What constitutes conservative therapy for anal sac disease?

- Manual expression of anal sac contents
- Anal sac irrigation with saline or dilute antiseptic
- Intraductal instillation of a corticosteroid antibiotic preparation
- Oral broad-spectrum antibiotics for cellulitis or abscessation

9. **List the indications for anal sacculectomy.**
   - Recurrent episodes of impaction, sacculitis, or abscessation
   - Neoplasia
   - Perineal fistulas (adjunctive surgical treatment)

10. **What is the patient positioning for anal sacculectomy?**
    Perineal position.

11. **What two types of procedures are used for anal sacculectomy?**
    1. **Open:** The anal sac is incised via a groove director and scalpel or scissors through its duct before complete removal by blunt dissection.
    2. **Closed:** A vertical incision is made over the anal sac, and it is bluntly dissected out intact.

12. **What are the major postoperative complications of anal sacculectomy?**
    - Fecal incontinence resulting from damage of the external anal sphincter muscle, pudendal nerve, or caudal rectal nerves
    - Chronic draining tracts resulting from retained glandular tissue
    - Tenesmus and dyschezia resulting from scar tissue formation

BIBLIOGRAPHY

1. Matthiesen DT, Marretta SM: Diseases of the anus and rectum. In Slatter D (ed): Textbook of Small Animal Surgery, 2nd ed. Philadelphia: W.B. Saunders, 1993, pp 627–644.
2. van Duijkeren E: Disease conditions of canine anal sacs. J Sm Anim Pract 36:12–16, 1995.

48. ADRENALECTOMY

Elaine R. Caplan, D.V.M., Dip. A.C.V.S., Dip. A.B.V.P.

1. **Where are the adrenal glands located?**
   Craniomedial to the ipsilateral kidney in the retroperitoneal space. The left adrenal lies between the aorta and the left kidney, and the right adrenal is between the caudal vena cava and the right kidney (from Latin, *ad,* near, + *ren,* kidney).

2. **What is the blood supply to the adrenal gland?**
   Branches of the aortic, phrenic, renal, accessary renal, lumbar, and phrenicoabdominal arteries. The right adrenal vein empties into the vena cava, and the left adrenal vein empties into the left renal vein, or both can empty into phrenicoabdominal veins.

3. **What substances are secreted by the adrenal cortex?**
   - Cortisol
   - Mineralocorticoids
   - Androgens
   - Estrogens

4. **What is secreted by the adrenal medulla?**
   Catecholamines (epinephrine and norepinephrine) are synthesized by hydroxylation and decarboxylation of phenylalanine and tyrosine.

5. List the indications for adrenalectomy.
- Hyperadrenocorticism caused by adrenocortical adenoma or carcinoma.
- Tumors of the adrenal medulla (pheochromocytoma).
- Pituitary-dependent hyperadrenocorticism.

6. What is the most common cause of hyperadrenocorticism in the dog?
Pituitary microadenomas, which secrete excessive ACTH and result in bilateral adrenal hyperplasia.

7. Which histopathologic tumor type is most commonly found in the adrenal gland of the dog?
The dog has a 50:50 chance of having an **adrenal adenoma** or **carcinoma.**

8. Which adrenal gland is most frequently affected with a tumor?
Right and left adrenal glands are equally affected.

9. List clinical presentations that are associated with canine adrenal medullary tumors (pheochromocytoma).

Hypertension (epistaxis, seizures, cerebrovascular accidents)	Tachycardia
	Murmur
Panting	Arrhythmias
Dyspnea	Dilated pupils
Tremors	Signs associated with partial obstruction
PU/PD	of the vena cava (ascites, rear leg edema,
Anorexia	distention of the cauda epigastric veins)

10. List clinical presentations that are associated with canine adrenal cortical tumors.

PU/PD	Anestrous	Calcinosis cutis
Pendulous abdomen	Obesity	Facial dermatosis
Hepatomegaly	Muscle atrophy	Facial nerve palsy
Skin atrophy	Comedones	Secondary bacterial infections
Hair loss	Excessive panting	Thromboembolism
Polyphagia	Testicular atrophy	Diabetes mellitus
Muscle weakness		

11. What clinical signs and associated organ findings can be seen in the ferret with an adrenal tumor?
- Bilaterally symmetric alopecia
- Enlarged vulva in spayed females
- Prostatic or paraurethral cysts in males
- Splenic enlargement
- Cardiomyopathy
- Concurrent pancreatic beta cell tumors

12. Which imaging modalities are helpful in the diagnosis of adrenal tumors?
- Survey radiography (adrenal calcification)
- Abdominal ultrasound
- CT
- Adrenal gland scintigraphy
- MRI
- Caudal vena cava venography (invasion by a pheochromocytoma)

13. What laboratory tests are used to diagnose canine adrenal cortical and medullary tumors?
Adrenal cortical tumors:
- CBC
- Serum chemistry
- Urinalysis
- ACTH response test

- Low-dose dexamethasone suppression test
- Urine cortisol-to-creatinine ratio

Pheochromocytomas:
- Indirect blood pressure profilometry
- Catecholamines and their metabolites (vanillylmandelic acid) in urine and plasma
- DHEAS (dehydroepiandrosterone sulfate)
- Plasma chromogranin A
- Nuclear scintigraphy using MIBG, NP-59, and 111-indium-pentetreotide and chemical shift resonance imaging techniques

14. How are adrenal tumors diagnosed in ferrets?
- Physical examination
- History
- Signalment
- Abdominal ultrasound
- Androgen steroid panel
- Abdominal exploratory surgery

15. What other diagnostic procedures can be performed (with caution) in dogs with adrenal tumors?

Ultrasound-guided or CT-guided aspiration and biopsy (complications of hemorrhage and pain).

16. What is the recommended preoperative treatment for pheochromocytoma patients?
- Phenoxybenzamine hydrochloride (α-adrenergic blocker).
- Propranolol (β-adrenergic blocker should be administered with phenoxybenzamine to avoid severe hypertension).

17. Why is preoperative treatment recommended?

Preoperative medical therapy minimizes adverse effects of catecholamines (cardiac arrhythmias and hypertension).

18. Which anesthetic agents should be avoided in patients with suspected pheochromocytoma?
- **Atropine**—tachycardia often already present.
- **Ketamine**—increases circulating catecholamine levels, heart rate, and blood pressure.
- **Xylazine**—increases the myocardial sensitivity to catecholamines and arrhythmias.
- **Halothane**—greater myocardial sensitivity to catecholamines and arrhythmias than isoflurane

19. What drug can be administered to treat acute hypertension associated with manipulating the pheochromocytoma during surgery?

Phentolamine.

20. List perioperative considerations for dogs with hyperadrenocorticism.
- Diabetes mellitus.
- Hypokalemia (muscle weakness, bradycardias, ventricular dysrhythmias, hypotension).
- Osteoporosis (careful handling of patients).
- Muscle weakness (hypoventilation during surgery).
- Blood loss.
- Postoperative mineralocorticoid or glucocorticoid replacement.

21. Describe two surgical approaches for adrenalectomy.
Ventral midline:
1. Facilitates a complete exploratory procedure to evaluate both adrenal glands and check organs for metastasis.

2. Can be combined with a paracostal celiotomy for better access to liver, lymph nodes, and bilateral adrenalectomies.

3. A potential for dehiscence in dogs with hyperadrenocorticism.

Retroperitoneal:

1. Avoids damaging an enlarged fatty liver.
2. Less likely to result in wound dehiscence.
3. Avoids pancreatitis from excessive manipulation to expose the right adrenal gland.
4. Allows for adequate exposure of the right adrenal gland.
5. Easier to deal with large quantities of fat in Cushing's disease patients.
6. Incomplete abdominal exploratory surgery to identify metastases.

22. Describe the surgical technique for adrenalectomy.

1. After a complete exploratory (especially liver and lymph nodes) procedure, the area around the adrenal is isolated with moistened laparotomy pads and self-retaining retractors.

2. Gentle dissection of the adrenals is performed with moistened sterile cotton swabs.

3. Hemostatic clips are used to ligate separately arteries and veins (avoiding blood supply to the kidney).

4. Temporary partial occlusion and venotomy of the vena cava may be required to remove tumor thrombus.

5. All biopsy specimens are submitted for histopathology.

23. What organs should be examined for potential metastases?

• Liver and regional lymph nodes for metastasis
• Adjacent vena cava, aorta, and ipsilateral renal artery and vein for tumor thrombus.

24. What suture material is recommended for abdominal wall closure after adrenalectomy for hyperadrenocorticism?

Nonabsorbable suture material.

25. Can the vena cava be occluded if necessary?

Yes. Vascular clamps are required so as not to damage the vessel wall. The caudal vena cava has been clamped for an hour in a ferret without causing clinical effects.

26. Name contraindications to adrenalectomy.

• Presence of extensive tumor metastasis.
• Invasion into the caudal vena cava and surrounding tissues, which makes complete excision unlikely.
• Concurrent diabetes mellitus (lack of catecholamines may result in difficulty regulating).

27. What is the prognosis for dogs with adrenocortical tumors?

Good with complete removal of benign adenomas; poor for carcinomas.

BIBLIOGRAPHY

1. Barthez PY, Marks SL: Pheochromocytoma in dogs: 61 cases (1984–1995). J Vet Intern Med 11:272–278, 1997.
2. Birchard SJ: Adrenalectomy. In Slatter D (ed): Textbook of Small Animal Surgery, 2nd ed., Philadelphia, W.B. Saunders, 1993, pp 1510–1514.
3. Duesberg CA, Nelson RW: Adrenalectomy for treatment of hyperadrenocorticism in cats: 10 cases (1988–1992). J Am Vet Med Assoc 207:1066–1070, 1995.
4. Scavelli TD: Adrenalectomy. In Bojrab MJ (ed): Current Techniques in Small Animal Surgery, 4th ed. Baltimore, Williams & Wilkins, 1998, pp 539–542, 764–767.
5. Weiss CA, Scott MV: Clinical aspects and surgical treatment of hyperadrenocorticism in the domestic ferret: 94 cases (1994–1996). J Am Anim Hosp Assoc 33:487–493, 1997.

49. PANCREATECTOMY

Elaine R. Caplan, D.V.M., Dip. A.C.V.S., A.B.V.P.

1. **When is surgery indicated for acute pancreatitis?**
   - Uncertain diagnosis, deteriorating patient.
   - Traumatic injury to parenchyma and excretory ducts.
   - Pancreatitis associated with infection and necrosis.

2. **List the surgical principles involved with severe pancreatitis and necrosis.**
   - Débridement and resection of necrotic tissue.
   - Preservation of major vessels, nerves, and ducts unaffected by disease.
   - Extensive lavage of abdominal cavity with warm sterile saline.
   - Drainage with sump drains or open peritoneal drainage.

3. **What is the postoperative care in patients with acute necrotizing pancreatitis?**
   - NPO for 2–5 days.
   - Broad-spectrum antibiotics.
   - Intravenous fluids, colloids, electrolytes, plasma (to replenish antiproteases).
   - Jejunostomy tube or total parenteral nutrition, if recovery is extended.
   - Aseptic bandage changes for drains or open peritoneal drainage.

4. **Name the short-term perioperative complications of acute necrotizing pancreatitis.**
   - Hypoproteinemia
   - Disseminated intravascular coagulation
   - Acute renal failure
   - Acute respiratory distress
   - Sepsis
   - Endotoxemia

5. **Name the long-term complications of acute necrotizing pancreatitis.**
   - Exacerbation of acute illness
   - Glandular fibrosis and pancreatic insufficiency

6. **What are complications of chronic pancreatitis and the surgical treatment for these complications?**

COMPLICATION	SURGICAL TREATMENT
Bile duct obstruction	Cholecystoenterostomy
Pyloric or duodenal obstruction resulting from fibrous tissue encroachment	Gastroduodenostomy, gastrojejunostomy, subtotal or total pancreatectomy*

*Subtotal or total pancreatectomy is less commonly performed because of technical difficulty and endocrine and exocrine insufficiency.

7. **What is a pancreatic anatomic difference between the cat and dog?**
   The cat has a common opening of the bile and pancreatic ducts.

8. **What is the prognosis for pancreatic abscess?**
   50% mortality rate; major complication is recurrence.

9. **List the goals of treatment for pancreatic abscess.**
   - Preoperative stabilization with fluids and electrolytes, antibiotics, and plasma.
   - Débridement of necrotic debris.

- External sump drain or OPD.
- Enteral hyperalimentation with gastrostomy tube or jejunostomy tube.

10. What is a pancreatic pseudocyst?
A collection of pancreatic fluid from ruptured ductules surrounded by a wall of granulation tissue; it may be associated with trauma or recurrent acute pancreatitis.

11. How is pancreatic pseudocyst treated?
Surgical drainage of cyst or partial pancreatectomy.

12. Which is the commonest malignant tumor of the pancreas in dogs and cats?
Exocrine pancreatic adenocarcinoma.

13. Why do patients with pancreatic adenocarcinoma develop abdominal effusion?
Effusion forms as a result of tumor metastatic lesions on the peritoneum or compression of the caudal vena cava.

14. How is exocrine pancreatic adenocarcinoma diagnosed?
- Abdominocentesis with cytologic evidence of malignant cells
- Exploratory surgery
- Biopsy
- Histopathology

Staging includes serum chemistry, CBC, urinalysis, thoracic amd abdominal radiography, and abdominal ultrasound.

15. What is the surgical treatment for exocrine pancreatic adenocarcinoma?
Tumors often metastasize to lymph nodes, liver, and peritoneum by the time of diagnosis. **Partial pancreatectomy** can be performed. Total pancreatectomy is not recommended. Biopsy all suspected metastatic lesions.

16. Does the presence of multiple small nodules on the pancreas indicate a poor prognosis?
Not necessarily; could be pancreatic nodular hyperplasia or pancreatic adenomas, both of which are benign.

17. Why is total pancreatectomy difficult and dangerous?
The blood supply to the right lobe of the pancreas is shared with the proximal part of the duodenum.

18. Describe methods for partial pancreatectomy and advantages of each.
- **Suture fracture technique**—suture is looped around tissue and ligature is tied, crushing parenchyma and ligating ducts and vessels. (Reduced operative time.)
- **Dissection and ligation technique**—ligature is tied around individual vessels and ducts, and tissue is removed after ducts and vessels are transected. (Fewer inflammatory changes.) Defect in the mesentery is sutured.

19. How do pancreatic wounds heal?
By fibrin deposition and polymerization, fibrous protein synthesis, and reepithelialization.

20. Where are the left and right lobes of the pancreas located?
- The left pancreatic lobe is in the deep leaf of the greater omentum.
- The right lobe is in the mesoduodenum.

21. What vascular supply might be affected when performing a partial pancreatectomy on the left pancreatic lobe?
Vessels of the gastrosplenic artery (potential interruption of blood supply to the spleen).

22. Are impaired endocrine and exocrine functions expected after extensive partial pancreatectomy?
Even after removal of 80–90% of the pancreas, no impairment of carbohydrate or fat metabolism is expected as long as the duct to the remaining portion is left intact.

23. Name 4 types of pancreatic islet cells.
1. A cells secrete glucagon.
2. B cells secrete insulin.
3. D cells secrete somatostatin.
4. F or P cells secrete pancreatic polypeptide.

24. Insulin-secreting islet cell tumors (insulinomas) result in hyperinsulinemia and hypoglycemia. List differential diagnoses for this disease in the dog.
- Hypoadrenocorticism
- Sepsis
- End-stage liver disease or cirrhosis
- Hunting dog hypoglycemia
- Starvation or cachexia
- Hepatic glycogen storage disease
- Portosystemic shunt
- Extrapancreatic tumors, including lymphoma
- Hepatoma
- Hepatocellular carcinoma
- Multiple myeloma
- Toxicities (ethanol, salicylates, propranolol)

25. What is Whipple's triad?
1. Clinical signs associated with hypoglycemia.
2. Fasting blood glucose <60 mg/dl at the time the animal is symptomatic.
3. Relief of clinical signs by administration of dextrose.

26. Compare common findings with insulin-secreting islet cell tumors for dogs and for ferrets.

DOGS	FERRETS
Seizures	**Hypersalivation**
Hind limb or generalized weakness	Weakness
Collapse	Lethargy
Muscle tremors	Collapse
Ataxia	Seizures **less** common
Slowly progressive and episodic	

27. How are B-cell islet cell tumors diagnosed?
- A high immunoreactive insulin level in a dog with hypoglycemia (<60 mg/dl) strongly suggests insulinoma.
- The most reliable diagnostic tool is abdominal exploratory surgery and biopsy with histopathology of suspicious lesions of the pancreas, liver, lymph nodes, duodenum, mesentery, omentum, and spleen.

28. What is the indication for methylene blue injection for insulinomas?
Administration (3 mg/kg, IV 30 minutes before exploratory surgery) helps identify abnormal tissue to resect neoplastic tissue completely, prolonging remission of clinical signs.

29. List complications of methylene blue injection.
- Inadequate uptake by islet cells
- Pseudocyanosis
- Regenerative anemia
- Acute renal failure

30. List complications after surgical removal of insulinoma.
- Pancreatitis
- Hyperglycemia (as a result of suppression of normal beta cells by tumor-derived insulin)
- Diabetes mellitus
- Hypoglycemia

31. What is the prognosis for dogs after surgery with insulinoma?
Mean survival is 12 months. Dogs with distant metastasis have shorter survival times.

32. List the features of Zollinger-Ellison syndrome resulting from a non–beta cell pancreatic tumor (gastrinoma) producing excessive gastrin.
- Excessive hydrochloric acid secretion from the parietal cells of the stomach.
- Hyperplasia and edema of the gastric mucosa.
- Duodenal ulceration from gastric hyperacidity.
- Villous atrophy and edema of the small intestine.
- Diarrhea with malabsorption.
- Steatorrhea resulting from acid inactivation of pancreatic lipase.

33. Why do dogs with gastrinoma have hypocalcemia?
Gastrin stimulates calcitonin secretion.

34. What is the most valuable nonsurgical diagnostic technique for gastrinoma?
Demonstration of elevated fasting gastrin concentrations and basal gastric acid secretion.

35. What is the best therapy for gastrinomas?
- Exploratory surgery, complete excision of tumor masses, and evaluation for metastasis.
- Medical management of hypergastrinemia and hyperchlorhydria with H_2-blockers, proton-pump inhibitors, and somatostatin analogues.

36. What is the prognosis in dogs with gastrinomas?
75% metastasize by diagnosis; survival averages 4.8 months; **highly malignant**.

BIBLIOGRAPHY

1. Harari J, Lincoln J: Surgery of the exocrine pancreas. In Slatter D (ed): Textbook of Small Animal Surgery, 2nd ed. Philadelphia, W.B. Saunders, 1993, pp 678–691.
2. Klausner JS, Hardy RM: Alimentary tract, liver, pancreas. In Slatter D (ed): Textbook of Small Animal Surgery, 2nd ed. Philadelphia, W.B. Saunders, 1993, pp 2099–2103.
3. Meleo KA, Caplan ER: Treatment of insulinoma in the dog, cat, and ferret. In Kirk RW (ed): Current Veterinary Therapy, 13th ed. Philadelphia, W.B. Saunders, 1999, pp 357–361.
4. Wheeler J, Bennett RA: Ferret abdominal surgical procedures: Part I. Adrenal gland and pancreatic beta-cell tumors. Comp Cont Educ Pract Vet 21:815–822, 1999.

50. SPLENECTOMY

Joseph Harari, M.S., D.V.M., Dip. A.C.V.S.

1. List the functions of the spleen.
- Hematopoiesis
- Storage of platelets and red blood cells
- Selective filtration of old, abnormal red blood cells
- Antibody (IgM) production by B cells
- Trapping and processing of bacteria

2. What are the most common splenic diseases in dogs and cats?
Dogs:
- Hemangiosarcoma
- Hyperplastic nodules
- Hematomas

Cats:
- Mast cell tumor
- Lymphosarcoma

3. What are indications for splenectomy?
- **Splenomegaly** resulting from neoplasia, torsion, immune-mediated thrombocytopenia and anemia, congestion, and lymphoproliferative diseases
- **Splenic infarct**

4. Why is splenectomy frequently performed?
Abnormalities of the organ are readily identified by palpation and diagnostic imaging; the organ is accessible following a midline celiotomy; minimal mesenteric attachments and identifiable vasculature promote uncomplicated ligations, resection, and removal (see figure).

5. What hematologic changes occur in normal dogs after splenectomy?
- Leukocytosis
- Regenerative anemia
- Increased Howell-Jolly bodies
- Nucleated red blood cells, target cell, and platelets
- Decreased red blood cell turnover
- Anemia in dogs with *Hemobartonella canis*

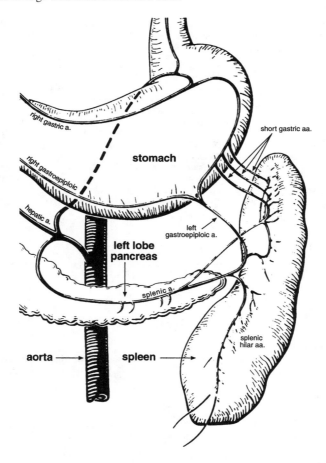

Vascular anatomy of the spleen and stomach illustrating major vessels for ligation. (From Hosgood G, Bone DL: Splenectomy in the dog by ligation of the splenic and short gastric arteries. Vet Surg 18:110–113, 1989, with permission.)

6. What are Howell-Jolly bodies?

Unimportant nuclear fragments found in newly released erythrocytes.

7. What are target cells?

Red blood cells with abnormal cellular membrane swelling, resulting from increased lipid content, which appear as a target; also called **codocyte;** clinically insignificant.

8. What laboratory changes have been documented in sick (e.g., torsion, congestion, neoplasia) dogs?

None consistently identified; 35% of aerobic bacterial cultures of splenic tissue were positive (*Staphylococcus*), although the clinical significance of this finding was unknown.

9. List complications of splenectomy.
- Hemorrhage
- Ventricular tachycardia
- Traumatic pancreatitis (rare)
- Gastric fistula (rare)

10. How is partial splenectomy performed?

Suturing (resection followed by a continuous oversew) or **stapling;** the latter reduces operative time and omental adhesions. Ultrasonic cutting devices and a carbon dioxide laser can also be used.

11. For total splenectomy, would ligation of the gastric and splenic arteries produce gastric necrosis?

No. Ligation of the splenic, short gastric, and left gastroepiploic arteries does not compromise stomach blood flow but does reduce operative time compared with splenic hilar vessel ligations.

12. What are the major clinical signs of splenic hemangiosarcoma?
- Acute collapse
- Pale mucous membranes
- Abdominal distention
- Hemoperitoneum

13. In dogs with splenic hemangiosarcoma, which two other organs need to be evaluated?

Liver and right atrium.

14. Which useful diagnostic tools can be used to evaluate a dog with suspected splenic neoplasia?

Abdominal and cardiac **ultrasonography** and **percutaneous aspiration cytology;** the latter may result in neoplastic cellular transplantation during fine-needle aspiration.

15. Although related to tumor staging, in general, what are the median survival times for dogs and cats with splenic hemangiosarcoma?
- **Dogs:** 2–3 months (chemotherapy may double these figures)
- **Cats:** 4–5 months

16. Which chemotherapeutic agents have been used to prolong recovery in dogs affected with splenic hemangiosarcoma?
- Doxorubicin
- Vincristine
- Cyclophosphamide

CONTROVERSY

17. What is the *law of two-thirds* for splenomegaly?

Two thirds of dogs with splenomegaly have splenic neoplasia, and two thirds of these patients have hemangiosarcoma. Mentioned, but not cited, is the addendum that two thirds of these dogs with hemangiosarcoma have microscopic regional and distant metastasis at the time of presentation. Contrary to this law, published data from samples submitted for histologic evaluation indicate that benign lesions, such as hyperplasia and hematoma, exceed hemangiosarcoma by nearly a 2:1 ratio. This disparity may exist because not all cases seen on the clinic floor have a subsequent gross and microscopic evaluation. Nonetheless, a "poor prognosis in an aging dog often becomes a self-fulfilling prophecy. If a clinician presumes that most cases of splenomegaly are hemangiosarcoma, the outcome may be unnecessarily adverse."

BIBLIOGRAPHY

1. Hosgood G, Bone DL: Splenectomy in the dog by ligation of the splenic and short gastric arteries. Vet Surg 18:110–113, 1989.
2. Morrison WB: Cancer in Dogs and Cats, 1st ed, Baltimore, Williams & Wilkins, 1998, pp 705–715.
3. Neath PJ, Brockman DJ: Retrospective analysis of 19 cases of isolated torsion of the splenic pedicle in dogs. J Sm Anim Pract 38:387–392, 1997.
4. Richardson EF, Brown NO: Hematological and biochemical changes and results of aerobic bacteriological culturing in dogs undergoing splenectomy. J Am Anim Hosp Assoc 32:199–210, 1996.
5. Spangler WL, Culbertson MR: Prevalence, type, and importance of splenic diseases in dogs: 1,480 cases (1985-1989). J Am Vet Med Assoc 200:829–834, 1992.
6. Spangler WL, Culbertson MR: Prevalence and type of splenic diseases in cats: 455 cases (1985–1991). J Am Vet Med Assoc 201:773–776, 1992.
7. Spangler WL, Kass PH: Pathologic factors affecting postsplenectomy survival in dogs. J Vet Intern Med 11:166–171, 1997.
8. Waldron DR, Robertson J: Partial splenectomy in the dog: A comparison of stapling and ligation techniques. J Am Anim Hosp Assoc 31:343–348, 1995.

51. THYROID AND PARATHYROID HYPERPLASIA AND NEOPLASIA

Sheldon Padgett, D.V.M., M.S., Dip. A.C.V.S.

1. What is the vascular supply to the thyroid gland in dogs?
The **cranial thyroid artery** (arising from the common carotid artery) is the primary arterial supply; the **caudal thyroid artery** (a branch of the brachiocephalic trunk) also supplies the gland. Each artery has a paired vein, which drains into the internal jugular vein.

2. Is the above anatomy also true for the cat?
No. The caudal thyroid artery is usually not present in the cat.

3. How many parathyroid glands are there in dogs and cats?
Four in both species.

4. Where are the parathyroid glands located?
A pair of external glands lie under the thyroid capsule at the cranial pole. A pair of internal glands are embedded in the thyroid parenchyma, in the caudal pole of the thyroid gland. Ectopic thyroid and parathyroid tissue has also been identified in dogs and cats between the proximal cervical area and mediastinum.

5. What are the indications for thyroid and parathyroid surgery?
Tumors.

6. What is the surgical approach for thyroid and parathyroid tumors?
Ventral midline, proximal cervical exploratory just distal to the larynx between the ventral strap muscles (sternocephalicus and sternohyoideus muscles) of the neck.

7. What are differences between thyroid tumors in dogs and cats?

Feline Thyroid Tumors	Canine Thyroid Tumors
Common	Rare
Mostly benign	Mostly malignant (locally
(adenomatous	invasive, pulmonary metastasis)
hyperplasia)	Nonfunctional
Functional	Euthyroid
Hyperthyroid	Present with:
Present with:	Ventral cervical mass (vascular)
Weight loss	Dysphagia
Hyperactivity	Dysphonia
Polyphagia	
Vomiting	
Polyuria and polydipsia	
Poor hair coat	
Elevated liver enzymes	
Elevated thyroxine (T_4) concentrations	

8. Do the differences between cats and dogs also apply to parathyroid tumors?
No. Parathyroid tumors are commoner in older dogs. They are usually functional adenomas, but adenocarcinomas can occur. Patients have clinical signs (polyuria and polydipsia, weakness, and lethargy) of hypercalcemia.

9. What are the therapeutic options for thyroid tumors in cats?
1. **Antithyroid medication** to block release of thyroid hormone.
Pro: No surgery (for patients unstable to undergo anesthesia, avoids complications of surgery).
Con: Lifelong daily medication, significant hematologic and gastrointestinal effects.
2. **Radioactive iodine** (^{131}I) to eradicate hyperplastic thyroid cells.
Pro: No surgery, spares non-hyperplastic tissue, usually curative.
Con: Availability of a nuclear medicine treatment facility, patient quarantine time varies with state law.
3. **Surgical removal** of hyperplastic tissue.
Pro: Widely available, can be curative.
Con: Complications with inadvertent parathyroidectomy, recurrence with incomplete excision.

10. What are the chances for unilateral versus bilateral involvement in feline hyperthyroidism?
Approximately 30% of hyperthyroid cats have unilateral involvement versus 70% that have bilateral involvement.

11. Can one accurately diagnose unilateral or bilateral involvement at surgery?
Not always. Approximately 15% of thyroid glands that look normal at the time of surgery contain adenomatous tissue. If a disease is truly unilateral, there should be atrophy of the normal gland because of the autonomous release of thyroid hormone from the hyperplastic gland.

12. How can one avoid the problems inherent in relying on gross evaluation of the feline thyroid?
Preoperative sodium pertechnetate (technetium) scanning demonstrates the location of hyperplastic thyroid tissue. Technetium scanning also demonstrates functional ectopic tissue and metastatic disease from thyroid adenocarcinomas.

13. What are the potential risks of surgical therapy for feline hyperthyroidism?

1. **Postoperative hypoparathyroidism (commonest).** If both external parathyroid glands are accidentally removed or the vascularity to the glands is disrupted, postoperative hypocalcemia can ensue. This can be severe and life-threatening.

2. **Anesthetic death.** Hyperthyroid patients commonly have compromised cardiac function because of tachycardia, hypertrophic cardiomyopathy, and myocardial sensitization to catecholamines.

3. **Damage to recurrent laryngeal nerve (rare).** The recurrent laryngeal nerve lies close to the thyroid gland; if damaged, decreased function can lead to voice change or laryngeal paralysis.

14. In what ways can the risks of treating feline hyperthyroidism be decreased?

1. **Hypoparathyroidism:**
   - Use meticulous surgical technique in preserving the external parathyroid gland and the associated vascularity.
   - If bilateral thyroidectomy is needed, staging the procedure (performing two unilateral thyroidectomies, allowing 2–3 weeks between) decreases incidence of postoperative hypocalcemia.
   - If both external parathyroid glands are inadvertently removed, one or both glands can be transplanted to a muscle belly and become functional in 2–3 weeks.

2. **Anesthesia:**
   - Attain euthyroid state before surgery with methimazole (hypertrophic cardiac changes are reversible).
   - Treat tachycardia with appropriate β-blocker before anesthesia.
   - Use an anesthetic protocol that minimizes catecholamine-induced arrhythmias (premedication with acepromazine, avoid ketamine and xylazine, thiobarbiturates for induction, avoid methoxyflurane and halothane as inhalent anesthetic).

3. **Nerve damage:**
   - Use meticulous surgical technique.

15. What is a method of increasing the visibility of parathyroid adenomas in dogs at the time of cervical exploratory surgery?

Infusion of methylene blue (3 mg/kg in 250 ml of 0.9% saline) approximately 20–30 minutes before surgical exposure can delineate the adenomas. The lesions may be small and multiple.

16. Discuss the most common complication after removal of parathyroid adenoma.

Postoperative hypocalcemia is due to the tumor's autonomous parathyroid hormone production leading to negative feedback on the normal parathyroid glands. Treatment is aimed at restoring and maintaining normal calcium levels until the other parathyroid glands start to function. Calcium and vitamin D supplementation is indicated.

BIBLIOGRAPHY

1. Feldman EC (ed): Feline hyperthyroidism (thyrotoxicosis). In: Canine and Feline Endocrinology and Reproduction. Philadelphia, W.B. Saunders, 1996, pp 118–166.
2. Flanders JA: Surgical therapy of the thyroid. Vet Clin North Am 24:607–621, 1994.
3. Klein MK, Powers BE, Withrow SJ, et al: Treatment of thyroid carcinoma in dogs by surgical resection alone: 20 cases (1981–1989). J Am Vet Med 206:1007–1009, 1995.
4. Padgett SL, Tobias KM, Leathers CW, et al: Efficacy of parathyroid gland autotransplantation in maintaining serum calcium concentrations after bilateral thyroparathyroidectomy in cats. J Am Anim Hosp Assoc 34:219–224, 1998.

52. RENAL NEOPLASIA AND CALCULI

Dennis Olsen, D.V.M., M.S., Dip. A.C.V.S.

1. How common are primary tumors of the kidneys?
- In **dogs,** 0.3–2.5% of all tumors.
- In cats, 0.6%–2.5% of all tumors (variability due to controversy regarding inclusion of lymphoma as a primary renal neoplasm).

2. Which are more common — primary tumors or metastases?
Metastases because of high blood flow through the kidneys and the rich capillary network.

3. List the most common types of tumors.
- Renal tubular adenocarcinomas (60–70% in canine; 40–68% in feline)
- Transitional cell carcinomas
- Squamous cell carcinomas
- Hemangiosarcoma
- Nephroblastoma
- Lymphoma (feline)

4. What is the biologic behavior of renal tumors?
Greater than 90% are malignant.

5. What is the general signalment of animals with renal tumors?
Older animals (except nephroblastoma); the only canine breed known to have a predisposition for renal neoplasia is the German Shepherd dog. No feline gender or breed dispositions.

6. Describe the clinical presentation of a renal tumor.
The classic triad of signs — hematuria, a palpable abdominal mass, and pain in the flank region — is rarely seen (<15% of cases).

Clinical signs are generally nonspecific, such as anorexia, weight loss, vomiting, and lameness secondary to hypertrophic osteopathy.

7. What are some diagnostic steps?
- **Careful palpation:** painful mass in the cranial aspect of the abdomen.
- **Hematologic changes:** mild anemia resulting from alterations in erythropoietin or chronic hematuria; polycythemia has also been seen.
- **Diagnostic imaging:** survey and contrast radiography, computed tomography, and ultrasonography.
- **Needle aspiration or biopsy:** with ultrasound.
- **Surgical exploration:** diagnosis and therapy (removal).

8. What types of therapy are available for renal tumors?
1. The treatment of choice for unilateral renal tumors that have not metastasized is **complete nephrectomy.** If possible, early venous ligation should be attempted to diminish the potential of releasing tumor emboli into the systemic circulation. The kidney and ureter as well as perinephric fat and, if necessary, sublumbar musculature should be removed.

2. Chemotherapy for lymphoma may be very effective but protocols used for other tumors generally have equivocal results.

9. What is the prognosis?
Many tumors have metastasized at the time of diagnosis, and metastatic disease is often the cause of death soon after diagnosis. Generally, if a dog survives surgical removal of the carci-

noma for 21 days, the median survival is approximately 7 months. Transitional cell carcinoma cases have a median survival of approximately 11 months.

10. How common are renal calculi (nephroliths)?
- **In dogs,** 1–4% of all urolith cases
- **In cats,** 2.8–5% of all urolith cases

11. Is there an association of nephroliths with uroliths in other locations?
Between 25% and 50% of dogs with nephroliths also have uroliths in another location of the urinary tract. Cats have uroliths in other locations 15% to 17% of the time.

12. List dog breeds that are at greater risk to develop kidney stones.
- Miniature schnauzers
- Shih Tzus
- Lhasa apsos
- Yorkshire terriers
- Female pugs
- Dalmatians
- Male basset hounds

13. What types of stones are commonly seen?
Mixed minerals, calcium oxalate, struvite, and urate. The most common type of feline nephroliths are calcium oxalate followed by calcium phosphate.

14. What are the clinical manifestations of nephrolithiasis?
Without obstruction or infection, renal calculi are asymptomatic and incidentally diagnosed while performing abdominal radiography or ultrasound for an unrelated condition. Complete obstruction results in hydronephrosis, which may cause abdominal pain. Unilateral renal calculi can exhibit recurrent urinary tract infection if the stone is infected. Bilateral urinary obstruction, even partial, often leads to reduced renal function and signs of uremia.

15. How is a diagnosis of nephrolithiasis confirmed?
Laboratory test results are variable: Pyuria, hematuria, bacteriuria, an active sediment containing casts and crystals, and impaired concentration of urine may be noted on urinalysis with infection or obstruction. Blood chemistry may show evidence of renal dysfunction with an obstruction. **Diagnostic radiography** (intravenous urograms) or ultrasonography confirms the presence of calculi within the kidney.

16. What procedures should be performed before definitive therapy?
- Nuclear scintigraphy to quantify kidney contribution to overall renal function
- Urinalysis, culture, and radiology can help in predicting the mineral composition of the stone

17. Discuss the treatment options.
Therapy of asymptomatic renal calculi that are incidentally found during diagnostics for unrelated conditions is controversial. It is prudent to evaluate renal function, to begin medical therapy based on abnormal lab results and stone composition, and periodically to monitor the stone. Surgical removal of nephroliths should be considered when there is continued risk for loss of renal function beyond that created by surgical intervention. Also, when stones are not amenable to medical dissolution and there is evidence of renal dysfunction, surgery should be considered. Shock-wave lithotripsy (fragmentation of stones) has the advantage of inducing less damage to the renal parenchyma than invasive surgery. Equipment for this procedure is not readily available in veterinary medicine.

18. What surgical techniques are available?
- Nephrolithotomy (percutaneous and via surgical laparotomy)
- Pyelolithotomy if the renal pelvis is dilated
- Nephrectomy in unilateral cases in which contralateral renal function is adequate

19. What is the technique for nephrolithotomy via laparotomy?
Temporary occlusion of arterial blood flow to the kidney. The convex surface is incised, and renal parenchyma is bluntly dissected to the level of the renal pelvis. The stone is removed and

all diverticuli are gently explored. A catheter should be inserted into the ureter and flushed to ensure patency. The kidney is then reapposed, the vascular occlusion released, and digital pressure applied until the blood flow has ceased and the clot has sealed the cut surfaces. A capsular suture can then be placed.

20. What is pyelolithotomy?
An incision into the renal pelvis for removal of stones. The renal blood supply need not be occluded and damage to the parenchyma is limited. After removal of the stone, the pelvis is flushed, and a catheter is used to ensure patency of the ureter. The renal pelvis is meticulously closed without placing sutures within the lumen.

21. What are the complications of nephrolithotomy?
- Loss (50%) of renal function secondary to damage inflicted on the renal parenchyma
- Failure to remove all of the stones from the kidney because of inaccessible location or increased patient risk
- Potential for recurrence if surgery is not complemented with appropriate medical therapy

22. How are bilateral conditions treated?
A choice is made between removal of the stones from both kidneys during one surgery or performing staged unilateral procedures. This decision is based on renal function, presence of infection, degree of urinary obstruction, and overall health. Staged unilateral surgery can be performed when urine flow is not obstructed. The kidney that is least likely to be compromised and will support the patient should be selected for the first procedure.

BIBLIOGRAPHY

1. Adams LG, Senior DF: Electrohydraulic and extracorporeal shock-wave lithotripsy. Vet Clin North Am Small Animal Pract 29:293–302, 1999.
2. Christie BA, Bjorling DE: Kidneys. In Slatter D (ed): Textbook of Small Animal Surgery 2nd ed. Philadelphia, W.B. Saunders, 1993, pp 1428–1442.
3. Ross SJ, Osborne CA, Lulich JP, et al: Canine and feline nephrolithiasis: Epidemiology, detection, and management. Vet Clin North Am Small Animal Pract 29:231–250, 1999.
4. Stone EA: Surgical therapy for urolithiasis. In Stone EA, Barsanti JA (eds): Urologic Surgery of the Dog and Cat. Philadelphia, Lea & Febiger, 1992, pp 174–181.
5. Withrow SJ: Tumors of the urinary system. In Withrow SJ, MacEwan EG (eds): Small Animal Clinical Oncology, 2nd ed. Philadelphia, W.B. Saunders, 1996, pp 380–392.

53. ECTOPIC URETERS

C. W. Smith, D.V.M., M.S., Dip. A.C.V.S.

1. What is an ectopic ureter?
A congenital anomaly in which one or both ureters empty beyond the bladder. The ureter may be intraluminal or extraluminal in position.

2. List common sites of ectopic ureter termination.

Vagina (most frequent)	Neck of bladder
Urethra	Uterus

3. What is the difference between an intraluminal and extraluminal ectopic ureter?
- **Extraluminal ureters** completely bypass the bladder.

- **Intraluminal ureters** course submucosally within the bladder wall before emptying beyond the bladder.
- **Intraluminal ureters** are more common.

4. What is the cause of ectopic ureter?
An abnormal differentiation of the mesonephric (embryonic kidney) and metanephric (definitive kidney) ducts.

5. List other urinary abnormalities that are associated with ectopic ureter.

Hydroureter	Ureteroceles
Hydronephrosis	Double ureteral openings
Functional bladder or urethral abnormalities	Vestibulovaginal abnormalities
Bladder hypoplasia	Ureteral trough

6. Is ectopic ureter an inherited condition?
This has not been established. A familial predisposition occurs in Siberian huskies, retrievers, and poodles. The mode of transmission is unknown.

7. Is there a gender predilection for ectopic ureter?
Possibly. The ratio of affected females to males is 20:1. Affected males, however, may be less commonly diagnosed because of a longer urethra, urethral-vesicular reflux, and external urethral sphincter pressures (all prevent dribbling).

8. What is the most common sign associated with ectopic ureter?
Constant or intermittent urinary **incontinence** after weaning. Normal voiding may occur with intermittent dribbling. Incontinence may occur less commonly in male compared with female dogs.

9. Does ectopic ureter occur in the cat?
Less frequently than in the dog.

10. How is ectopic ureter diagnosed?
Excretory urography is the method of choice for confirming ectopic ureters and defining associated urogenital abnormalities. The size and shape of the kidneys, ureters, and bladder; termination of the ureters; and any other urinary abnormalities are noted. Excretory urography is not 100% successful in demonstrating urinary lesions.

Ultrasonography was compared with excretory urography and the results found to be similar, although ultrasonography was more accurate in identifying normal ureteral anatomy.

11. What laboratory evaluations are important in patients with ectopic ureter?
- Complete blood count
- Chemistry profile
- Urinalysis and urine culture

12. How are patients with ectopic ureters treated?
The choice of the surgical procedure should be based on the functional capability of both kidneys or presence of infection or other pathologic changes in any portion of the urinary tract.
- **Ureterovesical anastomosis** should be considered in the following situations:
  Normal function of the kidney drained by an ectopic ureter
  Bilateral ureteral ectopia
  Hypofunction of both kidneys
- **Ureteronephrectomy** should be performed if the kidney drained by the ectopic ureter is nonfunctional or an intractable infection is present, provided the remaining kidney has adequate function.

13. What is neoureterostomy?

Formation of a new opening for intraluminal ectopic ureters. A ventral cystotomy incision is made near the urethra. Pressure applied to the urethra facilitates identification of the intraluminal ectopic ureter, which appears as a swelling or ridge within the bladder wall. A 3–5 mm longitudinal incision is made through the bladder mucosa into the lumen of the ureter. Small absorbable sutures are placed in a simple interrupted pattern to suture the ureteral mucosa to the bladder. A 3.5 or 5 French catheter is introduced into the distal ureter. Just distal to the new ureteral stoma, two nonabsorbable sutures (3–0 to 4–0) are passed from the serosal surface around the tube staying beneath the bladder mucosa. These sutures are tied, after removal of the catheter, to ligate the distal ureter.

14. What is a ureteroneocystostomy?

Reconnection into the bladder for extraluminal ectopic ureters. The ureter is resected and reimplanted into the bladder lumen. A stay suture is placed through the proximal end of the transected ureter. After a ventral cystotomy, an incision is made through the bladder mucosa, and a short oblique submucosal tunnel is created in the bladder wall. Using the stay suture, the ureter is pulled through the bladder wall into the lumen. The ureter is spatulated and sutured to the bladder mucosa with small absorbable sutures in a simple interrupted pattern.

15. Why is it important to handle the bladder gently?

The bladder responds to trauma by becoming edematous. Edema can occlude the ureteral openings.

16. What is the prognosis for surgical treatment of ectopic ureters?

30–55% of patients continue to show some degree of urinary incontinence after surgery. Repair of extraluminal ureters (terminating in urethra, uterus, or vagina) and patients with hydroureter have a poor prognosis.

17. Why would urinary incontinence persist after surgical correction?

Urethral sphincter incompetence may also be present. Cystometrographic studies and urethral pressure profiles can be used to detect functional abnormalities before surgery.

18. What drugs can be used to help control postoperative urinary incontinence?

- Phenylpropanolamine (α-adrenergic agonist) to increase urethral sphincter tone.
- Diethylstilbestrol to increase sensitivity of α-receptors and enhance urethral mucosal sealing, collagen content, and vascularity.

BIBLIOGRAPHY

1. Anderson CC, Cook CR: What is your diagnosis? Ectopic ureter. J Am Vet Med Assoc 214:1321–1322, 1999.
2. Bjorling DE, Christie BA: Ureters. In Slatter D (ed): Textbook of Small Animal Surgery, 2nd ed. Philadelphia, W.B. Saunders, 1993, pp 1443–1450.
3. Fossum TW: Surgery of the kidney and ureter. In Fossum TW (ed): Small Animal Surgery. St. Louis, Mosby, 1997, pp 461–480.
4. Lamb CR, Gregory SP: Ultrasonographic findings in 14 dogs with ectopic ureter. Vet Radiol Ultrasound 39:218–223, 1998.
5. Rawlings CA: Ureter. In Bojrab MJ (ed): Current Techniques in Small Animal Surgery, 4th ed. Baltimore, Williams & Wilkins, 1998, pp 445–449.

54. URETERAL TEARS AND CALCULI

Dennis Olsen, D.V.M., M.S., Dip. A.C.V.S.

1. How often are traumatic ureteral tears diagnosed?

Rarely in small animals because the ureter is well protected from injury by the sublumbar musculature and spine. The most common source of ureteral trauma is iatrogenic during surgical procedures of the female reproductive tract. Crushing trauma from clamps and sutures used during ovariohysterectomy have been implicated as a cause of ureteral necrosis and leakage.

2. What are the clinical manifestations of a ureteral tear?

- A clinical history of abdominal trauma, abdominal surgery, or urolithiasis should raise index of suspicion.
- Sterile urine in the retroperitoneum or peritoneum does not cause immediate clinical signs.
- Cellulitis, peritonitis, abdominal tenderness, and abdominal distention are detected 3–5 days after injury.
- Infected urine will result in a more acute presentation.

3. How are tears in the ureter diagnosed?

- Laboratory findings: inconclusive on early presentation
- Abdominocentesis: increased creatinine compared with serum concentrations (only if in abdominal cavity)
- Urinalysis: hematuria (maybe). May be gross or microscopic
- Radiography: hydroperitoneum, contrast leakage (only if in peritoneum)
- Exploratory laparotomy: direct visualization

4. What are the treatment options for a ureteral tear?

The ureter has remarkable regenerative capability, and even large full-thickness defects can heal if a properly sized stenting catheter is placed across the defect. Small tears in the ureter may heal completely without surgical intervention or catheter placement.

If a clamp or suture inadvertently placed during ovariohysterectomy is removed quickly (within 60 minutes), 90% of the resulting strictures resolve by 12 weeks. If the obstruction is removed by 1 week and the ureter is repaired, normal renal and ureter function can be regained. If the obstruction is 4 weeks or longer, renal function is completely lost.

5. List surgical techniques used for ureteral tears.

- Transureter stenting catheters
- Primary closure
- Nephroureterectomy
- Ureteroneocystostomy

6. What is renal descensus?

Mobilization and caudal displacement of the kidney to reduce tension on the ureter.

7. How common are ureteral calculi?

In a large retrospective study of dogs, ureteral calculi were seen with renal calculi in 0.3% of urolithiasis cases and ureteral calculi alone in 0.7%. In cats, incidence may be increasing.

8. What types of stones are commonly seen?

The mineral composition of ureteroliths reflects the composition of nephroliths. **Struvite** and **calcium oxalate** stones are the most common types found in dogs; in cats, calcium oxalate.

9. What are the clinical manifestations of ureteral calculi?

Depression, lethargy, anorexia, vomiting, dysuria. All may be due to pain.

10. How is a diagnosis of ureteral calculi confirmed?
- Radiography: dense calculi, enlarged kidney, hydronephrosis, and hydroureter (contrast)
- Ultrasonography: hyperechoic shadows, dilation of ureter
- Surgical exploration: visualization and palpation

11. What special procedures should be performed before to definitive therapy?
- Monitoring transit of calculus
- Evaluating renal function: nuclear scintigraphy (glomerular filtration) or contrast studies (iohexol)
- Evaluate entire tract for stones

12. What are the treatment options?
- Inducing diuresis
- Treatment with analgesics or muscle relaxants
- Lithotripsy—not in cats

13. Can ureteral calculi be medically dissolved?
Medical dissolution is unlikely to be successful because stones are not bathed in urine or are of nondissolvable composition.

14. What are the the principles of ureteral surgery?
1. Avoid disruption of ureteral vascularity.
2. Provide accurate apposition.
3. Avoid tension on the anastomosis site.

15. What surgical techniques are available?
- Nephroureterectomy: kidney function is lost
- Pyelotomy or ureterotomy
- Ureteroneocystostomy: mucosal apposition, mobilization of kidney or bladder

16. What is psoas cystopexy?
Cranial displacement and attachment of bladder to iliopsoas muscle to reduce tension on ureteral implantation site.

17. List complications of surgery.
- Uroabdomen and peritonitis
- Stricture formation
- Loss of functional renal tissue

18. What are some postoperative protocols?
1. Repeated contrast urograms or ultrasound examinations (or both) can be done to determine the presence of leakage, stricture formation, and recurrence of calculi.
2. Fluid and nutritional support may be required because of postoperative anorexia.
3. Proper antimicrobial therapy should be selected based on culture and sensitivity samples obtained from the site.
4. Renal function should be closely monitored to determine the degree of recovery.

BIBLIOGRAPHY

1. Adams LG, Senior DF: Electrohydraulic and extracorporeal shock-wave lithotripsy. Vet Clin North Am Small Animal Pract 29:293–302, 1999.
2. Bjorling DE, Christie BA: Ureters. In Slatter D (ed): Textbook of Small Animal Surgery, 2nd ed. Philadelphia, W.B. Saunders, 1993, pp 1443–1450.
3. Dupre GP, Dee LG, Dee JF: Ureterotomies for treatment of ureterolithiasis in two dogs. J Am Anim Hosp Assoc 26:500–504, 1990.
4. Kyles AE, Stone EA, Gookin J: Diagnosis and surgical management of obstructive ureteral calculi in cats: 11 cases (1993–1996). J Am Vet Med Assoc 213:1150–1156, 1998.

55. URINARY BLADDER CALCULI AND NEOPLASIA

Trevor N. Bebchuk, D.V.M.

1. What are common urinary calculi in the dog and cat?
- Calcium oxalate monohydrate and dihydrate
- Magnesium ammonium phosphate hexahydrate
- Ammonium and sodium urates
- Cystine
- Silicone dioxide
- Xanthine

2. Are there any breed-associated uroliths?

BREED	UROLITH	OCCURRENCE (%)
Dalmatian	Ammonium and sodium urate	98
Miniature schnauzer	Calcium oxalate	28
	Struvite	67
Bichon frise	Struvite	90
English bulldogs	Ammonium and sodium urate	35
	Cystine	42
Yorkshire terriers	Calcium oxalate	45

3. Which stone composition is commonest in the dog and cat?
- **Dogs**
  Struvite
  Calcium oxalate
- **Cats**
  Calcium oxalate
  Struvite

4. Is there an association between a specific type of urolith and urinary tract infection (UTI)?
Struvite uroliths are most commonly associated.

5. List the different types of urolith in order of radiographic density, from most radiodense to lease radiodense.
- Phosphate (apatite, struvite)
- Calcium oxalate
- Cystine
- Urates

6. Which types of calculi can be managed with dietary changes?
1. **Struvite uroliths** are the most responsive to dietary management (reduced protein, phosphorus, and magnesium). The diets also commonly have increased sodium chloride to stimulate thirst and polyuria.
2. **Ammonium urate uroliths** may also be managed by diet (purine-restricted alkalinizing diet with no supplemental sodium).
3. **Cystine urolithiasis** may also be managed with diet because the urine composition can be modified to contain less cystine.

7. What systemic metabolic conditions are associated with urolithiasis?
Dalmatian dogs have a decreased ability to oxidize uric acid to allantoin. This results in the excretion of high levels of uric acid in the urine, which predisposes Dalmatians to urate urolithi-

178

asis. Dogs with portal vascular anomalies or hepatic microvascular dysplasia are also predisposed to urate urolithiasis because the blood is shunted around the liver, preventing the conversion of uric acid to allantoin. Cystinuria leading to cystine uroliths is an inborn error of metabolism, but the precise mechanism of abnormal renal transport and the genetic mode of inheritance are unknown.

8. Is it important to know what types of calculi are present?
Yes. Different stones require different medical and surgical management and some may be evidence of a systemic metabolic abnormality. Also, the dissolution diets used for some stones (struvite) may predispose to the formation of others (calcium oxalate).

9. What tests can be used to determine the type of urolith present?
- **Urinalysis,** including visual analysis of crystals present. This may not be accurate, especially when dealing with stones of mixed composition.
- **Imaging studies,** radiographs, pneumocystography, double contrast radiography, and ultrasonography. These provide information on the size, shape, radiopacity, location, and number of stones detected, which may give clues to mineral composition.
- Surgical removal and stone submission for analysis, the only guaranteed means of accurate mineral composition analysis.

10. What potential problems can be associated with urolithiasis?
Obstruction of the renal pelvis, ureter, trigone, or urethra. If the obstruction is persistent, hydronephrosis, hydroureter and even urethral rupture may occur. **Chronic UTIs** may also be sequelae.

11. Is urolithiasis an emergency?
Yes, if the animal has a urinary tract obstruction as a result of lodging of the urolith in a ureter, bladder neck, or urethra (post–renal azotemia). This obstruction has systemic metabolic effects (uremia) and could lead to ureteral, bladder, or urethral rupture if urinary obstruction is severe and allowed to persist for several days.

12. What are the indications for cystotomy and urolith removal?
- Obstructive uropathy
- Calcium oxalate, calcium phosphate, silica, and sometimes cystine uroliths
- Uroliths that are refractory to medical dissolution
- Contraindications to medical management (nutritional concerns)
- Anatomica defects predisposing to UTI (urachal diverticulum)
- Male gender because medical dissolution of urinary calculi carries with it a greater risk of urethral obstruction

13. If a dog has urethral stones, what technique can be used to attempt to move them into the bladder for removal via cystotomy?
Retrograde urohydropropulsion. This technique should be employed if voiding urohydropropulsion has failed. A cystotomy is a much more benign procedure than urethrotomy or urethrostomy. This technique involves pulsatile sterile saline infusion into a urethral catheter with the catheter tip and inflated balloon located just distal to the stone. This urethra is distended and the stone flushed retrograde. If required, pressure can be placed on the urethra proximal to the stone per rectum to cause more urethral dilation. Heavy sedation or general anesthesia is necessary to perform this, and local anesthesia of the urethra with lidocaine gel may help prevent urethrospasm.

14. What are the surgical approaches to the bladder for urolith removal?
The bladder can be approached via a caudal ventral midline abdominal incision. In male dogs, the incision begins at the umbilicus and curves prepreputially. Branches of the caudal superficial

epigastric vessels are ligated, and the abdomen is entered on ventral midline. The bladder should be elevated out of the abdomen and isolated with moistened laparotomy sponges. A stay suture is then placed at the apex of the bladder at the cranial end of the proposed incision with another stay suture at the caudal end of the proposed incision. The dorsal or ventral bladder incision should be made in a relatively avascular area, and the trigone must be avoided.

15. What methods have been described for the closure of the urinary bladder?
The most frequently recommended is a **double closure** with a simple continuous pattern in the mucosal layer, taking care to place minimal suture material within the bladder lumen. The serosal and muscular layers are closed in a continuous inverting pattern, such as a Cushing or Lembert pattern.

Single-layer appositional techniques, such as simple interrupted and simple continuous patterns, have also been proposed. In normal canine bladders, the single-layer closure provides an equally good seal as the two-layer, inverting pattern. In a thickened bladder wall, it is often difficult to place an effective inverting pattern, and a single-layer appositional pattern is indicated. If anatomic defects that may predispose to UTI exist, they should be corrected before cystotomy closure.

16. Discuss the types of suture material that are best suited for urinary bladder surgery.
The ideal suture material would have strength at least as great as that of normal bladder tissue, and it would retain that strength for the 14–21 days it takes injured bladder tissue to retain 100% of prewound strength. It should be absorbable suture material to avoid acting as a nidus for stone formation. Two synthetic braided absorbable suture materials, **polyglycolic acid** (Dexon) and **polyglactin 910** (Vicryl), have sufficient tensile strength and maintain that strength for an adequate period, with all the strength lost by 28 days. They degrade over 3–6 weeks, but this may occur faster for polyglycolic acid in the face of UTI. Two monofilament suture materials, **polydioxanone** (PDS) and **modified polyglycolic acid** (Maxon), have 20% greater tensile strength than similar synthetic braided materials, less tissue drag, and prolonged decay. The first two properties are useful, but the prolonged decay may lead to a suture nidus and stone formation.

17. What techniques can be used to ensure that all uroliths are surgically removed from a bladder?
- **Preoperative radiography** notes the number and location of the radiodense uroliths.
- **During surgery, a catheter** can be placed into the urethra and saline flushed normograde to evaluate for the presence of stones in the urethra. Alternatively, a catheter can be placed retrograde in the urethra and a nonsterile assistant can flush sterile saline retrograde into the bladder. This helps to flush stones from the urethra into the bladder, where they can be removed.
- **Postoperative radiography** of the abdomen helps ensure stones were not retained in the bladder or urethra.

18. What is the incidence of bladder cancer in the dog and cat?
Less than 1% of all cancers. It is more common in the dog than the cat, and malignant tumors are more common clinically than benign ones. The most common histologic types are transitional cell carcinoma, followed by squamous cell carcinoma, and adenocarcinoma, however hemangiosarcoma has also been noted. Primary sarcomas are rare and young dogs can have a rare tumor called a **botryoid** or **embryonal rhabdomyosarcoma.** The most common benign lesions are fibromas, leiomyomas, and papillomas.

19. What is the biologic behavior of the most common tumors?
Malignant bladder carcinomas, especially transitional cell carcinomas, are locally invasive and, in greater than 50% of cases, metastasize to the regional lymph nodes and lungs.

20. What clinical signs are most commonly associated with bladder neoplasia?
- Chronic signs of hematuria, dysuria, and pollakiuria
- Hypertrophic osteopathy, especially in cases of botryoid rhabdomyosarcoma
- Any cystitis refractory to medical therapy (warrants further diagnostic evaluation)

21. Describe the techniques of urinary diversion to deal with nonresectable bladder neoplasia or tumors of the trigone region.

If a bladder tumor is not resectable and the trigone is involved, two different diversion techniques have been reported:

1. **Ureterocolonic anastomosis** or **trigonal-colonic anastomosis** has had limited success in dogs. Complications associated with this procedure include pyelonephritis, ureteral obstruction, and hyperchloremic acidosis. In a case series of 10 dogs, mean survival was only 4 months. When the morbidity of the procedure and metastatic rate are considered, this treatment is rarely indicated.

2. As a palliative technique, a **prepubic cystostomy catheter** can be placed, allowing for urine evacuation in cases in which the tumor is causing an obstruction and is not resectable.

22. Can bladder tumors be resected?

The bladder can be partially resected, but the trigone must be left for normal function to continue. Nearly 80% of the bladder can be removed with a return to normal or near-normal volume capacity. Tumors of the apex can be removed with wide margins, but tumors of the trigone present a bigger challenge. Transitional cell carcinomas frequently involve the trigone and ureters. Because of the high metastatic rate of the malignant carcinomas, an exploratory laparotomy, including examination of the sublumbar lymph nodes, should be made to identify metastases before tumor resection. Surgery tends to be palliative rather than curative for carcinomas.

23. What are options for bladder reconstructions?

The main reconstructive techniques for the bladder involve the isolation of a portion of the small intestine on its vascular supply and using this bowel segment to enlarge the bladder reservoir. In the dog, a **modified cup-patch ileocystoplasty** has been described in which a segment of ileum was used to reconstruct the bladder after removal of all but the bladder neck and trigone. The intestine should be denuded of its mucosa to prevent mucus production and secondary urinary obstruction and to allow uroepithelial migration from the remaining bladder neck.

24. What are the possible complications associated with bladder tumor excision?
- Urinary leakage resulting from small bladder volume or poor healing of the bladder closure because of incomplete tumor margins.
- **Subcutaneous surgical transplantation** of the tumor after surgical biopsy or excision. In this instance, instead of removing the tumor, the surgeon actually facilitates its spread. For this reason, a surgeon should use a different set of instruments and new gloves, for closure, and all contact between tumor and healthy tissues should be minimized.

25. Are there any chemotherapeutic options for bladder neoplasia?
- The use of **cisplatin**, or a combination of cisplatin and radiation, seems reasonable (cisplatin is excreted in its active form in the urine).
- Local infusion of chemotherapeutics is an option, but previous work suggests that the drug would not penetrate beyond the submucosa.
- **Doxorubicin and cyclophosphamide** have provided a longer median survival than surgery alone.
- A nonsteroidal antiinflammatory drug, **piroxicam,** may provide several months of palliation.

26. What adjuvant therapies can be employed with surgery for the treatment of bladder neoplasia?
- Chemotherapy
- Hyperthermic therapy
- Immunotherapy
- Radiation

BIBLIOGRAPHY

1. Anderson WI, Dunham BM, King JM, et al: Presumptive subcutaneous surgical transplantation of a urinary bladder transitional cell carcinoma in a dog. Cornell Vet 79:263–266, 1989.
2. Osborne CA (ed): Science of Canine Urolithiasis. Vet Clinics North Am Small Animal Pract 29:1–304,
   1999.
3. Schwarz PD, Egger EL, Klause SE: Modified "cup-patch" ileocystoplasty for urinary bladder reconstruction in a dog. J Am Vet Med Assoc 198:273–277, 1991.
4. Stone EA, George TF, Gilson SD, et al: Partial cystectomy for urinary bladder neoplasia: Surgical technique and outcome in 11 dogs. J Small Animal Pract 37:480–485, 1996.
5. Waldron DR: Urinary Bladder. In Slatter D (ed): Textbook of Small Animal Surgery, 2nd. Philadelphia,
   W.B. Saunders, 1993, pp 1450–1461.
6. Withrow SJ. Tumors of the urinary system. In Withrow SJ, MacEwen EG (eds): Small Animal Clinical
   Oncology. Philadelphia, W.B. Saunders, 1996, pp 380–389.

56. URETHROSTOMIES

C. W. Smith, D.V.M., M.S., Dip. A.C.V.S.

1. What is a urethrostomy?
Creation of a permanent or temporary (nonsutured) opening in the urethra.

2. What are the indications for urethrostomy in the dog?
- Calculi that cannot be removed by urethrotomy or retrograde flushing into the bladder.
- Recurrent calculi production that cannot be managed medically.
- Urethral strictures distal to the scrotum from calculi, trauma, or urethrotomy.
- Severe penile trauma or neoplasia of the prepuce or urethra when penile amputation is nec-
  essary.
- Congenital diseases (hypospadias, deficiency in penile or preputial length) that require am-
  putation of the penis or prepuce (or both) and formation of a more proximal urethral open-
  ing.

3. In the dog, at what levels can urethrostomy be performed?
- Prescrotal
- Scrotal
- Perineal
- Prepubic or antepubic

4. How is a site selected for a urethrostomy?
Based on the site of the obstruction and the surgeon's preference. If a choice exists and the
patient can be castrated, **scrotal urethrostomy** is preferred. Obstruction of the proximal urethra
above the scrotum requires perineal or prepubic urethrostomy.

5. List the advantages of a scrotal urethrostomy.
- Wide, superficial urethra
- Less cavernous tissue (hemorrhage)
- Direct exit for calculi
- Less urine scalding

6. How is scrotal urethrostomy performed?
With the dog in dorsal recumbency, the dog is castrated and the scrotum ablated leaving adequate skin for suturing to the urethra. A catheter is passed into the urethra to facilitate identifi-

cation and incision of the urethra. The retractor penis muscle is elevated and sutured laterally to expose the ventral aspect of the urethra. A 3–4 cm ventral incision is made in the urethra. The periurethral tissue is sutured to the subcutaneous tissue using small absorbable suture in a simple continuous pattern. This helps control the hemorrhage from the erectile tissue and prevents urine leakage. The urethra is sutured to the skin using monofilament nylon in a simple interrupted pattern.

7. What are advantages of a single-layer, simple continuous verus simple interrupted closure of a canine scrotal urethrostomy?
- Control of hemorrhage
- Strength of closure (incorporating tunica albuginea)
- Technical ease and speed

8. Discuss the complications that may occur with scrotal urethrostomy.
1. Hemorrhage commonly occurs when the dog gets excited or urinates and can persist intermittently for 7–10 days after surgery. It is usually self-limiting and not large in volume. **It can be a problem when the dog gets excited during discharge from the hospital.** Sedation is helpful to prevent this risk.
2. Licking and self-mutilation may occur and can be controlled with an Elizabethan collar.
3. Bruising and swelling of the skin around the urethrostomy may indicate leakage of urine into the subcutaneous tissues. If this occurs, an indwelling catheter may be necessary for 3–5 days, or surgical intervention may be indicated.
4. Stricture is a rare occurrence with scrotal urethrostomy.

9. What is an indication for a prescrotal urethrostomy in the dog?
Removal of urethral calculi, tumors, or strictures lodged caudal to the os penis.

10. What major complications can occur with prescrotal urethrostomy?
- Leakage of urine into the scrotum, which may lead to cellulitis
- Hemorrhage in unsutured incisions

11. Why is perineal urethrostomy seldom used in the dog?
- Urine scalding
- Profuse hemorrhage (cavernous tissues)
- Deep location of urethra (suture line tension)

12. What are the indications for perineal urethrostomy in the cat?
- Prevent recurrent urethral obstruction
- Obstruction not relieved by catheterization
- Relief of urethral strictures after multiple urethral obstructions and catheterizations

13. What are some preoperative considerations when performing a perineal urethrostomy?
Cats that have been obstructed are poor anesthetic risks. After unblocking, diuresis should be performed. If unblocking is impossible, antepubic urinary diversion by temporary cystostomy may be necessary to stabilize the ill patient before urologic surgery.

14. Describe the classic Wilson and Harrison technique for perineal urethrostomy.
The cat is positioned in dorsal or ventral recumbency. After placement of a purse-string suture in the anus, an elliptical incision is made around the scrotum and prepuce, and the cat is castrated. The penis is isolated, the ischiocavernous muscles are exposed, and the ischial attachments of these muscles are severed. The fibrous ventral band to the penis is identified and cut. Careful blunt dissection ventrally and digital elevation of the penis and pelvic urethra from the pelvic floor permit mobilization and posterior displacement of the penis and pelvic urethra. The loose tissue

near the penis is carefully excised to expose the retractor penis muscle, bulbocavernous muscle, and bulbourethral glands. The retractor penis muscle is transected near the external anal sphincter muscle, dissected from the urethra, and excised. **Careful dissection dorsal and lateral to the urethra is performed to avoid damage to the pelvic nerves.** The penile urethra is incised on its dorsal surface to the level of the bulbourethral glands. At this point, the urethral opening is about 4 mm in diameter. The incised pelvic urethra and two thirds of the penile urethra are sutured to the skin using small, monofilament nylon or synthetic absorbable suture material in a simple interrupted pattern. The remaining urethra and penis distal to the urethrostomy is excised. A mattress suture may be placed through the retained penile shaft to control hemorrhage. The remaining skin incision is closed routinely. The purse-string suture is removed.

15. Discuss the postoperative care for perineal urethrostomy.

The purse-string suture in the anus is removed, and analgesics are administered. Elizabethan collars are used to prevent licking and self-mutilation. Indwelling urinary catheters are avoided because of the increased risk of ascending infection and stricture formation. Maintaining hydration and alimentation is important. Electrolytes should be monitored, especially potassium. Clots and debris obstructing the new opening should be gently removed postoperatively (some clinicians apply a dollop of Panolog ointment in the urethral meatus to reduce swelling and prevent encrustation). Shredded paper is used in the litter pan. Ointment can be used to protect the perineum. Bladder function is monitored; it is manually expressed because bladder atony can occur after obstruction.

16. What are common complications of a perineal urethrostomy?

Inadequate mobilization and incising of the proximal urethra, causing tension on the suture line and stricture formation (closure of the orifice).

17. What are other problems after surgery?
- Hemorrhage
- Ascending cystitis resulting from underlying uropathy or alteration of urethral meatus
- Subcutaneous urine leakage and incisional dehiscence
- Urinary and fecal incontinence caused by dissection injury to nerves

18. Preservation of lower urinary function in cats to prevent postoperative dysuria may be enhanced by what procedure?

Minimal dissection dorsal to the urethra to avoid trauma to the pelvic plexus and pudendal nerve.

19. What are the indications for urethral prostheses in cats with recurrent urethral obstructions?

None; avoid them at all cost.

20. How are strictures after perineal urethrostomy managed?

Dilation is rarely successful. Surgery to remove the scarred area of the urethra, further mobilization of the urethra, and suturing of the urethra to the skin are necessary. If further mobilization cannot be done, antepubic urethrostomy is indicated.

21. What is the difference between prepubic and subpubic urethrostomy?

The urethra is exteriorized craniad to the brim of the pubis in a prepubic urethrostomy and caudad to the brim of the pubis with a subpubic urethrostomy.

22. Why is prepubic urethrostomy difficult in the dog?

When there is damage to the intrapelvic urethra requiring a prepubic urethrostomy, the urethra may be so short that separation of the prostate from the urethra may be necessary to gain urethral length. With a short urethra, kinking can lead to obstruction.

BIBLIOGRAPHY

1. Bradley RL: Prepubic urethrostomy. Prob Vet Med 1:120, 1989.
2. Dean PW, Hedlund CS: Canine urethrotomy and urethrostomy. Comp Cont Educ Pract Vet 12:1541–1554, 1990.
3. Ellison GW, Lewis DD: Subpubic urethrostomy to salvage a failed perineal urethrostomy in a cat. Comp Cont Educ Pract Vet 11:946–952, 1989.
4. Hosgood G, Hedlund CS: Perineal urethrostomy in cats. Comp Cont Educ Pract Vet 14:1195–1205, 1992.
5. Newton JD, Smeak DD: Simple continuous closure of canine scrotal urethrostomy. J Am Anim Hosp Assoc 32:531–534, 1996.
6. Smeak DD, Newton JD: Canine scrotal urethrostomy. In Bojrab MJ (ed): Current Techniques in Small Animal Surgery, 4th ed. Baltimore, Williams & Wilkins, 1998, pp 465–467.
7. Smith CW: Surgical diseases of the urethra. In Slatter D (ed): Textbook of Small Animal Surgery, 2nd ed. Philadelphia, W.B. Saunders, 1993, pp 1462–1473.
8. Wilson GP, Harrison JW: Perineal urethrostomy in cats. J Am Vet Med Assoc 169:1789–1793, 1971.

57. PYOMETRA

Robin Holtsinger, D.V.M.

1. Which two hormones are implicated in the pathogenesis of pyometra in cats and dogs?
Progesterone and estrogen.

2. How does progesterone affect the uterus?
Stimulates the growth and secretory activity of the endometrial glands, while decreasing myometrial activity.

3. Which bacteria is cultured most frequently from the uterus in pyometra?
Escherichia coli.

4. When is pyometra most frequently diagnosed?
- 1–4 weeks after estrus in intact female **cats**
- 4–8 weeks after estrus in intact female **dogs**

5. What conditions in male dogs have been associated with the development of pyometra?
- Pseudohermaphroditism
- Sertoli cell tumors

6. Name the most common acid-base abnormalities associated with pyometra.
- Respiratory alkalosis
- Metabolic acidosis

7. List the types of renal dysfunction that have been reported to occur in dogs with pyometra.
- Prerenal azotemia
- Primary glomerular disease
- Decreased renal tubular concentrating capacity
- Tubular interstitial disease
- Decreased glomerular filtration rate without concomitant azotemia
- Concomitant renal disease
- Combinations of these

8. What coagulation disorder is most frequently associated with pyometra?
Disseminated intravascular coagulation caused by circulating thromboplastins, tissue hypoperfusion or hypoxia, and vascular endothelial damage.

9. What histopathologic condition of the uterus typically precedes the development of pyometra?
Cystic endometrial hyperplasia. It develops secondary to progesterone influences and results from glandular proliferation and enlargement.

10. Why is the incidence of pyometra so much lower in queens than bitches?
Ovulation in queens is induced rather than spontaneous. Ovulation and subsequent corpus luteum formation and progesterone secretion usually occur only after mating. In this situation, queens are usually pregnant—they do not usually have prolonged exposure to progesterone during nonpregnancy, a feature of the canine cycle.

11. What is the most consistent clinical chemistry finding in patients with pyometra?
Elevated serum alkaline phosphatase is present in 50–75% of cases; occasionally, serum alanine transferase concentrations are mildly elevated. These changes reflect hepatocellular damage in response to toxemia or decreased hepatic circulation secondary to dehydration.

12. What is the recommended treatment for pyometra in dogs and cats?
The traditional therapy for pyometra in bitches and queens is surgical (**ovariohysterectomy**). Many of these patients are sick; although surgery should be performed as soon as possible after diagnosis, patients should be stabilized for surgery with intravenous fluids and broad-spectrum antibiotics. Medical management of pyometra should be reserved for metabolically stable, valuable breeding animals.

13. What intraoperative problems have been described in animals with pyometra?
- Hemorrhage
- Peritonitis
- Uterine torsion
- Entrapment of the pyometra in an inguinal hernia
- Uterine tumors

14. Name two common postoperative problems in pyometra patients.
Inappetence and hypothermia.

15. Name a common concurrent problem in patients with pyometra.
Urinary tract infection.

16. What are the commonest clinical signs noted by owners in cats with pyometra?
- Vaginal discharge (may not be noticed because of cats' grooming habits)
- Anorexia
- Lethargy

17. How is the diagnosis of pyometra confirmed?
Abdominal radiographs or abdominal ultrasonography.

18. What is a stump pyometra?
Uterine stump pyometra may occur after incomplete ovariohysterectomy during which a segment of the uterine body or horns and a portion of the ovarian tissue are not removed or if exogenous progestational compounds have been given.

19. What should you suspect if a postoperative pyometra patient develops a fever, neurologic signs, or lameness?
Bacterial septicemia with thromboemboli, polyarthritis, or both.

20. What is the treatment for bacterial septicemia?
Supportive care and appropriate antibiotic therapy based on bacterial culture and sensitivity testing.

21. What is the prognosis for patients with pyometra?
In general, good with ovariohysterectomy, if abdominal contamination is avoided, shock and sepsis are managed appropriately, and renal insult is reversed with aggressive fluid therapy and elimination of bacterial antigens.

BIBLIOGRAPHY

1. Hedlund CS: Pyometra. In Fossum TW (ed): Small Animal Surgery. St Louis, Mosby, 1997, pp 544–549.
2. Kenney KJ, Matthiesen DT, Brown NO: Pyometra in cats: 183 cases (1979–1984). J Am Vet Med Assoc 191:1130–1132, 1987.
3. Manfra Marretta S, Matthiesen DT, Nichols R. Pyometra and its complications. Prob Vet Med 1:50–62, 1989.
4. Wheaton LG, Johnson AL, Parker AJ: Results and complications of surgical treatment of pyometra: A review of 80 cases. J Am Anim Hosp Assoc 25:563–568, 1989.

58. EPISIOTOMY AND EPISIOPLASTY
Robin Holtsinger, D.V.M.

1. What is an episiotomy?
An incision of the vulvar orifice to allow access to the vestibule and the vagina.

2. What are the indications to perform an episiotomy?
- Surgical exploration of the vagina
- Excision of vaginal masses
- Repair of vaginal lacerations
- Modification of congenital defects or strictures
- Exposure of the urethral papilla
- Facilitation of manual fetal extraction

3. What is vulvar stenosis?
Abnormal fusion of the genital folds or genital swellings. Vulvar stenosis can occur in the body of the vestibule but more commonly in the vulva. Dogs have pain or difficulty mating. It is most commonly described in Collies and Shelties.

4. How is vulvar stenosis treated?
Via partial **epistiotomy** to enlarge the vulvar opening.

5. What causes a persistent hymen?
Failure of the paramesonephric ducts to unite or to cannulate with the urogenital sinus.

6. List the clinical signs associated with vaginal septa.
- Chronic vaginitis
- Urine pooling
- Difficulties in whelping or breeding

7. How are vaginal septa diagnosed?
- Digital vaginal examination
- Vaginoscopy
- Positive contrast vaginography

8. How are vaginal septa treated?
By episiotomy and resection of the bands at their attachments. Dogs without clinical signs need not be treated or may be treated by ovariohysterectomy alone.

9. List the clinical signs associated with vestibulovaginal stenosis.
- Urinary tract infection
- Urinary incontinence
- Chronic vaginitis
- Failure to mate

10. How is vestibulovaginal stenosis treated in the dog?
Vaginoplasty, in which the episiotomy incision is closed in a T fashion to enlarge the diameter of the vaginal lumen. This technique is technically demanding, and the results of surgery have been poor.

11. What is vaginal hyperplasia?
Excessive mucosal folding of the vaginal floor that occurs during the follicular phase of the estrus cycle. This mucosa becomes thickened and edematous and is prolapsed through the vulva. It arises just cranial to the urethral papilla.

12. What breeds are most commonly affected?
Brachycephalic breeds.

13. What is another condition that might be mistaken for vaginal hyperplasia?
Vaginal prolapse. This usually follows parturition and is characterized by complete eversion of the vagina. It is typically **donut-shaped.**

14. What is the treatment of choice for vaginal hyperplasia?
Episiotomy followed by resection of affected tissue. It is important to identify and catheterize the urethral papilla to protect it during excision. **Ovariohysterectomy** prevents future occurrences.

15. What are the commonest tumors of the vulva and vagina in the dog?
- **Leiomyomas** and **fibromas** are reported most frequently.
- **Leiomyosarcomas** and transmissible venereal tumors are the commonest malignant tumors.
- Benign tumors occur most frequently in intact animals, and malignant tumors are seen more commonly in ovariohysterectomized animals.

16. How are vulvar and vaginal tumors treated?
Surgically by **episiotomy** and local resection. Extensive tumors can be treated with **vulvovaginectomy** and **urethrostomy.** The entire vagina and vulva can be safely resected, whereas the distal one third to one half of the urethra can be removed, while still preserving urinary continence.

17. What is an episioplasty?
A reconstructive procedure that is most commonly performed to excise excess skin folds around the vulva that cause perivulvar dermatitis.

18. What is another disorder that necessitates episioplasty?
Vulvar hypoplasia or **infantile vulva,** which is recognized most frequently in spayed females. The infantile vulva is retracted into perineal skin folds, resulting in recurrent vestibulitis and cystitis.

19. Describe is the procedure for performing an episioplasty.
The patient is placed in sternal recumbency with the hind end elevated. After purse-string suture placement, the excessive skin folds are pinched between thumb and index finger to determine the amount of tissue to be removed to exteriorize the vulva. Two parallel crescent-shaped incisions are made around the folds. The skin and subcutaneous fat between the two incisions are excised. Sutures are preplaced at 9, 12, and 3 o'clock, and if the vulva is still recessed, additional tissue is excised. Hemorrhage is controlled, and the incision is closed in two layers.

20. What postoperative measures are taken to optimize surgical results?
- Antibiotics are continued as necessary for the pyoderma.
- An Elizabethan collar is placed until suture removal.
- Weight reduction is recommended.

21. When is episioplasty recommended in cats?
To treat conditions of skin fold pyoderma after perineal urethrostomy.

BIBLIOGRAPHY

1. Bilbrey SA: In: Proceedings ACVS Veterinary Symposium, 1996, pp. 486–488.
2. Hedlund CS: Episiotomy and episioplasty. In Fossum TW (ed): Small Animal Surgery. St Louis, Mosby, 1997, pp 544–549.
3. Pettit G: In Bojrab MJ (ed): Current Techniques in Small Animal Surgery. Philadelphia, Lea & Febiger, 1983, pp 352–359.
4. Thacher C, Bradley RL: Vulvar and vaginal tumors in the dog: A retrospective study. J Am Vet Med Assoc 183:690–696, 1983.

59. MASTECTOMY

Elaine R. Caplan, D.V.M., Dip. A.C.V.S., A.B.V.P.

1. What is the prevalence of mammary gland tumors (MGTs) in the bitch?
The most common tumors of the female dog.

2. What is the relationship of developing MGTs and ovariohysterectomy?
Risk of developing MGTs:
- 0.05% if spayed before the first estrous cycle
- 8.0% if spayed after the first estrous cycle
- 26% if spayed after the second cycle.

3. How are hormone receptors in dogs involved with MGTs?
- 40–60% of malignant MGTs contain estrogen and, less commonly, progesterone receptors.
- 70% of benign MGTs are receptor positive.

4. What is the likelihood that a MGT is malignant in the dog or the cat?
- 50% of dogs have metastatic disease at time of diagnosis
- 80% of cats have metastatic disease at time of diagnosis

5. How many pairs of mammary glands are present in the dog and cat?
- Five pairs in the dog.
- Four pairs in the cat.

Pairs are numbered cranial to caudal.

6. In which mammary glands do most tumors occur in the dog?
Mammary glands 4 and 5.

7. What is an inflammatory mammary carcinoma?
A poorly differentiated, fast-growing MGT that invades lymphatics and appears as an inflamed, edematous, and ulcerative mass.

8. How do you differentiate between an inflammatory carcinoma and mastitis?
- **Inflammatory carcinomas** are firm with diffuse swelling.
- **Mastitis** is more localized and usually seen after estrus or pseudocyesis.

9. List the elements of the diagnostic workup for a MGT?
- Physical examination, including rectal palpation to evaluate internal iliacs
- CBC
- Serum chemistry
- Three-view thoracic radiographs to evaluate lungs and sternal lymph nodes
- Abdominal radiographs
- Abdominal ultrasound
- Urinalysis

10. Why is a coagulogram recommended for a suspected inflammatory carcinoma?
Inflammatory carcinoma is associated with disseminated intravascular coagulopathy.

11. Is fine-needle aspirate and cytology a valuable tool to differentiate between a benign and malignant MGT?
No; it is an insensitive test, and results do not change surgical treatment. **Excisional biopsy** results in definitive diagnosis.

12. Is fine-needle aspirate and cytology ever beneficial in the diagnostic workup for MGT?
Yes; to evaluate lymph nodes for metastasis and for inflammatory carcinomas.

13. How are MGTs staged in dogs?

World Health Organization TNM Staging System:

T (TUMOR SIZE)	N (REGIONAL LYMPH NODE METASTASIS)	M (DISTANT METASTASIS)
T1: <3 cm T2: 3–5 cm T3: > 5 cm	N0: no histologic metastasis N1: nodal metastasis	M0: no distant metastasis M1: distant metastasis

14. What is the treatment of choice for MGTs?
Surgery.

15. List the types of mastectomies.
- **Lumpectomy**—removal of nodule or part of mammary gland.
- **Simple mastectomy**—removal of a single gland.
- **Regional mastectomy**—excision of involved and adjacent glands.
- **Unilateral mastectomy**—removal of all glands and subcutaneous and lymph tissues on one side of the midline.

- **Bilateral mastectomy**—staged or simultaneous removal of both mammary chains and associated tissues.

16. What are the treatment options for inflammatory carcinoma?
- Radiation
- Chemotherapy (doxorubicin, cyclophosphamide, or carboplatin).
Surgery is **not** indicated.

17. Does radical mastectomy result in better survival times compared with lumpectomy in the dog?
No difference in recurrence rate or survival time.

18. What is the goal of surgery in patients with MGTs?
Remove all tumor by the simplest surgical procedure.

19. What determines the surgical dose for canine MGTs?
- Size
- Fixation to surrounding tissue
- Number of lesions

20. What is the indication for nodulectomy and lumpectomy?
A 0.5-cm firm, superficial, nonfixed nodule.

21. When is mammmectomy performed?
- Lesion >1.0 cm
- Lesion centrally located within the gland
- Fixation to skin of lesion or fascia.

22. What are indications for unilateral or bilateral mastectomy?
Multiple tumors or several small tumors when this procedure is faster than multiple lumpectomies or mammectomies.

23. Is ovariohysterectomy routinely performed to decrease local recurrence for mammary gland tumors?
No.

24. What is tamoxifen, and is it generally used for canine MGTs?
An antiestrogen drug; no.

25. List significant prognostic factors for canine MGTs.
- Nuclear differentiation (grade)
- Histologic type
- Degree of invasion
- Tumor size
- Age at diagnosis
- Positive lymph nodes
- Hormone receptor activity
- Ulceration

26. Name common metastatic sites for malignant MGTs in the dog.
- Lung
- Sublumbar lymph nodes
- Liver
- Bone
- Kidney
- Heart
- CNS

27. How do MGTs differ in the cat?
- Prevalence is 17%.
- Positive association between progesterone drugs and development of mammary masses in cats.
- Lower number of progesterone and estrogen receptors compared with the dog.

28. To what organs do malignant MGTs metastasize in the cat?
- Lymph nodes
- Lungs
- Pleura
- Liver
- Diaphragm
- Adrenal glands
- Kidney

29. Does an enlarged, erythematous, necrotic mammary gland indicate inflammatory carcinoma in the cat?
No. This is a benign condition called **fibroepithelial hyperplasia,** which occurs 1–2 weeks after estrus. Ovariohysterectomy prevents its recurrence.

30. How does pulmonary metastasis appear on thoracic radiographs in a cat?
Interstitial densities or miliary lesions with pleural effusion.

31. What is the surgical dose for malignant feline MGT regardless of size?
- Complete unilateral mastectomy if one side is affected
- Staged or simultaneous bilateral mastectomy when tumors are bilateral.

32. Is ovariohysterectomy recommended in the cat at the time of MGT removal?
- Does not decrease recurrence rate.
- Perhaps useful with concurrent ovarian or uterine disease.

33. What is the prognosis for malignant MGTs in the cat?
Median survival time 11–12 months.

34. What are significant prognostic indicators in the cat?
Survival:
- Tumor >3 cm, 4–6 months
- Tumor 2–3 cm, 2 years
- Tumor <2 cm, >3 years

Nuclear differentiation:
- Well-differentiated tumor with few mitotic figures increases survival time.

BIBLIOGRAPHY

1. Hedlund CS: Mammary neoplasia. In Fossum TW (ed): Small Animal Surgery. St. Louis, Mosby, 1997, pp 539–544.
2. MacEwen EG, Withrow SJ: Tumors of the mammary gland. In Withrow SJ, MacEwen EG (ed): Small Animal Clinical Oncology, 2nd ed. Philadelphia, W.B. Saunders, 1996, pp 356–371.
3. Morrison WB: Canine and feline mammary tumors. In Morrison WB (ed): Cancer in Dogs and Cats. Philadelphia, Lippincott Williams & Wilkins, 1998, pp 591–598.

60. PROSTATIC DISEASES

MaryAnn Radlinsky, D.V.M., M.S., Dip. A.C.V.S.

1. What is benign prostatic hyperplasia (BPH)?

Spontaneous enlargement of the prostate gland that occurs in male dogs as they age. There is an increase in the number and size of epithelial cells, so that both hyperplasia and hypertrophy occur. An altered androgen-to-estrogen ratio has been postulated as a cause of BPH. Male dogs castrated early in life do not develop prostatic hyperplasia, and castration results in the regression of prostatic hyperplasia. Estrogen may enhance the sensitivity of the prostate to dihydrotestosterone, potentiating hyperplasia, and estrogen may also cause squamous metaplasia of the prostatic epithelium.

2. If BPH is a benign condition, why is it of clinical concern?

BPH-associated hyperplasia and hypertrophy cause prostatomegaly-related clinical signs:
- Constipation
- Tenesmus
- Dyschezia
- Ribbon-like stool
- Dysuria
- Strangury
- Hematuria
- Discharge from the penile urethra
- Decreased libido
- Reluctance to breed
- Hemospermia and locomotion abnormalities

3. How is BPH diagnosed?

A **presumptive diagnosis** of BPH may be based on the signalment, history, and physical examination findings in an otherwise healthy, male dog. Abdominal radiographs show prostatomegaly. Ultrasound evaluation reveals homogeneous enlargement of the prostate. Dogs with symmetric prostatic enlargement, history, clinical pathologic results, and radiographic and ultrasonographic findings consistent with BPH should respond to **castration.**

If alleviation of prostatomegaly and clinical signs does not occur after castration, repeat evaluation and prostatic fine-needle aspirate or preferably **biopsy** should be performed.

4. What are the treatment options?

- **Castration:** Permanent involution of the prostate takes a minimum of 2–3 weeks.
- **Hormone manipulations:** Synthetic progestins can alleviate signs associated with BPH in dogs, but relapses occur and side effects of the drug should be considered.

5. How common is prostate cancer?

- **Dogs:** 0.29 to 0.6%. Neoplasia represents approximately 5% of all prostatic diseases, but 15% of prostatic disorders prompting diagnostic evaluation.
- **Cats:** rare.

6. List common types of tumors.

- Adenocarcinoma (most common)
- Undifferentiated carcinoma
- Transitional cell carcinoma
- Squamous cell carcinoma

- Leiomyosarcoma
- Fibromyoma
- Leiomyoma

7. Is failure to castrate a predisposing factor for prostate cancer?
No.

8. What clinical signs may be associated with prostatic neoplasia?
1. Animals with prostatic cancer are usually 8–10 years of age with clinical signs of obstruction of the intestinal or urinary tract by the enlarged prostate gland or by local invasion of the tumor.
2. Signs include tenesmus, constipation, dyschezia, dysuria, hematuria, penile urethral discharge, and stranguria.
3. Metastatic lesions may cause pain or lymphatic or venous obstruction, leading to lumbar pain, pelvic limb lameness or weakness, and pelvic limb swelling.

9. What should be included in the diagnostic plan for prostatic neoplasia?
- Rectal examination
- Complete blood count
- Chemistry profile
- Radiography
- Ultrasound
- Ultrasound-guided fine-needle aspirates
- Prostatic biopsy

10. Discuss types of therapy available for prostatic tumors.
Most prostatic tumors have metastasized at the time of diagnosis. The goal of therapy becomes temporary control of the tumor. For tumors localized to the prostate gland, **prostatectomy** and **irradiation** are possible modes of therapy. Prostatectomy results in urinary incontinence from decreased maximum urethral closure pressure and detrusor instability. Radiation can be palliative, and orthovoltage may result in a median survival of 114 days. Chemotherapy combined with total or partial prostatectomy or intraoperative radiation results in 3–5 month survival. Best results are obtained if the tumor is localized to the prostate.

11. What is the prognosis of prostatic neoplasia?
Poor. Patients often die of local disease or metastasis 3–5 months after diagnosis, although survival to 29 months has been reported.

12. What is a prostatic cyst?
There are four different types of prostatic cysts:
1. Multiple cysts associated with BPH
2. Prostatic retention cysts (communication with urethra)
3. Cysts associated with squamous metaplasia (estrogen-dependent) of the prostate gland
4. Paraprostatic cysts

13. Because a prostatic cyst is just a collection of fluid, is there any clinical significance?
Cysts may cause any of the clinical signs associated with prostatomegaly or the presence of a caudal abdominal mass causing encroachment of the urinary or gastrointestinal tracts. Secondary ascending urinary tract infection resulting in abscessation may result in life-threatening sepsis.

14. How is a prostatic cyst diagnosed?
- Rectal examination
- Fine-needle aspiration
- Radiography
- Ultrasound

15. Discuss treatment options for prostatic cysts.
The goal of therapy is to remove, reduce, or drain the prostatic cyst. **Castration** is used to decrease prostatic secretion and should accompany any surgical manipulation for prostatic cysts.

Cystic prostatic hyperplasia responds to castration. Cysts associated with squamous metaplasia require removal of the source of estrogen (discontinuation of administration or castration for removal of testicular neoplasia). Retention cysts, large cysts associated with squamous metaplasia, and paraprostatic cysts are treated by cyst excision, excision and omentalization, excision and partial prostatectomy, and marsupialization.

16. What is marsupialization?

Creation of a permanent stoma for drainage of the cyst and an orifice for lavage (from the Latin, *marsupium*—pouch).

17. What is omentalization?

Packing of affected tissues with omentum to promote angiogenesis, enhance lymphatic drainage, create adhesions, and resolve chronic infection.

18. Are there any special postoperative concerns with the surgical treatment of prostatic cysts?
- Chronic urinary tract infections
- Recurrence if incomplete excision
- Urinary incontinence
- Abscessation

19. What causes infection of the prostate?

An ascending infection from the urinary or reproductive tracts; however, hematogenous seeding of the prostate is possible. The adjacent urethra has a normal flora with defenses against infection, including mechanical flushing of the tract with urination, zone of high positive pressure, surface characteristics of the mucosal lining, and normal urethral peristalsis. Zinc-associated antibacterial factors are present within prostatic secretions, providing a local defense within the prostate. Loss of any of these protective functions may result in urethritis, cystitis, and ascending prostatitis.

20. What are the most commonly isolated pathogens?
- *Escherichia coli* (most common)
- *Proteus*
- *Staphylococcus*
- *Streptococcus*
- *Pseudomonas*
- *Brucella canis*

21. What special concern is associated with *B. canis*?

B. canis has zoonotic potential, and dogs showing any signs should be tested and owners notified of results.

22. How serious is prostatic infection"

1. Signs vary from mild clinical abnormalities (pain, fever) to lethargy, anorexia, vomiting, sepsis, shock, and death.

2. Chronic prostatitis may be asymptomatic, or the dog may have intermittent episodes of dysuria and hematuria.

3. Infertility may also be the presenting complaint.

23. How is prostatitis diagnosed?
- Pain during rectal palpation
- Leukocytosis with a left shift
- Elevated serum alkaline phosphatase, alanine aminotransferase, bilirubin, prothrombin time, activated partial thromboplastin time, and fibrin degradation products
- Hematuria, bacteriuria, and pyuria
- Prostatomegaly with mineral densities (radiography)
- Fibrosis, mineralization, cavitation, and hyperechogenicity (ultrasonography)

24. What are the treatment options for dogs with prostatitis?
Antibiotics with a high pKa (erythromycin, clindamycin, and potentiated sulfas) or a high lipid solubility (chloramphenicol, macrolides, potentiated sulfas, and fluoroquinolones).

25. Describe the surgical techniques that are available for prostatic abscessation.
Drainage via passive or active drains, partial prostatectomy, or omentalization. The gland should be isolated from the abdomen with laparotomy sponges, and dorsal dissection should be minimized to protect the nervous and vascular supply. A urinary catheter placed before surgery allows identification and preservation of the urethra. After drainage and culture of the abscess, any defects in the urethra may be sutured, or urinary diversion with an indwelling urethral catheter or tube cystostomy and closed collection system should be instituted.

The cavities within each lobe or in the entire prostate are digitally dissected and copiously lavaged. Omentalization is the most common surgical technique. The omentum is passed through bilateral incisions in the ventrolateral prostate to encircle the prostatic urethra. Care is taken to make the incisions large enough for easy passage of the omentum and to avoid compression of the urethra. Alternatively, Penrose drains or closed suction drains may be place in the prostate and the caudal abdomen bandaged after surgery.

26. What is subtotal prostatectomy?
Intracapsular **electroscalpel** dissection of the prostate proceeds with sequential half-moon incisions, ultimately retaining 2–3 mm of parenchyma adjacent to the urethra. Alternatively, a **laser** (neodymimum-yttrium-aluminum-garnet) may be used to ablate all ventrolateral parenchyma, leaving the dorsal and periurethral parenchyma intact. An **ultrasound surgical aspirator** may also be used to perform intracapsular subtotal prostatectomy in dogs. The advantage of the aspirator is the preservation of nerves and vessels within the prostate.

27. What is total prostatectomy?
The neurovascular structures and as much urethra as possible must be preserved, followed by prostatic excision and urethral anastomosis. Most dogs are incontinent after prostatectomy.Total prostatectomy for prostatic abscessation is technically difficult and rarely performed.

28. Are there any special postoperative concerns with surgical treatment of prostatic abscesses?
* Urinary incontinence
* Urinary tract infection
* Recurrent abscessation

29. What is the prognosis?
Approximately 50%; dogs with sepsis, shock, or cardiopulmonary failure have a poor prognosis.

BIBLIOGRAPHY

1. Basinger RR, Robinette CL, Hardie EM, et al: The prostate. In Slatter D (ed): Textbook of Small Animal Surgery. Philadelphia, W.B. Saunders, 1993, pp 1349–1367.
2. Caney SM, Holt PE: Prostatic carcinoma in two cats. J Small Animal Pract 39:140–143, 1998.
3. Harari J, Dupuis J: Surgical treatments for prostatic diseases in dogs. Semin Vet Med Surg 10:43–47, 1995.
4. Kincaid LF, Sanghvi NT: Noninvasive ultrasonic subtotal ablation of the prostate in dogs. Am J Vet Res 57:1225–1227, 1996.
5. Rawlings CA, Mahaffey MB, Barsanti JA, et al: Use of partial prostatectomy for treatment of prostatic abscesses and cysts in dogs. J Am Vet Med Assoc 211:868–871, 1997.
6. White RAS, Williams JM: Intracapsular omentalization: a new technique for management of prostatic abscesses in dogs. Vet Surg 24:390–395, 1995.

61. ECTOPIC AND NEOPLASTIC TESTICLES

Holly S. Mullen, D.V.M., Dip. A.C.V.S.

1. What are ectopic testicles?
Testicles located somewhere other than in the scrotum; also called **undescended testicles.**

2. What is cryptorchidism?
A developmental defect characterized by the failure of one (unilateral cryptorchid) or both (bilateral cryptorchid) testes to descend into the scrotum.

3. Where may ectopic testicles be located?
- **Intraabdominal**—between the kidney and inguinal ring.
- **Subcutaneous**—between inguinal and prescrotal areas.

4. The testicles descend into the scrotum?
The **gubernaculum** (from the Latin, *helm*, or something that guides), a fetal ligament attached to the caudal epididymis and testis and the bottom of the scrotum guides the descent of the testes into the scrotum; it atrophies at the time of birth.

5. What is monorchidism?
The rare condition of having only one testicle. The ductus deferens, cremaster muscle, testicular artery, and vein are usually present on the affected (missing) side.

6. How does monorchidism occur?
- **Congenital testicular agenesis**—testicle never develops.
- **Congenital testicular hypoplasia**—testicle develops, then undergoes regression before birth, probably because of intrauterine torsion of the testicle.

7. What is anorchidism?
Having no testicles. This usually refers to castrated males because congenital anorchidism has not been reported.

8. Is cryptorchidism an inherited trait?
Definitely in some breeds; probably in most.
In **dogs,** it is a sex-linked autosomal recessive occurring most frequently in small-breed dogs.
In **cats,** it is presumed to be a similar trait, although less common.

9. Which is more common, unilateral or bilateral cryptorchidism?
- **Dogs—Unilateral.** right side retained twice as frequently.
- **Cats**—both sides retained with the same frequency.

10. Are there breed predispositions for cryptorchidism?
- **Dogs**
  Miniature schnauzer
  Poodle
  Pomeranian
  Chihuahua
  Yorkshire terrier
  Siberian husky
  Shetland sheepdog
- **Cats**
  Persian

11. At what age should the testicles be descended?
At, or shortly after, birth. Evidence suggests that testicles not located in the scrotum by 2–3 months of age should be considered permanently undescended.

12. What are some characteristics of the retained testicle?
- Smaller than normal size
- Loss of exocrine function (infertile) because of exposure to body heat
- Normal endocrine function (produces testosterone)
- More prone to neoplasia and torsion than normal testicle

13. Can the scrotal testicle of a unilateral cryptorchid be considered normal?
No. There is a higher incidence of disturbed function and increased incidence of testicular neoplasia of more than one histologic type even in the scrotal testicle.

14. Is there any medically effective therapy to bring down a retained testicle?
No.

15. How accurate is palpation for detection of a retained testis?
Not very. Palpation of retained abdominal testicles is almost impossible. Prescrotal testicles are felt easily, but retained inguinal testicles can be reliably palpated only about 50% of the time in cats and slightly more often in dogs.

16. What physical examination finding helps in determining the intact nature of a young adult stray male cat with an empty scrotum?
Examine the penis. **Penile barbs,** or spines, are present. Barbs develop only when testosterone is present in the body. The cat is bilateral cryptorchid.

17. What is a method of detecting a retained, unpalpable testicle in a dog or cat with an empty scrotum who is showing signs of testosterone influence?
HCG stimulation test — to see if there is an increase in endogenous testosterone production (usually from a retained testicle, but cannot rule out a tumor).

18. Describe the best method for castration of a unilateral cryptorchid.
Dog
Make a prescrotal incision for normal testicle removal; it may be possible to retrieve a caudad inguinal retained testicle from same incision. If not, make incision directly over retained inguinal testicle. If an abdominal testicle, make a parapreputial skin incision on the affected side, lateral to the tip of the prepuce; separate muscle layers and enter the peritoneum; 90% of the time the testicle is found at this point in the abdomen.
Cat
Make a scrotal incision for the normal testicle; make a caudad abdominal skin incision, and expose the inguinal ring on affected side. If the ductus deferens exiting the ring is seen, follow it until the testicle is found in the subcutis. If no ductus, make a caudad abdominal, ventral midline incision, and look along the dorsolateral abdominal wall.

19. Describe the best method for castration of a bilateral cryptorchid.
Dog
Make a lateral parapreputial skin incision, reflect the prepuce, and enter the abdomen through a ventral midline linea incision that starts at about the tip of the prepuce; look laterally along the right and left dorsal abdominal wall.
Cat
Use the same approach as for a unilateral cryptorchid.

20. What structure may be confused for the ductus deferens and injured during abdominal castration?
Ureter.

21. What can the surgeon do if he or she is having trouble locating a retained abdominal testicle?
Find the ductus deferens at the level of the prostate and follow it down to the testicle.

22. Do cats have a prostate, and, if so, is it easily identified?
Yes, and no.

23. How common are testicular tumors in the dog and cat?
- **Dog**—testicular tumors make up 5–15% of all tumors.
- **Cat**—very rare.

24. List the tumor types that have been reported in the testicles.
- Sertoli cell
- Interstitial (Leydig) cell
- Granulosa cell
- Sarcoma
- Seminoma
- Hemangioma
- Embryonal carcinoma
- Metastatic (rare)

25. What are the three most common testicular tumor types in the dog?
Sertoli, seminoma, and interstitial cell tumors occur with equal frequency in descended testes. In retained testes, 60% of tumors are **Sertoli** cell, and 40% are **seminomas**. Two or more tumor types can occur in the same testicle.

26. How do these three tumors behave in the dog?
1. **Sertoli**—10–20% metastasize, 20–50% cause feminization (of these, 15% develop estrogen-induced bone marrow suppression).
2. **Seminoma** — <5% metastasize, do not feminize.
3. **Interstitial**—unlikely to metastasize, rarely may cause feminization.

27. What tumors are commonest in cats?
Not enough information exists to be sure. One study suggests **Sertoli** and **interstitial cell** tumors, followed by carcinoma and seminoma. All have been reported to metastasize except interstitial cell tumor.

28. How common are testicular tumors in undescended testicles?
Occur **13 times** more frequently (and in younger dogs) in retained testicles. They are **twice** as common in **inguinal** verus abdominal testicles.

29. List clinical signs of testicular neoplasia.
- Scrotal asymmetry
- Testicular firmness
- Feminization
- Acute abdomen associated with torsion of a retained abdominal testicular tumor
- Palpable testicular mass
- Painful testicle
- Abdominal or inguinal mass (retained testicle)

30. Name the differential diagnoses for testicular tumors.
- Testicular torsion
- Trauma (hematoma)
- Scrotal hernia

- Orchitis
- Epididymitis
- Spermatocele
- Scrotal neoplasia (rare)

31. Name some signs of hyperestrogenism in a dog with a feminizing testicular tumor.
- Attraction to other males
- Contralateral testicular atrophy
- Prostatomegaly (BPH)
- Gynecomastia
- Pendulous prepuce
- Bone marrow suppression
- Alopecia
- Pigmentary changes

32. Besides estrogen, are other feminizing hormones secreted by neoplastic testicles?
Progesterone from a Sertoli cell tumor has been reported to cause nonpruritic alopecia in a dog.

33. What is the best treatment for testicular neoplasia?
Castration. If there is any suggestion of feminization, check a complete blood count for effects of bone marrow suppression.

BIBLIOGRAPHY

1. Boothe HW: Testes and epididymides. In Slatter D (ed): Textbook of Small Animal Surgery, 2nd ed. Philadelphia, W.B. Saunders, 1993, pp 1325–1336.
2. Crane SW: Orchiectomy of descended and retained testes in the dog and cat. In Bojrab MJ (ed): Current Techniques in Small Animal Surgery, 4th ed. Baltimore, Williams & Wilkins, 1998, pp 517–523.
3. Millis DL, Hauptman JG, Johnson CA: Cryptorchidism and monorchidism in cats: 25 cases (1980–1989). J Am Vet Med Assoc 200:1128–1130, 1992.
4. Richardson EF, Mullen HS: Cryptorchidism in cats. Comp Cont Educ Pract 15:1342–1345, 1993.

III. Orthopedic Surgery

62. PRINCIPLES OF FRACTURE REPAIR

Robert M. Radasch, D.V.M., M.S., Dip. A.C.V.S.

1. What is the goal of fracture fixation?
An early return to normal limb function.

2. How is this goal obtained?
- Functional or anatomic reconstruction of damaged bone column.
- Maintenance of proximal and distal joint alignments.
- Preservation of neurovascular elements, periosseous soft tissue, and bone structures.
- Rigid (early) fracture stability.

3. Which bones in dogs are most frequently fractured (or presented for treatment)?
According to the Veterinary Medical Data Bank at Purdue (1980–1990):
- Pelvis 22%
- Femur 19%
- Radius/ulna 10%
- Tibia/fibula 9%
- Humerus 8%
- Hind/forefeet 6%
- Scapula 2%

4. List the common factors that determine location and pattern of a fracture.
- Nature and magnitude of the disruptive forces (compression, bending, shear, tension, torsion).
- Material properties (cortical or cancellous) of the bone, porosity, rate of bone loading, and orientation of the bone's microstructure.
- Age, size, and shape of bone.
- Concomitant bone defects or disease.

5. What are the five basic forces that cause bone fractures?
1. Compression
2. Tension
3. Bending
4. Shear (transverse)
5. Torsion

6. What typical fracture pattern develops in a bone subjected to these loads?

LOADING MODE	FRACTURE PATTERNS
Compression	Short oblique*
Tension	Transverse
Shear	Short oblique
Bending	Transverse, or short oblique with butterfly fragment on compression surface†
Torsion	Oblique spiral fracture
Combined	Complex fracture with comminutions, fissures, and fracture lines

*Occasionally, a transverse fracture occurs in a vertebral body or growth plate.
†Combined bending and compressive loading accentuates the obliquity of fracture lines on the compression surface, resulting in a butterfly fragment.

7. Most fractures occurring *in vivo* are a result of which forces?
A combination of three or more loading forces.

8. Which disruptive forces most commonly affect repaired diaphyseal fractures during the postoperative period?
Bending, compression, and **torsional** disruptive forces are present as a result of normal weight bearing and muscular contractions. Depending on the bone and fracture location, tensile and shear forces may also be present.

9. What is strain?
Change in bone dimension (as a result of loading) compared with the bone's original dimension (**strain = change length/original length**).

10. How much strain can a bone tolerate before fracture?
Cancellous bone does not fracture until strain exceeds approximately 7%, whereas cortical bone fractures if strain exceeds 2%.

11. Define the interfragmentary strain theory.
Pluripotential cells located at a fracture are sensitive and responsive to the degree of deformation or strain present at the fracture gap. Different cell lines withstand varying levels of strain, beyond which the cells are incapable of survival.

12. How much strain can granulation tissue, cartilage, fibrous tissue, and bone tolerate and still heal?

Granulation tissue—100%	Cartilage—10%
Fibrous tissue—20%	Bone—2%

13. What factors should be considered when choosing an implant system to repair a fracture?
- Patient factors (e.g., age, health) and characteristic of the fracture (transverse, spiral, etc.)
- Owner compliance and patient's environment
- Available orthopedic equipment and expertise of surgeon
- Expense of treatment

14. What is the fracture-assessment score?
A scale of 1 through 10 representing **mechanical** (size of dog, character of fracture, number of affected limbs), **biologic** (patient and tissue healths), and **clinical** (postoperative care) factors that affect treatment outcome. Low numbers (< 4) reflect guarded prognosis and imply selection of technically demanding techniques and implants. High numbers (>8) suggest a good prognosis for easily treatable and recoverable injuries and involve less complex procedures.

15. List common implant systems used to repair long bone fractures.

• Intramedullary (IM) pins	• Linear external fixators
• Rush pins	• Circular external fixators
• Cerclage/hemicerclage and Kirschner wires	• Interlocking nails (IN)
	• Plate and screws

16. What are the capabilities of primary fixation devices to neutralize disruptive fracture forces?

	DISRUPTIVE FORCE				
FIXATION DEVICE	TENSION	COMPRESSION	SHEAR	BENDING	TORSION
Cast/splint	−	−	−	+	+
Single IM pin	−	−	±	+	−
Multiple IM pins	−	−	±	+	±
Bone plate	+	+	+	+	+
Plate—rod	+	+	+	+	+
IN	+	+	+	+	+
Linear external fixator	+	+	+	+	+
Circular external fixator	+	+*	+	+	+

† = effective; − = ineffective; ± = potentially effective.
*Narrow, tensioned wires permit controlled axial micromotion.

17. What are the functions of auxiliary implants?
Cerclage/hemicerclage, Kirschner wires (K-wires), and (lag) screws provide fragmentary alignment and are susceptible to disruptive forces, and **require** protection (from failure) by use of primary implants.

18. How do bone fractures heal?
- **Indirect union** occurs with unstable (pins, wires) implants and is composed of fracture gaps filled with (in sequence) a hematoma, granulation tissue, fibrocartilage, cancellous bone, and cortical bone. A periosteal callus is visible radiographically.
- **Direct bone** union occurs with a stable implant (plate) producing cortical contact or small (200 μ) gaps. Bone formation develops directly through haversian remodeling without fibrocartilage formation. Radiographs reveal little callus and loss of fracture lines.

19. How do fractures heal after stabilization with an external fixator?
Combination of endosteal and periosteal callus formation based on the character of the fracture and degree of stabilization (type of fixator).

20. What is dynamization?
The technique of manipulating and destabilizing the implant system, used to repair a fracture. This allows controlled **axial load sharing** by the fracture, while preventing excessive bending and rotational disruptive forces. Dynamization is believed to stimulate early fracture callus.

21. What implant systems can be dynamized?
Virtually any system by removal of screws or pins. Because of their external location, **linear** and **circular fixators** lend themselves best to this process.

22. How are open fractures classified?
- **Grade I**—bone fragments penetrate the muscle and skin from within, minimal soft tissue damage.
- **Grade II**—external trauma causes a penetrating wound of the soft tissues with exposure of the bone, moderate soft tissue damage.
- **Grade III**—external trauma causes a penetrating wound of the soft tissue and exposure of bone, severe soft tissue and bone damage.

23. How likely are grade I, II, and III open fractures to develop postoperative osteomyelitis?
- Grade I and II open fractures, if properly managed, are no more likely to develop osteomyelitis than a closed fracture.

- Grade III open fractures, because of the extensive soft tissue damage, vascular impairment, and contamination, are likely to develop osteomyelitis.

24. Can open reduction and internal fixation be performed if bacterial contamination of a fracture is present?

Yes. Bone heals in the face of infection if adequate stability is provided (and proper medical therapy initiated).

25. What is biologic osteosynthesis?

Also referred to as **biologic fracture fixation** or **bridging osteosynthesis**; it involves a limited surgical approach to a comminuted fracture with minimal manipulation of the fracture fragments. This concept is based on the preservation of the surrounding soft tissue envelope (favoring the local biology) and distribution of interfragmentary motion to a level that favors bone healing. Spatial realignment of the limb (joint surfaces) is achieved and the fracture buttressed with an appropriate implant, such as a pin-plate combination, IN, or an external fixator. Anatomic reconstruction is sacrificed; however, healing times are reduced and complications are minimized.

26. Does an end-threaded trocar pin have any advantages over a smooth trocar pin?

No. The end-threaded trocar pin was initially developed to have improved holding power in cancellous bone. Because the thread is cut into the pin shank (negative-profile), however, no improvement in holding power is offered by the pin. Where the threads are cut into the pin shank, a significant loss of strength occurs and predisposes the pin to cycle and break at that point.

27. When using an IM pin to repair a fracture, what diameter of pin should be selected?

The ability of an IM pin to resist bending is directly proportional to its radius raised to the fourth power. Filling the medullary cavity at the fracture site maximizes the resistance to bending and horizontal shear forces; however, it can result in damage to the medullary blood supply. It is generally recommended to choose an IM pin diameter that fills approximately 60–70% of the medullary cavity.

28. What is a Rush pin and how is it used?

A form of IM pin that is designed to be driven into bone with special instruments. A true Rush pin has a beveled or **sled** point. The pin enters the bone distal to the fracture, crosses the fracture, deflects and glides off the opposite inner cortex traveling up the medullary cavity, and becomes seated in the proximal end of the bone. This provides three-point fixation under spring-loaded tension. Rush pins are generally used for metaphyseal fractures of long bones. The pins were developed by physicians (Rush family) in the 1930s in Mississippi.

29. What is stack pinning?

An IM pinning technique in which multiple small-diameter pins are placed down the medullary cavity rather than a single larger pin.

30. Biomechanically, does stack pinning have any benefit over using a single IM pin?

Probably not. Stack pinning improves rotational stability (contact between pins and endosteal cortex). Clinical studies have shown a greater than 50% complication rate and generally unsatisfactory results with the use of stack pinning.

31. What are the fundamental principles used for proper cerclage wire applications?

- Length of the fracture is two times the diameter of the bone.
- Wires should be used only if the full cylinder of bone can be reconstructed.
- No more than two fragments and two fracture lines should be present.
- 18- or 20-gauge wires should be used.
- Wires should be tight and avoid soft tissue entrapment.

- Wires should be perpendicular to the long axis of the bone.
- Wires should be 0.5 cm from fracture ends and spaced 1 cm apart.
- At least two to three wires should be used.

32. List the basic types of knots used to tighten a cerclage wire.
  - Looped knot
  - Twist knot
  - Granny knot

33. Is one form of knot better than another?
Yes. Generally, **loop** and **twist** knots work well in clinical cases, and granny knots do not.

34. What are the advantages of each type of knot used to tighten a cerclage wire?
  - **Looped knot:** 40–60% more static tension than twist knot, more bone compression, less soft tissue irritation.
  - **Twist knot:** Resists knot slippage and distraction better than looped, requires greater tensile force to break.

35. What is the tension band principle?
An engineering principle in which tensile or distractive forces are converted into compressive forces at the fracture site. It is most often accomplished by the use of 2 K-wires or pins and a figure-eight wire, placed across an osteotomy or fracture in which the pull of muscles, tendons, or ligaments results in distraction of bone fragments.

36. Name three functions of a bone plate.
(1) Compression, (2) neutralization, or a (3)buttress of the fracture.

37. Do different types of plates serve as a compression plate, neutralization plate, or a buttress plate?
No. Any dynamic compression plate can be used as a compression, neutralization, or buttress plate. The difference is how the plate and screws are applied and the type of fracture.

38. What type of fracture should be stabilized by a compression, neutralization, or a buttress plate?
  - **Compression plate**—a transverse or short oblique fracture
  - **Neutralization plate**—comminuted fracture anatomically reconstructed
  - **Buttress plate**—bone loss present or anatomic reconstruction cannot be obtained.

39. What are the ways in which the bending stiffness and strength of a plated fractured bone can be maximized?
  - Spanning the length of bone with the plate
  - Using wide and thick plates
  - Using the largest screws possible
  - Filling all holes of the plate with a screw
  - Using a plate-rod construct

40. The tension band principle also applies to bone plating. Plates placed on the tension band surface of long bones are intended to convert tensile forces into compressive forces. What is the tension band surface of the femur, tibia, humerus, and radius?
  - **Femur:** craniolateral surface
  - **Tibia:** craniolateral surface
  - **Humerus:** craniomedial surface
  - **Radius:** cranial surface

41. What is the minimum number of screws placed on each side of a fracture when using a bone plate?
Enough screws should be used so that six cortices on each side of the fracture are engaged by screws. Three screws could be used if each screw engages two cortices.

42. What is a plate-rod construct?

The combination of a bone plate and an IM pin that occupies approximately 50% of the marrow cavity. Generally, plate-rod constructs are used when a plate must buttress a section of bone because anatomic reconstruction was not or could not be performed.

43. What biomechanical advantages does a plate-rod construct have over a buttress plate?

1. Combining an IM pin with a bone plate reduces the bending strain in the plate by twofold.
2. The IM pin increases the fatigue life of the plate by ten times.

44. What is an IN?

A large-diameter pin with holes to accept screws. The nail is placed into the medullary cavity of a fracture bone and locked to the bone by inserting screws through the holes in the IN and corresponding holes drilled into the cis-cortices and trans-cortices of the bone.

45. What biomechanical advantages does an IN have over an IM pin or plate?

1. An IN is placed along the neutral axis of the bone similar to an IM pin instead of eccentrically located similar to a bone plate.
2. An IN provides superior bending stiffness, resistance to torsional forces, axial stability, and lower implant failure rates than IM pins or bone plates.

46. The holes in an IN are mechanically the weakest part of the nail. What rule of thumb should be followed when placing a nail to prevent the IN from breaking at a screw-hole?

A screw-hole in the nail should be 2 cm or more away from the fracture to minimize the stress riser effect, nail fatigue, and breakage.

47. List the factors that affect stiffness and strength of an external fixator.

- Frame geometry
- Number and size of pins
- Pin design (threaded verus nonthreaded, negative verus positive profile pins)
- Spatial orientation of fixation pins
- Number of pins inserted into each bone fragment
- Distance between bone and clamps (**working** length of pin)
- Distance between clamps
- Orientation of clamps
- Size, number, and length of interconnecting rods
- Material property of interconnecting rod (metal verus acrylic or epoxy)
- Method of pin insertion (hand chuck verus slow and fast power insertion)

48. Which three implant systems provide excellent biomechanical stability, biologic preservation, and complementary support?

1. IN and screws
2. IM pin and plate construct
3. IM pin and external fixation (connected)

49. What does the term *KE fixator* refer to?

Kirschner-Ehmer external fixation splint, developed in Seattle in the 1940s by Ehmer, a Washington State veterinarian, and the Kirschner manufacturing company.

50. What diameter of acrylic tubing equals the strength of a medium external fixator stainless steel interconnecting rod?

2 cm (approximately ¾ inch).

51. What damaging physical phenomenon occurs when using acrylic to form an interconnecting external fixation rod?

As acrylic polymerizes, it creates an **exothermic reaction,** which can generate high temperatures at the pin-bone interface, creating thermal necrosis of bone. This can result in premature pin loosening. **Bathing** the acrylic bar or fixation pins in saline-cooled sponges minimizes heat conduction from the acrylic to the fixation pin and bone.

52. What type of pin offers the best resistance to *pull out* when applying an external fixator?

A positive-profile, end-threaded pin. This is a pin in which the threads have been *rolled onto* the pin shank.

53. Is external fixation pin insertion speed important?

Yes. If a smooth or threaded pin is inserted at a high RPM, heat generation at the bone-pin interface occurs, causes thermal necrosis of the bone, and leads to premature pin loosening and pin tract drainage.

54. If using power equipment, what speed of pin insertion should be used?

Less than 150–200 RPMs.

55. What is *predrilling,* and what benefit does it have?

A technique used for external fixation pin insertion to reduce microfracturing of bone and minimize thermal necrosis during pin insertion. A drill bit (smaller in diameter than the threaded ESF pin) is used to predrill a hole through the bone before fixation pin insertion. After the hole has been predrilled, the external fixation pin is inserted by hand or slow speed power.

56. When choosing a transfixation pin, what rule in pin diameter selection should be followed?

The diameter of the transfixation pin should not be greater than 20–30% of the bone diameter. Use of a larger diameter pin may lead to a stress riser effect and fracture of the bone at the pin insertion site.

57. What is a circular external fixator?

An apparatus that consists of full cylindrical rings, partial rings, and arches connected to each other using all-thread, linear motors or hinges. It has commonly been referred to as the **Ilizarov apparatus.** The rings are connected to the bone by the use of narrow wires, which are placed under tension.

58. Who was Ilizarov?

A preeminent Russian orthopedist (1921–1992) who developed the external fixator (in Siberia) to treat complex and infected fractures as well as shortened, deformed limbs. After his successful treatment in 1967 of Olympic high jumper Valerie Brumel's chronically infected nonunion fractures of both legs, Ilizarov's reputation soared into national medical prominence.

59. Do circular external fixators have any benefit in the treatment of fractures?

Yes. In highly comminuted fractures, circular fixators enhance the rate of healing. Because it is usually placed on the bone in a closed fashion, it maximizes the principle of biologic osteosynthesis.

60. What unique and advantageous biomechanical characteristics do circular external fixators possess?

Circular external fixators are attached to the fractured bone with narrow-tensioned wires. These wires allow controlled (<1mm) axial micromotion at the fracture site during weight bearing, which stimulates early bone healing by distraction osteogenesis.

61. What is an olive wire?

A narrow-diameter pin (similar to a K-wire) with a bead on its shank. It is used with circular external fixators as a transfixation wire holding the device to the bone. Use of olive wires imparts resistance to bone translation. It can also be used to move bone segments or fragments to improve bone alignment.

62. List the parameters of a circular external fixator that can be altered to change the degree of rigidity (or elasticity) in a fracture.

Ring diameter and wire length	Diameter of transfixation wires
Number of rings above and below the fracture	Wire tension
	Position of the bone within the rings
Spatial orientation of rings in relationship to the fracture	Number of wires used
	Angle of wire intersection

63. What are major complications of fracture repair?

- Nonunion
- Malunion
- Delayed union
- Acute or chronic osteomyelitis
- Fracture disease

64. What is fracture disease?

A set of soft tissue complications secondary to a fracture or the results of a fracture repair:
1. Adhesions (periosseous) preventing the normal gliding motion of muscles and tendons.
2. Excessive periarticular capsular fibrosis resulting in reduced joint range of motion.
3. Disuse atrophy of articular cartilage leading to secondary degenerative joint disease.

65. What is stress protection or stress shielding?

A sequela to the use of an excessively rigid implant, such as a bone plate. The rigid implant prevents the bone from responding to normal physiologic stresses as a result of a mismatch of stiffness between the implant and bone resulting in thinning of the surrounding cortical bone. It is particularly common in toy breeds, in which forelimb bone plate repair has been performed. It can result in near-complete bone resorption under a plate and a secondary pathologic fracture. Any implant system can result in stress protection.

66. How can stress protection be avoided?

- Use of limited contact plates
- Reducing construct stiffness by removing bone screws or fixator pins during healing (6 weeks postsurgery)

67. What is the *triple A* score for postoperative evaluations of fracture repair?

- **Activity** (osteogenesis, bone healing)
- **Alignment** (apposition of fragments)
- **Appliance** (apparatus or implant stability)

BIBLIOGRAPHY

1. Anderson MA, Palmer RH, Aron DN: Improving pin selection and insertion technique for external skeletal fixation. Comp Cont Educ Pract Vet 19:485–493, 1997.
2. Aron DN, Palmer RH, Johnson AL: Biological strategies and a balanced concept for repair of highly comminuted long bone fractures. Comp Cont Educ Pract Vet 17:35–42, 1995.
3. De Young DJ, Probst CW: Methods of internal fracture fixation—general principles. In Slatter D (ed): Textbook of Small Animal Surgery, 2nd ed. Philadelphia, W.B. Saunders, 1993, pp 1610–1631.
4. Durall I, Diaz MC: Early experience with the use of an interlocking nail for the repair of canine femoral shaft fractures. Vet Surg 25:397–406, 1996.

5. Egger EL: External skeletal fixation-general principles. In Slatter D (ed): Textbook of Small Animal Surgery, 2nd ed. Philadelphia, W.B. Saunders, 1993, pp 1641–1656.
6. Hulse D, Hyman W: Reduction in plate strain by addition of an intramedullary pin. Vet Surg 26:451–459, 1997.
7. Hulse DA, Johnson AL: Fundamentals of orthopedic surgery and fracture management. In Fossum TW (ed): Small Animal Surgery. St. Louis, Mosby, 1997, pp 705–765.
8. Lewis DD, Bronson DG, Samchukov ML: Biomechanics of circular external skeletal fixation. Vet Surg 27:454–464, 1998.
9. Pardo AD: Methods of internal fracture fixation—cerclage wiring and tension band fixation. In Slatter D (ed): Textbook of Small Animal Surgery, 2nd ed. Philadelphia, WB Saunders, 1993, pp 1631–1640.
10. Piermattei DL, Flo GL (eds): Fractures: Classification, diagnosis and treatment. In: Handbook of Small Animal Orthopedics and Fracture Treatment, 3rd ed. Philadelphia, W.B. Saunders, 1997, pp 24–146.
11. Radasch RM: Biomechanics of bone and fractures. Vet Clin North Am Small Animal Pract 29:1045–1082, 1999.
12. Schwarz P: Fracture biomechanics. In Bojrab MJ (ed): Disease Mechanisms in Small Animal Surgery, 2nd ed. Philadelphia, Lea & Febiger, 1991, pp 1009–1026.

63. MANDIBLE AND MAXILLARY FRACTURES

Kristi M. Sandman, D.V.M.

1. What are the common causes for jaw fractures in the dog and cat?
- Trauma
  - Vehicular trauma
  - Fights with other animals
  - Kicks
  - Gunshot wounds
  - **High-rise** syndrome in cats
- Pathologic
  - Periodontal disease
  - Oral neoplasia
  - Metabolic derangements

2. Where do fractures of the mandible commonly occur?
- In **dogs:**
  - Premolar
  - Molar
  - Symphyseal
- In **cats:**
  - Symphyseal

3. What are important preanesthetic considerations for an animal with a jaw fracture?
- Patent airway
- Hemorrhage from facial and oral injuries
- Cardiac dysrhythmias
- Brain trauma
- Pneumothorax and hemothorax
- Pulmonary contusions
- Diaphragmatic hernia

4. What is the primary goal of jaw fracture repair?
Restoration of proper dental occlusion.

5. Why would it be advantageous to perform a pharyngostomy to administer anesthesia for repair of jaw fractures?
In mandibular and maxillary fracture repairs, frequent closure of the mouth (without tube interference) during surgery is necessary to assess proper dental occlusion. Temporary **tracheostomy** is also an option.

6. Name some other important principles of jaw fracture repair.
- Stable anatomic or functional fixation of fracture fragments
- Avoidance of soft tissue entrapment and dental trauma
- Assessment of tissue viability
- Avoidance of excessive soft tissue elevation from bone surfaces
- Coverage of exposed bone with soft tissues
- Rapid restoration of oral functions

7. What are common complications of mandible fracture repair?

Dog
- Dental malocclusion
- Osteomyelitis
- Nonunion and malunion
- Appliance failure

Cat
- Dental malocclusion
- Soft tissue infection
- Temporomandibular degenerative joint disease
- Nonunion

8. List treatment options for jaw fractures.
- Tape muzzles
- Circumferential wiring
- Interarcade wiring
- Dental composite
- Interosseous wiring
- Partial mandibulectomy
- Interdental wiring
- Acrylic splints
- External skeletal fixation
- Intramedullary pinning
- Bone plating

9. How does one select among treatment options?

Fracture-Assessment Score

SCORE	FIXATION
0–3	Closed reduction and external fixator application
	Plate and screw fixation
	Tape muzzle for vertical ramus
4–7	Interfragmentary wire
	Bone plate and screws
	External skeletal fixation
8–10	Tape muzzle
	Interdental wiring
	Interfragmentary wiring
	Cerclage wires (symphyseal fractures)

10. What is the fracture assessment score?
Use of information from the patient's mechanical, biologic, and clinical parameters to assist in appropriate implant selection for the fracture repair. A low number represents mechanical, biologic, and clinical factors that do not favor rapid bone healing and return to function. High numbers represent factors that favor rapid bone healing and return to function.

11. Where is the tension side of the mandible?
The alveolar margin.

12. Which neurovascular structures are associated with jaw fractures?
The maxillary branch of the **trigeminal nerve** innervates the cutaneous muscles of the head and nasal and oral cavity and muscles of mastication. It passes rostrally through the alar canal and can be damaged with maxillary fractures. The mandibular **alveolar nerve** passes through the mandibular canal and is sensory to the teeth of the mandible. The mandibular **alveolar artery**

supplies the cortical and alveolar bone and teeth of the mandible and passes along with the mandibular alveolar nerve in the canal. Often these structures are damaged in mandibular fractures, although clinical signs may not be evident.

13. Which fractures may be amenable to tape muzzles?
- Minimally displaced or nondisplaced fractures
- Highly comminuted fractures with the opposite hemimandible intact
- Vertical ramus fractures
- Adjunctive treatment to internal reduction

14. What are tape muzzles?
Nonelastic tape (0.5–2 inches) encircling the muzzle and skull. Tape muzzles are an inexpensive, practical, and noninvasive method generally well tolerated by animals.

15. What is the best treatment method for articular fractures of the temporomandibular joint?
Removal of the mandibular condylar head to create a pseudarthrosis (similar to femoral head ostectomy in the hip joint).

16. Do all maxillary fractures require surgical treatment?
No. If there is not severe displacement, healing quickly occurs. Maxillary fractures that should be surgically treated include lesions causing malocclusion, large areas of oronasal communication, facial deformity, and obstruction to airflow through the nasal cavity.

17. How does the direction of obliquity in longitudinal fractures of the mandible affect the stability of the fracture?
The combined effects of the masseter, pterygoid, and temporalis muscles tend to displace caudad fragments dorsally. This force is resisted by the rostral fragment if the fracture line is dorsocaudal to rostroventral.

18. Which of the following interdental fixations is strongest: metal, metal with acrylic reinforcement, or acrylic alone?
Metal with acrylic reinforcement.

CONTROVERSY

19. How should teeth in the fracture line be handled?
Generally, a stable tooth in the fracture line should remain in place and be extracted only if there are clinical complications. Teeth help with anatomic alignment and stability of the fracture repair.

Increased infection may occur when damaged or loose teeth are retained in the fracture line, and early antibiotic therapy is recommended by some clinicians. Diseased teeth should be removed from the fracture site to facilitate healing in animals with pathologic fractures secondary to periodontal disease.

The answer may also depend on the clinician: Orthopedic surgeons tend to treat the bone fractures primarily and address dental problems later, whereas veterinary dentists focus on dental lesions in the initial assessment.

BIBLIOGRAPHY

1. Bennett JW, Kapatkin AS, Manfra Marretta S: Composite for the fixation of mandibular fractures and luxations in 11 cats and 6 dogs. Vet Surg 23:190–194, 1994.
2. Davidson JR, Bauer MS: Fractures of the mandible and maxilla. Vet Clin North Am 22:109–119, 1992.
3. Kern DA, Smith MM, Grant JW, et al: Evaluation of bending strength of five interdental fixation apparatuses applied to canine mandibular. Am J Vet Res 54:1177–1182, 1993.

4. Manfra Marretta S, Schrader SC, Mathiesen DT: Problems associated with the management and treatment of jaw fractures. Prob Vet Met 2:220–245, 1990.
5. Umphlet RC, Johnson AL: Mandibular fractures in the cat, a retrospective study. Vet Surg 17:333–337, 1988.
6. Umphlet RC, Johnson AL: Mandibular fractures in the dog, a retrospective study of 157 cases. Vet Surg 19:272–275, 1990.

64. FRACTURES OF THE SCAPULA

Joseph Harari, M.S., D.V.M., Dip. A.C.V.S.

1. How common are fractures of the scapula?

They have been reported to range from 0.5–2.4% of all fractures identified at veterinary teaching hospitals.

2. What is the anamnesis for the injury?

Vehicular trauma in most cases, affecting young (<4 years of age), intact male dogs with most of the lesions involving the left scapula.

3. What other injuries can occur concurrently?

- Thoracic trauma (pulmonary contusions, pneumothorax)
- Other forelimb or hindlimb orthopedic injuries
- Soft tissue wounds
- Nerve (brachial plexus, spinal cord) damage

4. Are scapular fractures easily diagnosed?

No. Many lesions are overlooked because of
- Difficulty in palpation of a bone surrounded by extensive muscular elements.
- Missing a lameness in a patient who is completely nonambulatory or ambulatory with a mild injury.
- Misinterpretation of radiographs because of malpositioning or superimposition of other structures.

5. Which radiographic projections are useful in diagnosis?

- Lateral view with the affected limb cranially extended
- Caudocranial view (patient is in dorsal recumbency and limb is pulled cranially)
- Distoproximal view (patient is in dorsal recumbency and leg is pulled caudally)
Patient is heavily sedated or anesthetized for all views.

6. Which (indirect) radiographic projection has been used frequently to diagnose a scapular fracture retroactively?

Lateral and ventrodorsal projections of the thorax.

7. How are scapular fractures classified?

Traditional scheme based on **location**	**Biomechanical** scheme
• Body	• Stable extraarticular
• Spine and acromion	• Unstable extraarticular
• Neck including glenoid region	• Intraarticular

8. How are scapular fractures treated?
1. Stable extraarticular lesions can be treated with cage rest or bandage (e.g., Velpeau, Spica) support.
2. Unstable extraarticular and intraarticular lesions are usually treated with internal implants, such as wires, pins, bone plate (stainless steel or plastic), and screws.

9. What types of stainless steel plates are useful for repair of scapular fractures?
Small fragment or miniplates with angled (L) or T configurations.

10. Which orthopedic principle needs to be followed for repair of supraglenoid tubercle or acromion fractures and avulsions?
Tension band principle with figure-8 wire and pins or bone screw with or without pin to counteract the distractive forces of the biceps brachii tendon of origin or acromial head of deltoideus muscle.

11. What type of bone plate is useful for stabilizing horizontal fractures of the scapular body?
Semitubular plates inverted and placed cranially or caudally along the base of the scapular spine.

12. How are articular (glenoid) fractures classified?
As Y or T fractures based on the configuration of the lesion.

13. Which surgical approach is useful for glenoid or articular fractures?
Craniolateral approach with osteotomy of the acromion and tenotomy of the infraspinatus muscle.

14. What is the metacromion?
A caudally projecting protuberance on the feline scapular spine located 1–2 cm proximal to the acromion and overhanging the infraspinatus muscle.

15. What important structures need to be identified and preserved during repair of glenoid fractures?
Suprascapular artery, vein, and nerve.

16. What is the prognosis after treatment of scapular fractures?
Although based on the degree of injury, bone healing is favored by periosseous muscular coverage and vasculature and cancellous bone in the body of the scapula. Complex articular fractures may warrant a guarded prognosis because of the severity of bone trauma and subsequent implant failures. Scapulohumeral arthrodesis may be an alternative, although lameness persists. Amputation has also been performed after failed surgeries or in animals with severe irreparable injuries.

BIBLIOGRAPHY

1. Cook JL, Cook CR: Scapular fractures in dogs: Epidemiology, classification, and concurrent injuries. J Am Anim Hosp Assoc 33:528–532, 1997.
2. Harari J, Dunning D: Fractures of the scapula in dogs. Vet Comp Orthol Traum 6:105–108, 1993.
3. Johnston SA: Articular fractures of the scapula in the dog. J Am Anim Hosp Assoc 29:157–164, 1993.
4. Jerram RM, Herron MR: Scapular fractures in dogs. Comp Contin Educ Pract Vet 20:1254–1259, 1998.
5. Roush JK, Lord PF: Clinical application of a distoproximal (axial) radiographic view of the scapula. J Am Anim Hosp Assoc 26:129–132, 1990.

65. FRACTURES OF THE HUMERUS

Spencer A. Johnston, V.M.D., Dip. A.C.V.S.

1. Do fractures of the humerus occur less commonly than fractures of the femur?
Yes. Because many fractures occur as a result of dogs and cats being struck by automobiles, the proximity of the front legs to vital structures (skull and thorax) results in a high incidence of fatalities when forelimbs are injured.

2. What is the most likely diagnosis for lameness and a swollen elbow in a puppy after a fall?
A **Salter-Harris IV fracture** of the lateral aspect of the humeral condyle.

3. Why does this fracture occur?
Because of the shape of the distal humerus and relationship of the radial head to the humeral condyle. The lateral aspect of the humeral condyle is offset from the axis of the humerus. This is also the portion of the humeral condyle that articulates with the radial head. When excessive force is transmitted up the radius (as the puppy lands), the force is transferred to the humeral condyle. The shearing force is sufficient to cause a fracture through the middle of the condyle and the lateral epicondylar crest.

4. Does the humerus contain medial and lateral condyles?
No. According to Miller's *Anatomy of the Dog,* the humerus has only one condyle, with medial and lateral epicondyles.

5. What is the best way to repair these fractures?
With a lag screw placed from the lateral aspect of the humeral condyle to the medial aspect of the humeral condyle and an antirotational pin placed from the lateral epicondyle into the shaft of the humerus. Although repair of these fractures with interfragmentary pins instead of a lag screw has been described, it is not the optimal method of fixation.

6. If the fracture is not severely displaced, can a soft padded bandage or splint be used to provide stabilization (then refer it in 3–6 weeks if it does not heal)?
Only if you want to doom the patient to a lifetime of discomfort resulting from a severely dysfunctional joint. Although this fracture involves the articular surface, the prognosis is good if repair is done soon after the injury. Left untreated, there is irreversible damage to the articular surface, loss of identifying interdigitation of the fracture fragments, and periarticular fibrosis. Attempts to reestablish articular congruity and provide a functional joint this long after injury are usually frustrating. Arthrodesis or amputation may be the only options.

7. How soon should these fractures be repaired?
Within 3–5 days of the injury, sooner if possible.

8. Do these fractures occur only in young dogs?
No, they can occur in older patients, usually cocker or Brittany spaniels. This may be due to incomplete ossification of an intracondylar growth plate in this breed, predisposing the dog to fracture secondary to minimal trauma.

9. How does a T or Y fracture differ from a fracture of the lateral aspect of the humeral condyle?
T or Y fractures involve fracture of the medial and lateral epicondylar crests as well as the articular surface. There is communication with the supratrochlear foramen from both the medial and lateral sides.

10. Are these fractures difficult to repair?
Yes. Repair can be achieved by a variety of methods but basically requires reconstruction of the condyle with a lag screw, then attachment to the humeral shaft by pins or plates. If comminution is present, it is difficult to obtain satisfactory alignment and reduction.

11. Why is that so difficult?
Because of the exposure, difficulty in obtaining reduction, and amount of bone available for implant placement. Attachment of the flexors (medially) and extensors (laterally) distract fractured portions of the condyle, and visualization may be impaired by blood clots and torn and swollen tissues. Because of the proximity to the articular surface and shape of the humerus, plating techniques are limited by the ability to contour the plate and place screws with sufficient purchase to secure the plate. Pins are easier to place but have limitations with respect to rotational stability. One should not try to repair these fractures, unless one has a real love, talent, and patience for orthopedic surgery.

12. What type of approach is used to repair these fractures?
An approach to the lateral aspect of the humeral condyle and epicondyle is usually sufficient to allow repair of uncomplicated fractures of the lateral aspect of the humeral condyle. If greater exposure is necessary, **osteotomy of the olecranon** process allows access to the caudad compartment of the elbow and visualization and manipulation of the medial aspect of the humerus. This is frequently necessary when repairing T or Y fractures. **Tenotomy of the triceps tendon** can be performed for exposure of T or Y fractures in immature patients.

13. Do all fractures of the distal humerus involve the articular surface?
No. **Supracondylar fractures,** which involve the distal portion of the humerus but do not involve the articular surface, can also occur. Supracondylar fractures occur more commonly than condylar fractures in cats, but not in dogs.

14. List examples of biologic fixations of comminuted humeral fractures.
- Intramedullary pin and plate combination
- Interlocking nail (with screws)
- Intramedullary and external fixation (connected externally)

15. List the advantages of biologic fixations.
- Biomechanical stability
- Decreased soft tissue dissection (infection, avascularity)
- Technical ease and reduced operative time
- Complementary implants

16. Discuss some factors that must be considered when selecting a method of repair for humeral shaft fractures.
The **location** of the fracture, the **configuration** and degree of comminution of the fracture, the size of the bone, and the **forces** that will be acting on the fracture repair (bending, rotation, shear, compression) must all be considered when choosing a method of fixation.
1. The humerus is a highly contoured bone that does not lend itself readily to fixation. It is difficult to fill the medullary cavity with pins because the medullary cavity is relatively broad proximally and has a relatively narrow isthmus in the distal one third.
2. The contour of the bone sometimes makes plate application problematic because of the need to contour the plate in three planes to adapt to the surface of the bone (at least when the plate is applied on the lateral side).
3. The contour of the bone can also make cerclage wire application problematic because the tapering nature of the proximal and distal portions of the humerus predispose the wire to slipping as it is tightened.

4. The narrowing of the distal humerus and division into lateral and medial epicondyles sometimes make interlocking nail application difficult because the width of the medial epicondyle can limit the size of nail used.

5. It is difficult to avoid overlying muscle with external fixator pins, and care must be taken to avoid the radial nerve when transfixation pins are applied to the distal one third of the bone.

6. The muscle mass of the humerus also requires that the clamps be placed at a relatively far distance from the axis of the humerus, making the external fixator relatively weak.

7. In addition to the above-listed factors, the approach to the humerus is more difficult than the approach to the other long bones because of the overlying musculature and proximity of nerves.

17. Discuss specific problems with the surgical approaches to the humerus.

The **lateral approach** to the shaft of the humerus requires ligation or avoidance of the cephalic and axillobrachial veins; elevation of the deltoideus, superficial or deep pectoral muscles, and lateral head of the triceps; and retraction of the brachialis muscle and radial nerve.

The **medial approach** provides access to the midportion and distal portion of the humerus, which have straight and flat surfaces and lend themselves to plate application. The brachial artery and vein, along with the median, musculocutaneous, and ulnar nerves, must be avoided. Identification of these structures in traumatized tissue is not always easy. This approach does not provide good access to the proximal one third of the bone.

18. Are there differences to humeral fracture repair in dogs and cats?
Cats

Cats have supracondylar fractures more frequently than condylar fractures. Cats also have a straighter humerus than dogs, and this makes fixation with an intramedullary pin easier than in dogs. The distal humerus of the cat is slightly different from the dog. The **median nerve** and **brachial artery** pass through the **supracondylar foramen.** Also, the **ulnar nerve** lies under the medial head (short portion) of the triceps muscles.

Dogs

Condylar fractures are commoner than supracondylar fractures. Fixation with an intramedullary pin is more difficult in dogs.

19. What nerve is of greatest concern with fractures of the humerus?

The **radial nerve** is most commonly injured with fractures of the distal portion of the humerus, where the nerve courses cranially and laterally along with the brachialis muscle. Long oblique fractures in this area or comminuted fractures with long sharp fragments of bone are most commonly associated with radial nerve injury. The radial nerve is important because the ability to extend the elbow is necessary for front limb ambulation. Although damage to the ulnar, median, and musculocutaneous nerves can occur, loss of these nerves does not cause severe limb dysfunction.

20. How is radial nerve injury identified?

Lack of pain sensation in the dermatome (dorsal surface of the paw) associated with the radial nerve. Sometimes the nerve is found to be transected at the time of surgery.

21. Why is the appearance of a dog with a humeral fracture sometimes misleading?

Dogs have a dropped elbow and do not extend the carpus (either drag the paw or are willing to place pressure on the dorsum of the paw). Nerve sensation should be evaluated.

22. If the radial nerve is transected, should the leg be amputated?

Not necessarily. It is important to determine at what level the injury has occurred. If the nerve is transected distal to the branches of the triceps, the dog will still have the ability to extend and fix the elbow. In this case, injury to the distal portion of the nerve results in lack of extensor functions, and the major defect is an inability to extend the carpus. Many dogs develop an ability to swing the limb forward, extending the carpus and placing the palmar surface of the foot appropriately. If the radial nerve is transected proximal to the branches innervating the triceps, amputation should be considered.

23. Do fractures of the proximal humerus occur commonly?

No. **Salter-Harris fractures** (usually type I or II) do occur through the proximal physis.

24. What about fractures of the proximal humerus in mature dogs?

Although these can occur secondary to trauma, the possibility of pathologic fracture associated with osteosarcoma or other tumor should always be considered. This is particularly true if the signalment (large-breed dog, middle-aged or older) is associated with a history of no or minimal trauma.

25. Can external coaptation be used for fractures of the humerus?

No. The proximal location of the humerus does not lend itself to external coaptation, with the exception of a spica (over the body) splint. A spica splint is not good for long-term management, but it is useful for short-term immobilization to provide comfort to the patient while awaiting definitive repair.

26. Should spica bandages be used postoperatively to reduce weight bearing?

No. It is best to avoid the combination of internal fixation and external coaptation because this can lead to decreased range of motion of the elbow or shoulder. If a fracture repair is somewhat tenuous, weight bearing can be avoided by placing the patient in a carpal sling (carpal flexion bandage), which allows motion of the elbow and shoulder, yet prevents the stress of weight bearing on the fracture repair.

BIBLIOGRAPHY

1. Bardet JF, Hohn RB, Rudy RL: Fractures of the humerus in dogs and cats: A Retrospective study of 130 cases. Vet Surg 12:73–77, 1983.
2. Cook JL, Tomlinson JL, Reid AL: Fluoroscopically guided closed reduction and internal fixation of fractures of the lateral portion of the humeral condyle: Prospective clinical study of the technique and results in ten dogs. Vet Surg 28:315–321, 1999.
3. Dueland RT, Johnson KA, Roe SC: Interlocking nail treatment of diaphyseal long-bone fractures in dogs. J Am Vet Med Assoc 214:59–66, 1999.
4. Guerin SR, Lewis DD, Lanz OI: Comminuted supracondylar humeral fractures repaired with a modified type I external skeletal fixator construct. J Small Animal Pract 39:525–532, 1998.
5. Hulse D, Hyman W, Nori M: Reduction in plate strain by addition of an intramedullary pin. Vet Surg 26:451–459, 1997.
6. Marcellin-Little DJ, DeYoung DJ: Incomplete ossification of the humeral condyle in spaniels. Vet Surg 23:475–487, 1994.
7. Piermattei DL, Flo GL: Brinker, Piermattei, and Flo's Handbook of Small Animal Orthopedics and Fracture Repair, 3rd ed. Philadelphia, W.B. Saunders, 1997, pp 261–287.
8. Vannini R, Smeak DD, Olmstead ML: Evaluation of surgical repair of 135 distal humeral fractures in dogs and cats. J Am Anim Hosp Assoc 24:537–554, 1988.

66. FRACTURES OF THE RADIUS AND ULNA

Joseph Harari, M.S., D.V.M., Dip. A.C.V.S.

1. How common are radial and ulnar fractures?

Estimates range from 8–18% of all fractures in dogs and cats.

2. What are some important anatomic considerations for repair of radial and ulnar fractures?
- The radius is the major weight-bearing bone of the forearm and is more frequently repaired than ulnar fractures.
- Open injuries occur frequently because of paucity of soft tissue (muscle) coverage in the mid and distal aspects of the bones.
- Fractures in the distal third of the radius heal poorly, especially in small dogs.
- The cranial or convex aspect of the radius is the tension side; the concave caudal border is the compression side.
- Limb shortening and angulation can occur secondary to proximal or distal physeal trauma.
- Hanging the limb during surgery promotes limb alignment.

3. Name some indications for repair of ulnar fractures.
- Fractures of the olecranon
- Monteggia lesions
- Severely displaced shaft fractures in large dogs with concurrent radial injury
- Styloid fractures and avulsions.

4. Which orthopedic principle forms the basis for repair of olecranon and styloid fractures?
    Tension band stabilization with pins, screws, or wires to counteract the distractive forces of the triceps muscle proximally or lateral collateral ligament distally.

5. What is a Monteggia lesion?
    Fracture of the proximal aspect of the ulna combined with cranial dislocation of the radial head; first described in people in 1814 by Monteggia, an Italian surgeon.

6. How is a Monteggia fracture-dislocation treated?
    The ulnar fracture can be repaired with intramedullary pins, cerclage or figure-8 wires, and bone plate and screws. The radial head dislocation is stabilized with annular ligament repair or transfixation to the ulna with pins, screw, or wire.

7. If necessary, how are ulnar shaft fractures treated?
    Intramedullary pin, with or without cerclage wires or bone plate and screws applied caudolaterally.

8. How are radial shaft fractures treated?
- External support with a cast for minimally (>50% overlap) displaced, interlocking, or incomplete fractures in young animals with good healing capabilities. Mason metasplints (provide only caudal support) are not recommended.
- Bone plate and screws applied in a neutral, compression, or buttress fashion along with cancellous bone grafting.
- Alternatively, biologic osteosynthesis using external skeletal fixation with minimal surgical invasiveness and cancellous grafting.

9. How are plates applied to mid or distal radial diaphyseal fractures?
    Traditionally, plates are applied to the cranial (tension) surface after a craniomedial surgical approach. More recently, medial plate application has been used successfully because of thick mediolateral bone diameter, use of more screws placed per fragment, avoidance of extensor tendons, and biomechanical stability.

10. Why are fractures of the distal aspect of the radius and ulna in small dogs predisposed to the high complication rates of inadequate bone healing (non-union and delayed union)?
- Biomechanical instability of fracture site
- Decreased intraosseous vascular supply

- Reduced soft tissue coverage and extraosseous blood supply
- Persistent cartilage formation at the fracture site
- Weak implant holding capabilities of the bones
- Excessive periosseous dissection during surgery
- Reduced stimulation of osteogenesis because of limited weight bearing by patients

11. What kind of external fixators can be applied to radial and ulnar fractures?

Acrylic or stainless steel (circular or linear). Types II (medial and lateral bars or columns attached to through-and-through pins) and Ib (unilateral, biplanar) are the most popular.

12. What option should be considered for fixation of proximal and distal metaphyseal radial fractures?

Hooked or **T plates** for internal fixation; temporary transarticular fixation with skeletal fixators, including stabilization of the ulna proximally. Cross pins, cerclage wire, and casting or Rush pinning have been less frequently described for distal shaft and metaphyseal injuries. Experimentally created distal radial osteotomies have also been stabilized with orthopedic staples (bent 1.6-mm Kirschner wires).

13. Which external fixator pins are useful for treatment of radial fractures in small dogs?

Acrylic or miniature external fixator pins; these are small (1–2 mm shank diameter), double trochar pins with a threaded end and a central roughened area to enhance acrylic gripping.

14. Limb disuse after external fixation or splinting of radial and ulnar fractures in small dogs produces what radiographic features?

Osteopenia (disuse atrophy) of the distal ulna and, possibly, the carpal and metacarpal bones.

CONTROVERSIES

15. Which fixation method, internal with a bone plate and screws or external with a skeletal fixator, is preferred for treatment of radial fractures?

The answer may be more related to clinical experience, opinion, and prejudice than scientific data. Plates require more extensive dissection, provide immediate stability, do not require extensive postoperative management, can induce osteopenia from stress protection, can conduct cold environmental temperatures, and require a second surgery for removal.

External skeletal fixation provides less rigid stability, is more biologic for healing, is less invasive, is often more difficult to apply (yet easier to remove) from the side to a flat curved bone, and requires more intensive postoperative care.

Costs between external and internal fixation may be similar.

16. Is intramedullary pinning of radial fractures an acceptable treatment option?

Intramedullary pinning of radial fractures has consistently been associated with more complications in healing than either bone plating or external skeletal fixation. Causes of failure include inadequate stabilization and iatrogenic trauma to the carpus during retrograde placement. Many practitioners persist in using this technique. Few references to support the procedure are documented in the veterinary literature.

BIBLIOGRAPHY

1. Binnington AG, Miller CW: Fractures of the radius and ulna. In Brinker AO, Olmstead ML (eds): Manual of Internal Fixation in Small Animals, 2nd ed. Berlin, Springer, 1998, pp 142–148.
2. Egger EE: Fractures of the radius and ulna. In Slatter D (ed): Textbook of Small Animal Surgery, 2nd ed. Philadelphia, W.B. Saunders, 1993, pp 1736–1756.
3. Larsen LJ, Roush JK: Bone plate fixation of distal radius and ulna fractures in small and miniature breed dogs. J Am Anim Hosp Assoc 35:243–250, 1999.
4. Muir PM: Distal antebrachial fractures in toy-breed dogs. Comp Cont Educ Pract Vet 19:137–145, 1997.

5. Piermattei DL, Flo GL: Handbook of Small Animal Orthopedics, 3rd ed. Philadelphia, W.B. Saunders, 1997, pp 321–343.
6. Sardinas J, Montavon PM: Use of a medial bone plate for repair of radius and ulna fractures in dogs and cats. Vet Surg 26:108–113, 1997.
7. Schwarz PD, Schrader SC: Ulnar fracture and dislocation of the proximal radial epiphysis (Monteggia lesion) in the dog and cat. J Am Vet Med Assoc 185:190–194, 1984.
8. Thomson MJ, Read RA: Comparative strengths or orthopaedic staples versus a 2.7 mm T plate in the stabilization of distal radial osteotomies. Vet Comp Orthop Traum 11:100–104, 1998.

67. TRAUMATIC INJURIES OF THE CARPUS AND METACARPUS

Joseph Harari, M.S., D.V.M., Dip. A.C.V.S.

1. What is the carpus?
A compound joint composed of seven bones arranged in two transverse rows, plus a small medial sesamoid bone.

2. Where is the greatest joint movement in the carpus?
The antebrachiocarpal joint.

3. What are common injuries of the forepaw?
- Traumatic luxations or subluxations
- Hyperextension
- Shearing lesions
- Fractures involving the numerous bones and joints of the region

4. List diagnostic tests that are useful in delineating the location and severity of the injury.
- Physical examination to determine the degree of weight bearing
- Palpation to evaluate dorsal/palmar and medial/lateral instabilities
- Stressed lateral and oblique radiographic projections to examine joint stability (including position of accessory carpal bone), fractures, and periosteal reactions

5. What problems of forepaw surgery should be addressed and managed to reduce complications?
Decreased visibility and increased operative time can occur secondary to constant hemorrhage from highly traumatized vascularized tissues; a forelimb tourniquet is useful in reducing blood flow.

Postoperative swelling secondary to the injury and surgery affecting lymphatic and venous drainage can be controlled by heavily padded limb bandages for 24–72 hours, before application of casts or splints.

6. How should a tourniquet be applied?
Ideally, exsanguination of the limb by elevation or an Esmarch bandage should be performed for 5 minutes before application of a pneumatic cuff proximally with pressures not exceeding 100 mm Hg above systolic pressure for less than 3 hours.

Realistically, sterilized elastic bandage is tightly applied to the forelimb for 60–90 minutes, and incisions are made through the bandage. Although controversial, some surgeons recommend concurrent intravenous corticosteroid medication (e.g., methylprednisolone, prednisolone sodium succinate) to mitigate cellular derangements associated with tissue ischemia, reperfusion injury, and subsequent edema all related to the initial trauma, to surgery, or to the tourniquet.

7. What is an Esmarch bandage?

Named after a German surgeon (Johann Friedrich August von Esmarch, 1823–1908) and originally composed of rubber tubing, it now refers to a circumferential wrap of the distal aspect of the limb applied in a proximal direction to expel blood from the operative field.

8. Which ligamentous injuries occur most frequently in the carpus?

INSTABILITY	LESION
Lateral subluxation of radiocarpal joint	Tearing of medial (radial) collateral ligament
Dorsomedial middle carpal joint subluxation	Tearing of dorsomedial ligaments and joint capsules and palmar supporting structures
Hyperextension of the carpus	Tearing of palmar ligaments and fibrocartilage

9. How are ligament sprains classified?

- **First degree**—mild injury; minimal pathology; treatment not usually necessary.
- **Second degree**—moderate injury; damaged fibers and hematoma present; external splintage required.
- **Third degree**—severe injury; interstitial disruption or bone avulsion; surgical stabilization required.

10. What is a common clinical feature of carpal hyperextension or palmar carpal breakdown?

Plantigrade stance following a history of falling or jumping.

11. Which joint space is most frequently affected in hyperextension injury?

Carpometacarpal or middle carpal (both reported).

12. What surgical treatments are recommended for palmar carpal breakdown?

Pancarpal or partial carpal arthrodesis of the middle and distal joints, with bone plates, screws, intramedullary or cross pins, and external skeletal fixation. Additionally, cartilage débridement, autogenous cancellous bone grafting, and external supports are mandatory.

13. Which carpal bones are most frequently fractured and treated surgically?

- Radiocarpal chip or slab fractures associated with jumps or falls in athletic dogs
- Accessory carpal bone fractures in racing greyhounds

14. What are some characteristics of accessory carpal bone fractures in greyhounds?

- Strain-avulsion fractures associated with ligamentous or tendinous attachments and classified type I (most common) through V based on location of the fracture.
- Most frequently identified in the right carpus and associated with stresses of racing in a counterclockwise direction.

15. How are these injuries usually treated to obtain performance levels similar to the pre-trauma state?

Open reduction and stabilization with bone screws.

16. Discuss the usual treatment of shearing injuries of the carpus.

Most frequently, the medial aspect of the joints is affected and necessitates stabilization because of the normal slightly valgus deviation of a weight-bearing carpus. Treatments include débridement and open wound management of contaminated lesions, synthetic collateral suture replacement, and temporary immobilization with external splints or external fixation. Healing may take 1–3 months, including multiple rechecks.

Pancarpal arthrodesis or limb amputation may need to be performed in severely injured patients, in cases of failed stabilization, or because of financial constraints of the owner.

17. When is internal fixation with small pins or bone plate and screws recommended for treatment of metacarpal fractures?
- Fractures of the weight-bearing digits (metacarpals III and IV)
- Fractures of all four metacarpal bones
- Grossly displaced or malunion injuries
- Single bone (large) fractures in performance animals.

Internal fixation with plates improves axial alignment of the bones more so than pin fixation or external coaptation; because progressive healing occurs with all stabilization methods, the clinical significance of plates versus pins may be irrelevant except in the treatment of severely displaced or malaligned lesions. Third metacarpal bone fractures have been described with dorsally applied pancarpal arthrodesis plates being less than 50% of the bone length. Clinical recovery occurred without the need for surgery.

18. Which sesamoids have been reportedly associated with clinically significant fractures?
The second and seventh proximal sesamoids in racing greyhounds and young rottweilers.

19. What is the treatment for these fractures involving carpal laxity sesamoids?
Surgical excision.

20. Nontraumatic carpal laxity syndrome has been described in which breeds?
- Immature German shepherds, Great Danes
- Doberman pinschers

21. What is the treatment for nontraumatic carpal laxity syndrome?
Light, temporary support wraps and housing on soft surfaces with mild exercise. Most animals recover within 1–2 months.

22. What is the clinical significance of periosteal bone formation (enthesophyte) on the proximal aspect of the radial styloid process?
Unknown. Historical evidence of trauma, localized pain, and joint instability are inconsistent findings. This location is the origin of the short radial collateral ligaments.

CONTROVERSIES

23. Should injuries of the middle and distal carpal joints be treated with pancarpal or partial arthrodesis?
Panarthrodesis produces highly satisfactory clinical results with most dogs having improved and near-normal gait function; conversely, the normal radiocarpal joint is destroyed, and bone plating equipment is required.

Partial carpal arthrodesis may be technically easier to perform than pancarpal fusion, does not require a bone plate and screws, and maintains the integrity and motion of the radiocarpal joint preserving normal limb function; conversely, unrecognized lesions (chronic or acute) of the radiocarpal joint and the theoretical possibility of increased stress, as a result of fusion of the middle and distal joints, may cause subsequent proximal joint breakdown and necessitate panarthrodesis.

24. Where should a plate be applied for pancarpal arthrodesis?
Technically and ideally, plate application should be performed on the palmar or tension side of the forepaw; realistically the dorsal surgical approach is technically easier to accomplish because of reduced neurovascular and tendon structures. In this latter instance, external support (splints, casts) is mandatory for 2–4 months, until bone healing is apparent clinically and radiographically.

BIBLIOGRAPHY

1. Guilliard MJ: Enthesiopathy of the short radial collateral ligaments in racing greyhounds. J Small Anim Pract 39:227–230, 1998.

2. Johnson KA: Carpal injuries. In Bloomberg MS, Dee JF (eds): Canine Sports Medicine and Surgery, 1st ed. Philadelphia, W.B. Saunders, 1998, pp 100–119.
3. Muir P, Norris JL: Metacarpal and metatarsal fractures in dogs. J Small Anim Pract 38:344–348, 1997.
4. Piermattei DL, Flo GL: Handbook of Small Animal Orthopedics, 3rd ed., Philadelphia, W.B. Saunders, 1997, pp 344–394.
5. Whitelock RG, Dyce J: Metacarpal fractures associated with pancarpal arthrodesis in dogs. Vet Surg 28:25–30, 1999.
6. Willer RL, Johnson KA: Partial carpal arthrodesis for third degree carpal sprains. Vet Surg 19:334–340, 1990.

68. PELVIC FRACTURES

C. W. Smith, D.V.M., M.S., Dip. A.C.V.S.

1. What is the pelvis?
Ossa coxarum (ilium, ischium, pubis, and acetabulum), sacrum, and first caudal vertebrae.

2. How are fractures of the pelvis classified?
Based on location:
- Sacroiliac joint
- Ilium
- Acetabulum
- Ischium
- Pelvic symphysis/pubis

3. How common are pelvic fractures?
Approximately 20%–30% of all fractures involve the pelvis.

4. When pelvic fractures and displacement occur, how many bones are affected?
The pelvis is similar to a rectangular box. For displacement to occur with pelvic fractures, the pelvis must be broken in at least three places.

5. What other evaluations are performed on patients with pelvic fractures?
- **Abdominal**—bladder, urethra.
- **Thoracic**—pulmonary and cardiac contusions, pleural space.
- **Neurologic**—voluntary leg movement; deep pain perception; patellar, femoral, anal sphincter reflexes.
- **Other long bones and vertebrae**—polytrauma.
- **Rectal palpation**—canal compromise, perforations.

6. What radiographic evaluations are necessary for proper diagnosis and treatment of pelvic fractures?
Ventrodorsal, lateral, and **oblique** views. The oblique view is important in assessing acetabular fractures.

7. List some biologic and mechanical characteristics of pelvic fractures.
- Excellent healing resulting from periosseous vascularity and cancellous bone content
- Effective muscular support of bones
- Difficult reduction of fragments because of muscular contractions
- Transient nerve damage
- Difficult anatomic reduction and stabilization of small fragments
- Closed injuries most common

- Clinical recoveries usually within 4–6 weeks
- Implants not removed
- Low rates of infections

8. Which pelvic fractures are considered nonsurgical?
- Fractures with little or no displacement and intact acetabula
- Fracutres with minor disruption of pelvic ring continuity
- Fractures affecting non–weight-bearing structures (pubis, ischium)

9. How are nonsurgical pelvic fractures managed?
- Cage rest
- Limited activity
- Well-padded area
- Monitoring defecation and urination
- Sling support of the animal in rising and ambulation

10. List pelvic fractures that are considered surgical?
- Acetabular
- Disruption of the weight-bearing arch (sacroiliac joint, ilium, acetabulum)
- Markedly decreased size of pelvic canal
- Unstable hip segment
- Compromised sciatic nerve or urethra

11. When is the best time to repair pelvic fractures?
Within 3–4 days pending resolution of other more pressing, life-threatening problems (e.g., pulmonary contusions, pneumothorax, traumatic myocarditis, hypovolemia, acid-base and electrolyte disorders).

12. In repairing fractures, which areas of the pelvis are of major consideration?
- Sacroiliac joint
- Ilium
- Acetabulum
If these are reduced and stabilized, other bones often are realigned or have little effect on weight bearing.

13. What specific nerve injuries can occur with pelvic fractures?
- **Sciatic**—sacroiliac luxations, ilial shaft fractures, acetabular fractures, ischial fractures. Signs: foot knuckling, paw dragging, loss of skin sensation on caudolateral distal limb.
- **Obturator**—pubic fractures. Signs: no limb adduction.
- **Femoral**—sacroiliac luxation. Signs: lack of stifle extension, patellar reflex.
- **Pudendal/pelvic**—sacral fractures. Signs: incontinence.

14. When is reduction stabilization of fracture-dislocation of the sacroiliac joint necessary?
- Unstable hemipelvis
- Inability to stand or ambulate
- Persistent pain and nerve deficits (a return to function may not occur after repair)

15. What approaches are recommended for the reduction and stabilization of the sacroiliac joint?
- **Dorsolateral**—gluteal roll down, better visualization of sacrum.
- **Ventrolateral**—gluteal roll up, digital palpation of sacrum.

16. How are sacroiliac luxations stabilized?
Two-point fixation with pins and screws.

17. What are the commonest problems associated with screw stabilization of sacroiliac luxations?

Accurate reduction and placement of the screw is challenging because, in the average-size dog, the area for purchase of the sacral body with a screw is about 1 cm. Common errors include **incomplete reduction** and **screw misplacement,** including inadequate depth (<60% of sacral body width).

18. List possible locations of misplaced screws in stabilization.
- Lumbar articular process
- Lumbosacral disk space
- Seventh lumbar vertebra
- Missing the sacrum completely

19. What fixation methods are useful for ilial shaft fractures?
- Plate and screw fixation following a lateral approach to the ilium and a gluteal roll up.
- Bone screw fixation applied in lag fashion across long oblique fractures.
- Pin and wire fixation for oblique fractures in small patients.

20. What neurovascular structures are encountered when performing a lateral approach (gluteal roll up) to the ilium?
- Lateral circumflex femoral artery and vein located just craniad to the acetabulum.
- Cranial gluteal artery, vein, and nerve located midway.
- Iliolumbar artery and vein located at the caudal ilial spine.

21. When can acetabular fractures be treated conservatively?

Acetabular fractures, especially in young animals, with no displacement on lateral and ventrodorsal radiographs, can be treated with cage rest. Application of an Ehmer sling or a non–weight-bearing bandage may be helpful. There is risk that with early weight bearing, displacement of the fracture may occur; recheck radiographs should be performed early (<7 days) during convalescence.

22. What approach is used to repair acetabular fractures?
- Dorsal approach via trochanteric osteotomy (Gorman approach)
- Dorsal approach via gluteal myotomies (limited exposure)

23. What two muscles are cut to permit better exposure to the posterior acetabulum and ischium and used to retract the sciatic nerve?

External rotators—gemellus and internal obturator muscles.

24. What treatment is recommended for comminuted fractures of the acetabulum with ventral coxofemoral luxation?

Femoral head and neck excision. Reconstruction of the acetabular weight-bearing surface is usually unsuccessful, and ventral luxation recurs because of the damaged acetabular fossa (collapse and failure of the medial buttress).

25. What fixation methods are best for stabilization of acetabular fractures?

Acetabular plates, reconstruction plates, and **screw stabilization**. For small dogs, a combination of two screws and figure-8 wire fixation with a Kirschner wire across the fracture to prevent rotation can be successful. Screw and wire fixation with polymethyl methacrylate has been described.

26. What is the treatment of choice for acetabular fractures that cannot be reconstructed?

Femoral head and neck excision.

27. When are pubic fractures managed surgically?
- Soft tissue impingement of the urethra.
- Tearing of the prepubic tendon and herniation of abdominal viscera.

28. When are ischiatic fractures managed surgically?
Fracture and distal displacement of the ischiatic tuberosity (attachment of biceps femoris, semitendinosus, and semimembranosus muscles) producing pain and lameness. Treatment is by tension band fixation using pins and a dorsal wire.

29. How are pelvic malunions that cause compromise of the pelvic canal treated?
Carefully with:
- Pubic symphysiotomy and distraction with implants
- Ilial osteotomy
- Triple pelvic osteotomy

30. In cats with acquired pelvic stenosis secondary to trauma, what is the prognosis after pelvic osteotomy?
Surgical widening is effective if obstipation and tenesmus are less than 6 months' duration and megacolon is not present.

CONTROVERSY

31. What is the treatment of choice for a caudal one third acetabular fracture?
Some surgeons have suggested that because most of the weight-bearing (cranial two thirds) joint surface is intact, open reduction and stabilization may not be necessary for displaced segments. Others recommend stabilization of any acetabular fracture because of the high incidence of degenerative joint disease in patients in whom stabilization is not performed. Osteoarthritis occurs after natural and surgical trauma to the joint.

BIBLIOGRAPHY

1. Betts CW: Pelvic Fractures. In Slatter D (ed): Textbook of Small Animal Surgery, 2nd ed. Philadelphia, W.B. Saunders, 1993, pp 1769–1786.
2. Bookbinder PF, Flanders JA: Characteristics of pelvic fractures in the cat. Vet Comp Orthol Traum 5:122–127, 1992.
3. Boudrieau RJ, Kleine LJ: Nonsurgically managed caudal acetabular fractures in dogs: 15 causes (1979–1984). J Am Vet Med Assoc 193:701–705, 1988.
4. Houlton J, Dyce J: Management of pelvic fractures in the dog and cat. Waltham Focus 4:17–25, 1994.
5. Hulse DA: Pelvic fractures—conservative and surgical management. Vet Med Rep 2:267–278, 1990.
6. Kuntz CA, Waldron D: Sacral fractures in dogs. J Am Anim Hosp Assoc 31:142–150, 1995.
7. Lewis DD, Stubbs WP: Results of screw/wire/polymethylmethacrylate fixation of acetabular fractures. Vet Surg 26:223–234, 1997.
8. Piermattei DL, Flo GL: Brinker, Piermattei, and Flo's Handbook of Small Animal Orthopedics and Fracture Repair, 3rd ed. Philadelphia, W.B. Saunders, 1997, pp 395–421.
9. Schrader SC: Pelvic osteotomy for obstipation in cats with acquired pelvic canal stenosis. J Am Vet Med Assoc 200:208–209, 1992.
10. Verstraete FM, Lambrechts NE: Diagnosis of soft tissue injuries associated with pelvic fractures. Comp Cont Educ Pract Vet 14:921–930, 1992.

69. FRACTURES OF THE FEMUR

Spencer A. Johnston, V.M.D., Dip. A.C.V.S.

1. What is the capital physis?

The growth plate of the femoral head. It separates the neck from the epiphysis of the femoral head.

2. In which dogs does fracture through the capital physis occur?

Young dogs (usually <10 months) in which the growth plate has not yet completely closed. Once the dog is skeletally mature, fractures tend to occur through the femoral neck instead of the closed physis.

3. When should these fractures be repaired?

As soon as possible after the initial injury to prevent further trauma to the growth plate—this usually means within 3–5 days or earlier.

4. How are these fractures repaired?

Typically, by placing **multiple (two to four) Kirschner wires** from the femur into the capital physis. These wires are placed in a divergent fashion to provide stability. Alternatively a lag screw can be placed from the lateral aspect of the femur into the femoral head, perpendicular to the growth plate. If a lag screw is used, an additional Kirschner wire can be placed to aid in preventing rotation. Placement of a lag screw prevents further growth of the femoral neck, although the growth potential from the capital physis is probably severely compromised by the initial injury. In cats and small dogs, the amount of available bone for purchase by the implants is limited. Because these patients typically do well with femoral head and neck excision, that procedure is commonly chosen as the most practical method of treatment.

5. Are these fractures difficult to repair?

Yes. Exposure can be difficult, and landmarks for alignment and reduction can sometimes be difficult to identify, particularly if the fracture is more than a few days old. The bone is soft in this area and tends to lose identifying features if there is motion between the metaphysis and capital physis. There is only a small amount of bone for purchase of implants into the epiphysis.

6. What surgical approach is used?

A craniolateral approach to the hip provides satisfactory exposure. If additional exposure is needed, partial tenotomy of the deep gluteal muscle can be performed.

7. What is the prognosis associated with this type of fracture?

Relatively good overall, although the prognosis is worse if the patient is less than 4 months old. Studies suggest that long-term function is satisfactory, although most (>70%) patients develop osteoarthritis in that joint. The radiographic appearance of these fractures a few weeks after treatment typically demonstrates a unique remodeling of the femoral neck, called an **apple core** appearance. This is due to increased vascularity to the femoral neck associated with healing. This appearance is common and does not indicate failure of repair or future collapse of the femoral neck.

8. How do femoral neck fractures differ from capital physeal fractures?

The amount of bone available for repair. There is usually more bone available for purchase by the implants in the case of a femoral neck fracture compared with a capital physeal fracture. The method of fixation is essentially the same (lag screw or multiple small pins). Screw fixation is preferred with femoral neck fracture because compression of the fracture fragments aids in stability of the repair. The greater amount of bone available for screw purchase also makes screw application technically easier.

9. What approach is used to repair a midshaft femoral fracture?

Craniolateral approach most commonly. This allows exposure of the entire lateral aspect of the femur. If it is necessary to expose the distal portion of the femur, a branch of the caudal femoral artery needs to be identified and ligated.

10. What is the best way to repair a midshaft femoral fracture?

The **location** and **configuration** of the fracture, the degree of **comminution,** the **size** of the bone, the **forces** that will be acting on the fracture repair (bending, rotation, shear, compression), the degree of **soft tissue disruption,** and the **signalment** of the patient must all be considered when choosing a method of fixation. Plates provide the most stable repair, but this does not mean all midshaft femoral fractures need to be plated. Pins and wire are satisfactory for oblique fractures if the shaft can be reconstructed. Interlocking nails are an alternative to plates for comminuted fractures and provide greater stability than intramedullary (IM) pins but less stability than plates. External fixators can also be used, alone or in combination (connected or tied-in externally) with an IM pin. Pin-and-plate constructs are useful for treating highly comminuted diaphyseal fractures.

11. What is a pin-and-plate combination?

Use of an IM pin to realign major femoral segments followed by plate application for rigid stability in the treatment of comminuted shaft fractures.

12. List the advantages of the pin-and-plate combination.

- Biomechanical stability and protection of implants (similar to interlocking nails and screws or IM pins and external fixators)
- No need for fragmentary reconstructions (high strain) and soft tissue dissections (reduced surgery time)
- Technical ease of plate application, including use of lengthening plate and monocortical or bicortical screws
- Biologic healing with callus formation

13. Discuss some common mistakes with internal fixation of a femoral fracture.

Misuse of **IM pins** and **cerclage wire.** For IM pins and cerclage wire to be used satisfactorily as the sole method of treatment, the fracture must be able to be reconstructed so that the forces of weight bearing are transmitted by the bone and not the pin. This means nearly anatomic alignment and reduction. IM pins counteract bending but do not neutralize rotational forces. IM pins are not useful for transverse fractures, and use of a single IM pin for repair of a comminuted, transverse, or short oblique fracture may result in rotational instability, leading to nonunion. The common mistakes with cerclage wire are insufficient size or improper application (number and locations of wires) to counteract rotational forces; also the fractures may not be properly reconstructed to allow transmission of forces across the fracture without disrupting the repair.

14. What is the landmark for introduction of an IM pin into the proximal aspect of the femur?

The pin is placed into the **trochanteric fossa.** This can be identified by finding the greater trochanter with the tip of the pin, then walking the pin off the medial aspect of the greater trochanter. Care is taken to align the pin with the shaft of the bone, before driving the pin distally. Initial penetration of the proximal femur by the pin may be difficult, but once the medullary cavity is entered, the pin should advance easily.

15. When repairing a femoral fracture with pins, how much of the femoral shaft should be occupied by the pin?

Because the femur is a curved bone that is wider proximally and distally and has an isthmus in the midportion, it is not possible to fill the entire medullary cavity with pins. Instead the size of the pins depends on the width of the isthmus, and this area should be filled to the greatest degree. Although there were once concerns regarding disruption of the endosteal blood supply by large implants, this can be reestablished quickly after trauma of pin placement, and, in the interim, blood supply increases from periosteal and muscular sources. Filling the medullary cavity provides strength to resist bending and shear forces. Because there is a natural curvature to the femur, it may be easier to fill the shaft of the femur with multiple pins instead of one large pin. Practically speaking, 80% or more of the medullary cavity should be filled at the isthmus.

16. How far distally should an IM pin be placed into the femur?

Because of the natural curvature of the canine femur, IM pins typically exit just proximal to the femoral trochlea. If the fracture is overreduced (so that there is a gap at the caudad aspect of the fracture site, effectively straightening the femur), an IM pin can be seated more deeply into a condyle. It is important to maximize seating of the pin for fractures of the distal diaphysis. It is less important to risk penetration of the articular surface if the fracture is in the midshaft or proximal one third.

17. How can joint penetration be avoided or identified?

Use the proximal aspect of the femoral trochlea and the patella as landmarks. By having a pin of identical length available and using these landmarks, an IM pin can be driven the appropriate distance without penetrating the joint. Once the pin is driven, the joint can also be extended and flexed to determine if there is any crepitus (rubbing of the pin on articular cartilage). If there is doubt regarding penetration of the pin into the joint, it is best to perform a small arthrotomy for direct visualization. The morbidity associated with arthrotomy is minimal compared with a pin entering the joint and damaging the patella.

18. Should pins with threaded ends be used to increase holding power and prevent migration?

No. Because IM pins are seated in cancellous bone, a threaded pin does not provide any increased resistance to migration compared with a smooth pin. A disadvantage to the use of threaded pins is breakage at the pin-thread junction.

19. To which side of the femur should a bone plate be applied?

Typically, to the lateral aspect because this is the tension side and has less overlying musculature and neurovascular elements than other regions of the bone.

20. Discuss problems associated with applying external fixators.

There is a tendency for soft tissue irritation at the pin insertion sites because muscle penetration, trauma from injury, and motion around the pins, particularly near the stifle. Also, to avoid the soft tissues, the clamps and connecting bar are placed relatively far from the axis of the bone, a biomechanical disadvantage. Problems with soft tissue morbidity and weak constructs can be avoided by using new SK fixators, which are stronger than traditional KE fixators.

21. Can a femur fracture be repaired with a cast?

No. One of the principles of casting is to immobilize the joint above and below the fracture. This cannot be done effectively for a long enough period of time with a cast, even if it is placed in a spica (up and over the body) fashion.

22. Can a fracture of the distal femoral growth plate be treated with a Robert Jones bandage?

No. It is difficult to keep a Robert Jones bandage up high enough on the femur to immobilize any femoral fracture. The bandage tends to make the leg act as a fulcrum so that it bends at the fracture site. Attempted treatment in this manner is not effective and results in malalignment; the delay in repair makes internal fixation more difficult and the development of quadriceps contracture more likely.

23. How should fractures of the distal femur be treated?

With internal fixation, ranging from a single IM pin to plating. Most frequently, these fractures are repaired with a cross-pinning technique or pins placed in Rush pin fashion (inserted into the distal fragment, across the fracture line, and bouncing off the opposite cortex). Use of reconstruction plates has also been described for repair of these fractures.

24. Are these Salter-Harris I or II fractures?

They tend to be **Salter-Harris II fractures in dogs** and **Salter-Harris I fractures in cats.** This difference is due to the amount of undulation of the growth plate in each species. Dogs have a greater undulation, and it is more difficult to have a clean separation through the growth plate without including some of the metaphysis.

25. Does it matter if it is a Salter-Harris I or II fracture?

Not clinically; only in rounds or examinations.

26. To which side (metaphyseal or epiphyseal) are the cells with growth potential attached?

Physeal fractures as originally described by Salter and Harris were thought to occur between the hypertrophic zone and the zone of provisional calcification. Growth potential remains with the epiphyseal fragment, and this surface should not be disrupted during repair. One study of naturally occurring physeal fractures in dogs suggests that more severe disruption of the physis actually occurs, limiting growth potential after fracture repair.

27. Discuss complications with fractures of the distal femur.

Because the fracture occurs through the growth plate, the potential for loss of bone growth exists, although shortening of the limb does not seem to be a common problem. A more serious complication is the development of fracture disease (**quadriceps contracture**), in which fibrous change of the quadriceps mechanism eventually results in an inability to flex the stifle. This typically occurs within 1 month of fracture repair.

28. How can quadriceps contracture be prevented?

It is always difficult to predict which patients will develop this devastating complication, and specific recommendations for prevention are difficult to make. **Minimal disruption** of muscle during surgery is beneficial. **Rigid internal fixation** with early return to function, and **passive range of motion exercises** to help maintain joint and muscle pliability are beneficial. Avoiding immobilization of the stifle after fracture of the distal femur is prudent, although some surgeons prefer **temporary** early postoperative splintage of the joint in flexion to overcome extensor rigidity.

29. Can internal fixation be combined with external coaptation (spica bandage or a Schroeder-Thomas splint) for treatment of a femur fracture?

Only if you want to treat quadriceps contracture.

CONTROVERSIES

30. Should anatomic reconstruction be the goal of all femoral fracture repairs?

Anatomic reconstruction is important for articular fracture repair. For shaft fractures, current concepts of fracture repair suggest that the entire fracture environment must be considered during repair and that there is frequently a trade-off between disruption of vascular supply and obtaining rigid fixation. If satisfactory stability can be obtained with a treatment (interlocking nails, external fixators, buttress plates, pin-and-plate combinations) providing **minimal disturbance of the fracture environment,** it may be preferred versus obtaining anatomic alignment and reduction at the expense of disrupting the fracture environment. Some surgeons use anatomic reconstruction for noncomminuted lesions wherein cortical realignment for **load sharing** can be obtained, whereas comminuted fractures are treated **biologically** with minimal dissection or implantation at the fracture sites.

31. When using IM pins to repair a long oblique midshaft femoral fracture, should the pins be placed in a normograde or retrograde fashion?

According to some surgeons, **normograde** (starting from the proximal end of the bone and driven distally). Pins started at the fracture site and retrograded proximally can exit from or near the femoral head, are difficult to cut because of location, and can impinge on the sciatic nerve. Others believe that during **retrograde** pinning, adduction of the proximal segment and placement in the caudomedial aspect of the femoral canal avoids proximal bone and joint problems.

BIBLIOGRAPHY

1. Aron DN, Palmer RH, Johnson AL: Biologic strategies and a balanced concept for repair of highly comminuted long bone fractures. Comp Cont Educ Pract Vet 17:35–50, 1995.
2. DeCamp CE, Probst CW, Thomas MW: Internal fixation of femoral capital physeal injuries in dogs: 40 cases (1979–1987). J Am Vet Med Assoc 194:1750–1754, 1989.
3. Dueland RT, Johnson KA, Roe SC: Interlocking nail treatment of diaphyseal long-bone fractures in dogs. J Am Vet Med Assoc 214:59–66, 1999.
4. Gibson KL, van Ee RT, Pechman RD: Femoral capital physeal fractures in dogs: 34 cases (1979–1989). J Am Vet Med Assoc 198:886–890, 1991.
5. Johnson JM, Johnson AL, Eurell JA: Histological appearance of naturally occurring canine physeal fractures. Vet Surg 23:81–86, 1994.
6. Lorinson D, Millis DL, Bright RM: Determination of safe depth of pin penetration for repair of distal femoral physeal fractures in immature dogs: A comparison of normograde and retrograde pin placement. Vet Surg 26:467–471, 1997.
7. Piermattei DL, Flo GL: Brinker, Piermattei, and Flo's Handbook of Small Animal Orthopedics and Fracture repair, 3rd ed. Philadelphia, W.B. Saunders, 1997, pp 469–515.

70. FRACTURES OF THE TIBIA AND FIBULA

Joseph Harari, M.S., D.V.M., Dip. A.C.V.S.

1. How common are tibial fractures?
10%–20% of all fractures in dogs and cats.

2. What are the causes of tibial fractures?
- Vehicular trauma
- Gunshot injuries
- Falls
- Fights

3. List the most common types of tibial fractures.
- Closed diaphyseal spiral
- Closed diaphyseal oblique

4. What are some important anatomic considerations for repair of tibia and fibula fractures?
- Surgical treatments are usually restricted to the tibia because it is the main weight-bearing bone, and fibular fractures often become realigned after reduction of the tibial lesion.
- The main vascular supply is the caudal tibial artery located at the caudolateral proximal third of bone.

- A generous amount of intramedullary vascularity, proximal cancellous bone, and a periosseous muscular envelope contribute to progressive fracture healing.
- Despite tissue paucity distally, delayed healing of distal fractures is not common compared with radial fractures in small dogs.
- The medial approach to the tibial shaft is most frequently used for repair of diaphyseal or metaphyseal fractures.
- Although tensile forces have been recorded along the cranial and lateral aspects of the bone, external fixators and bone plates have been traditionally applied to the medial bone surface.
- The proximal growth plates contribute 40% to bone length, and the distal growth plates contribute 60%.

5. Which postinjury and surgery protocol is extremely useful in reducing soft tissue swelling and providing bone and limb support for tibial fractures?

Application of a Robert Jones bandage.

6. Which proximal tibial injuries can occur frequently in immature patients?

Avulsion of the tibial tuberosity (apophysis) and fracture-separation of the proximal tibial physis.

7. How are these apophyseal and physeal injuries repaired?

The tibial tuberosity is stabilized with pins and figure-8 wire or bone screw using the tension band technique to counteract the distractive bones of the patellar tendon. Physeal separations are stabilized with angled cross pins.

8. What is an apophysis?

A traction physis that is the site of origin or insertion of muscle groups; it contributes to bone shape and not longitudinal growth. The name is derived from the Greek *apo* (from) and *pausis* (growth) (i.e., an offshoot or growth from the bone).

9. How are diaphyseal fractures treated?

TREATMENT OPTIONS	REASONING
Closed repair	Incomplete, interlocking, aligned, or highly comminuted fractures in young patients. Natural, biologic repair
Open repair	Minimal dissection only (to preserve tissues, vascularity) for grafting, realigning major fragments, pin placement. Wide dissection for application of bone plates for stability
External skeletal fixation	Minimal surgical invasiveness, staged disassembly, postoperative care important, various frames
Intramedullary IM pin	Normograde pinning, axial alignment, combined with fixator or wires
Interlocking nail	Special instrumentation, stable, less dissection than plate
Bone plating	Extensive dissection, stable, early recovery, minimal postoperative care, complications necessitate second surgery
Kirschner and cerclage wires	Ancillary devices, placement errors lead to complications with healing

10. List the factors on which decision making regarding fracture treatment is based.

- Nature of the injury (patient-fracture assessment score)
- Clinical expertise or prejudice of the surgeon
- Postoperative environment
- Owner's finances

11. What are advantages of autogenous, cancellous grafting during repair of tibial diaphyseal fractures?
Enhancement of fracture healing by osteoinduction, osteoconduction, and osteogenesis.

12. What is an alternative to a fresh, autogenous cancellous graft?
Commercially prepared demineralized bone matrix containing bone morphogenetic proteins.

13. What is biologic osteosynthesis?
A more **normal** (**biologic**) repair of comminuted fractures characterized by minimal dissection to preserve tissues and vascularity; stabilization is with an external fixator and IM pin, plate, or interlocking nail in place of anatomic reconstruction with bone plate, screws, pins, and wires.

14. What is a clamp-on-plate?
A small (3–4 mm length) plate with two pairs of crimp arms that encircle a long bone already aligned with an IM pin. They require minimal dissection and provide less stability than standard plates.

15. Which important neurovascular elements need to be preserved during a medial approach to the tibial diaphysis?
- Cranial branch of the medial artery and vein
- Saphenous nerve

16. Which fibular fractures require stabilization?
Proximal (head) and distal (lateral malleolus) fractures involving attachment sites of lateral collateral ligaments and causing varus instabilities.

17. How are these fractures repaired?
Following the tension band principle with the use of pins and figure-8 wires or screws to counteract the distractive forces of the lateral collateral ligaments.

18. How are proximal and distal tibial metaphyseal fractures repaired?
- T plates
- Rush pins
- Static or dynamic cross pins

19. How are distal tibial physeal fractures repaired?
With the placement of cross pins retrograde through the medial and lateral malleoli.

20. What is a useful pre-operative and intraoperative protocol for application of an external fixator to an injured tibia?
Use of a hanging limb preparation—attachment of the paw to an intravenous stand or ceiling hook while the patient is placed in dorsal recumbency and the table lowered to produce a 2–4 cm gap between the table surface and body.

21. List the advantages of the hanging limb preparation.
- Limb alignment and parallelism of proximal and distal joints
- Circumferential access to the bone
- Lack of manual assistance required to stabilize or support the limb
- Reduction of muscular contraction

22. In which breed of dogs have spontaneously occurring distal tibial articular fractures been described?
Racing greyhounds; open anatomic reduction and rigid screw fixation were performed, although few dogs returned to racing.

23. What are some general healing rates for tibial fractures?

TYPE OF FRACTURE	HEALING TIME (MO)
Physeal fractures	1
Diaphyseal fractures treated with	
Casts	1
Pins and wires	1–2
External fixator	2–3
Bone plate and screws	2–4

NOTE. Variably based on the nature of injury, patient age, and method of fixation.

24. What are some trends in healing rates of tibial fractures?

Closed wounds or closed reductions were associated with shorter healing rates compared with open wounds or open fracture repair.

CONTROVERSY

25. How should an IM pin be placed for repair of a tibial diaphyseal fracture?

Normograde, in a slightly caudolateral direction, medial to the patellar tendon midway along the craniomedial edge of the tibial plateau. This positioning avoids damage to the craniad cruciate ligament, femoral condyle, and joint capsule.

Less frequently described options:

- Craniomedially directed retrograde pins seated below the articular surface.
- IM pin exiting (retrograde pinning) or entering (normograde pinning) the cranial border of the tibial tuberosity.

BIBLIOGRAPHY

1. Aron DN, Johnson AL: Biologic strategies and a balanced concept for repair of highly comminuted long bone fractures. Comp Cont Educ Pract Vet 17:35–49, 1995.
2. Boone EG, Johnson AL: Fractures of the tibial diaphysis in dogs and cats. J Am Vet Med Assoc 188:41–45, 1986.
3. Coetzee GL: Long bone fracture fixation with an intramedullary pin and C-clamp-on plate in dogs. Vet Comp Orthol Traum 12:26–32, 1999.
4. Dudley M, Johnson AL: Open reduction and bone plate stabilization, compared with closed reduction and external fixation, for treatment of comminuted tibial fractures in dogs. J Am Vet Med Assoc 211:1008–1012, 1997.
5. Dueland RT, Johnson KA: Interlocking nail treatment of diaphyseal long-bone fractures in dogs. J Am Vet Med Assoc 214:59–66, 1999.
6. Harari J, Seguin B: Closed repair of tibial and radial fractures with external skeletal fixation. Comp Cont Educ Pract Vet 18:651–665, 1996.
7. Johnson AL, Boone EG: Fractures of the tibia and fibula. In Slatter D (ed): Textbook of Small Animal Surgery, 2nd ed. Philadelphia, W.B. Saunders, 1993, pp 1866–1875.
8. Montavon PM, Dee JF: Distal tibial articular fractures in racing greyhounds. Vet Comp Orthop Traum 6:146–152, 1993.
9. Pardo AD: Relationship of tibial intramedullary pins to canine stifle joint structures: A comparison of normograde and retrograde insertion. J Am Anim Hosp Assoc 30:369–374, 1994.
10. Piermattei DL, Flow GL: Handbook of Small Animal Orthopedics, 3rd ed. Philadelphia, W.B. Saunders, 1997, pp 581–606.

71. TRAUMATIC INJURIES OF THE TARSUS AND METATARSUS

Joseph Harari, M.S., D.V.M., Dip. A.C.V.S.

1. What is the tarsus?

In the **dog,** a complex structure composed of seven bones arranged in two transverse rows and supported by collateral ligaments, intertarsal ligaments, plantar ligaments, and fibrocartilage. In the cat, 14 bones with more than 20 joint surfaces.

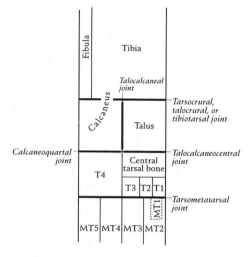

Relationships of bones and joints in the canine hock.

2. What are the components of the collateral ligaments?

The long part of the medial collateral ligament originates on the medial malleolus and firmly attaches to the first and central tarsal bones. The short parts run under the long section and attach caudally to the talus and the first tarsal and metatarsal bones. The long part of the lateral collateral ligament passes from the lateral malleolus to the base the fifth metatarsal and attaches, along its course, to the calcaneus and fourth tarsal bone. The underlying short parts attach to the tuber calcaneus and talus.

3. What are the functions of these components?

1. The long parts stabilize the joint in extension.
2. The short parts stabilize the joint in extension and flexion.

4. What are the most common injuries of the tarsus?

Traumatic luxations and subluxations of one or several joints, bone fractures, and shearing wounds.

5. List the diagnostic procedures useful in determining the nature of a tarsal injury.

- Physical examination of gait during weight bearing
- Palpation to detect instability
- Oblique and stressed radiographs to identify fractures and instabilities

6. Which surgical protocol is useful in reducing intraoperative hemorrhage and surgical time during surgery of the tarsus?

Use of a tourniquet.

7. Which joint of the tarsus is responsible for the greatest degree of movement?

Talocrural joint (also called **tarsocrural** or **tibiotarsal joint**).

8 Tarsocrural luxation is often associated with which lesions?

- Rupture of collateral ligaments
- Joint capsule tearing
- Fractures of the malleoli

9. How are collateral ligament instabilities treated?

Prosthetic ligament replacement using synthetic, nonabsorbable suture placed in a figure-8 pattern under screws and washers or through bone tunnels. Placement follows the origins and insertions of short and long components of the collateral ligaments.

10. For tarsocrural arthrodesis, what is the dorsal angle for stabilization of the joint?

In general, the hock angle of the contralateral (normal) limb is the best example to follow.
- For dogs, 135°
- For cats, 120°

11. How is tarsocrural arthrodesis performed?

Bone screws, multiple pins, bone plate, or external skeletal fixation (linear or circular). In all cases, cancellous bone graft, cartilage débridement, and external support (except for external fixation) should be performed.

12. What are the clinical results of pantarsal arthrodesis?
- Pantarsal arthrodesis with a dorsally applied plate provides the greatest stability to the limb for return of near-normal function.
- Implant failures are common.
- Incomplete bone fusion of the middle and distal joints may be apparent radiographically.
- Clinical outcomes are variable and do not match the success of pancarpal arthrodesis.

13. Which surgical protocol is useful when applying a bone plate dorsally on the tension side (rather than the theoretically preferred compression side) of the tarsus during panarthrodesis?

Use of lengthening plates, in dogs, which lack central screw-holes and are resistant to bending stresses.

14. In comparing the biomechanical properties of an acrylic versus metal external fixator for hock arthrodesis, which findings are noted?

The acrylic external fixator is biomechanically comparable to the stainless steel external fixator, and application of metatarsal pins in a dorsal-to-plantar direction is superior in maintaining joint reduction.

15. Name the most common shearing injury of limbs.

Medial aspect of the tarsometatarsal area.

16. With shearing injuries of the medial tarsus, which technique, prosthetic collateral ligament placement or transarticular external fixation, is superior with regards to patient recovery?

Neither of the techniques is better in terms of healing rates, regaining limb function, or final clinical outcome. Both treatments produce nearly 75% excellent or good recovery rates within 2–3 months.

17. Which joint spaces make up the proximal intertarsal joint?

Laterally the calcaneoquartal and medially the talocalcaneal joint spaces.

18. Which breeds are predisposed to proximal intertarsal luxation or subluxation?

The Shetland sheepdog and the collie.

19. How is calcaneoquartal arthrodesis performed?

A laterally applied bone plate or tension band wire technique.

20. How is a talocalcaneal luxation treated?

A bone screw placed from talus to calcaneus.

21. Which treatment is recommended for tarsometatarsal luxation or subluxation?

Arthrodesis with pins or a laterally applied bone plate.

22. What are important characteristics of tarsal injuries in cats?
- The degree of soft tissue trauma greatly influences final clinical outcome.

- Collateral ligament and intertarsal injuries can be easily treated.
- Tarsocrural luxations have a poor prognosis.

23. Which bones of the tarsus are frequently fractured?
The calcaneus and the central tarsal bone.

24. Which breed most frequently sustains tarsal fractures?
Greyhound

25. Which principle must be critically followed during repair of calcaneal fractures?
The **tension band principle** must be used to counteract the distractive forces of the common calcaneal tendon (Achilles' tendon); implants used can be pins and figure-8 orthopedic wire or a laterally applied bone plate. Cancellous grafting and external support with the hock in extension are also useful in promoting bone healing.

26. What is the Achilles' tendon?
The confluence of structures attaching to the tuber calcanei, including the tendons of the gastrocnemius muscle, superficial digital flexor muscle, biceps femoris muscle, semitendinosus muscle, and gracilis muscle.

27. How are central tarsal bone fractures treated?
Internal repair with bone screws is recommended based on the grade (I–V) or severity of injury (available bone stock). Highly comminuted fractures are externally coapted. Synthetic (titanium) replacement has also been described.

28. Which is the most common type of central tarsal bone fractures in racing greyhounds?
Type IV fracture, composed of dorsal and medial slabs.

29. In racing greyhounds, which hind limbs have the highest incidence of distal paw fractures?
Fractures of the right tarsus (central bone) and the third metatarsal; these have been related to stresses from multiple turns, racing counterclockwise on circular or elliptical tracks.

30. What orthopedics principles are useful for treating metatarsal fractures?
- Similar to metacarpal fractures, intramedullary pinning and bone plating (large dogs) are reserved for multiple (three or more bones), displaced, or weight-bearing (third and fourth metatarsal) bone fractures.
- Fractures of the lateral or medial bones proximally should be stabilized if valgus or varus deformation of the tarsometatarsal region exists.

BIBLIOGRAPHY

1. Beardsley S, Schrader SC: Treatment of dogs with wounds of the limbs caused by shearing forces. J Am Vet Med Assoc 207:1071–1075, 1995.
2. Boemo CM: Injuries of the metacarpus and metatarsus. In Bloomberg MS, Dee JF (eds): Canine Sports Medicine and Surgery. Philadelphia, W.B. Saunders, 1998, pp 150–164.
3. Diamond DW, Besso J: Evaluation of joint stabilization for treatment of shearing injuries of the tarsus in 20 dogs. J Am Hosp Assoc 35:147–153, 1999.
4. Dyce J, Whitelock RG: Arthrodesis of the tarsometatarsal joint using a laterally applied plate in 10 dogs. J Small Anim Pract 39:19–23, 1998.
5. Gorse MJ, Earley TD: Tarsocrural arthrodesis: Long-term functional results. J Am Anim Hosp Assoc 27:231-235, 1991.
6. Muir P, Norris JL: Metacarpal and metatarsal fractures in dogs. J Small Anim Pract 38:344–348, 1997.
7. Muir P, Norris JL: Tarsometatarsal subluxation in dogs: Partial arthrodesis by plate fixation. J Am Anim Hosp Assoc 35:155–162, 1999.
8. Piermattei DL, Flo GL: Handbook of Small Animal Orthopedics and Fracture Repair, 3rd ed. Philadelphia, W.B. Saunders, 1997, pp 607–658.
9. Schmökel HG, Hartmeier GE: Tarsal injuries in the cat. J Small Anim Pract 35:156–162, 1994.
10. Taylor RA, Dee JF: Tarsus and metatarsus. In Slatter D (ed): Textbook of Small Animal Surgery, 2nd ed. Philadelphia, W.B. Saunders, 1993, pp 1876–1887.

72. PHYSEAL FRACTURES

Randy J. Boudrieau, D.V.M., Dip. A.C.V.S.

1. What are the basic principles of treatment for physeal fractures?
- Preservation of the blood supply
- Accurate anatomic reduction
- Stable skeletal fixation

2. What are the primary concerns with a physeal fracture?
Prevention of **angular deformities** and **limb shortening.** Client communication is critical so that potential long-term problems are anticipated because 100% success is unlikely. A reasonable expectation must be proposed so that appropriate corrective surgery may be performed to prevent or treat a leg deformity or shortening.

3. How does longitudinal bone growth occur?
By **endochondral ossification** (the process by which cartilage is resorbed and replaced by bone).

4. Discuss the anatomic basis of endochondral ossification at the physis or growth plate.
The physis is traditionally divided into four zones:
1. **Reserve zone**—located adjacent to the epiphysis and composed of scattered chondrocytes and abundant cartilage matrix. Random cell division and matrix production occur in this zone.
2. **Proliferating zone**—chondrocyte division occurs in a linear fashion (cells closest to the epiphysis, at the base of each cell column, are true germinal cells of the physis). Cellular division occurs in columns extending away from the epiphysis. Additionally, these cells change shape from round or oval to broad and flat as they move away from the epiphysis; matrix production is maximum.
3. **Hypertrophic zone**—the flattened chondrocytes gradually enlarge to a more cuboidal shape ($8\times$ increase in volume). There is a corresponding decrease in the amount of matrix surrounding these cells; biochemical changes begin to occur in the matrix that prepares it for subsequent calcification.
4. **Provisional calcification zone**—seeding of the matrix with amorphous calcium phosphate leads to hydroxyapatite crystal formation and subsequent calcification of the longitudinal septa of the matrix. The cartilage matrix calcification provides a template for subsequent vascular invasion and a scaffold for bone deposition from the metaphysis or formation of the primary spongiosa (woven bone). The primary spongiosa consequently undergoes further remodeling to secondary spongiosa (lamellar bone). The latter becomes the trabecular architecture of the metaphysis and gradually becomes the more dense cortical bone of the diaphysis.

5. Describe the blood supply to both sides of the physis.
The epiphysis and the metaphysis are supplied separately. The **epiphyseal vessels** supply the nutritional needs to the reserve and proliferative zones of the physis. The metaphysis is supplied by the **metaphyseal vessels** and their anastomosis with the terminal branches of the medullary circulation (originating from the nutrient artery). The metaphyseal vessels provide the access for subsequent ossification of the calcification zone and the primary spongiosa.

6. Why should one care about the anatomic configuration of the physis and its blood supply?
Understanding the anatomy helps delineate fracture location through the physis and determines prognosis (continued or arrested growth, shortened limb or angular deformity). Interruption of the epiphyseal blood supply results in necrosis of the germinal cells and cessation of growth (irreversible); interruption of the metaphyseal blood supply results in a temporary cessation of ossification, which resumes once the blood supply is restored (reversible).

7. Where is fracture through the physis most likely to occur?
The **cartilaginous physis** is weaker than surrounding bone and ligaments, making it most susceptible to injury. The weakest area of the physis is the junction between the hypertrophic and proliferative zones. The hypertrophic zone has the largest difference of cell-to-matrix ratio that weakens its structure. There is a difference in mechanical or material properties at this level between these two zones that results in an area of stress concentration. The result is a fracture that occurs **through the hypertrophic zone.**

8. Why is the specific fracture location in the physis significant?
A fracture through the hypertrophic zone does not affect the reserve or proliferating zones, preserving proliferation of the germinal cells, which permits further longitudinal bone growth.

9. Does knowledge of the anatomy and vascular supply have any bearing on the Salter-Harris classification of physeal fractures?
Yes. It helps to determine the prognosis or potential for remaining longitudinal bone growth.

10. What is the Salter-Harris classification scheme?
Classification of physeal fractures based on anatomic location and correlated with prognosis.

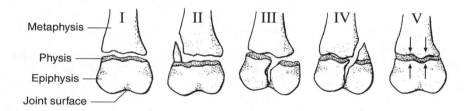

11. Describe the types of Salter-Harris fractures.
- **Type I**—fracture or separation through the hypertrophic zone.
- **Type II**—fracture or separation through a portion of the hypertrophic zone and metaphysis.
- **Type III**—fracture or separation through a portion of the hypertrophic zone and epiphysis (intraarticular).
- **Type IV**—fracture or separation through a portion of the hypertrophic zone, metaphysis, and epiphysis (intraarticular)
- **Type V**—a crushing injury of the physis.

12. Where are the most common physeal fracture locations for each of the individual Salter-Harris categories?

TYPE	LOCATION
I	Femoral head (capital physis)
II	Distal femur
III	Proximal tibia
IV	Distal humerus
V	Distal ulna

13. Is there a Salter-Harris type VI fracture?

Salter and Harris did not originally describe this fracture classification; in a subsequent publication, they added it as a variant of the Salter-Harris type V fracture. In this instance, trauma to the physis results in some bridging of new bone across one side of the growth plate (effectively resulting in cessation of growth in that area and an angular or rotational deformity). One iatrogenic example is with the use of a large-diameter pin to stabilize (bridge) the physis.

14. What is the prognosis for continued longitudinal bone growth based on each of the Salter-Harris classifications from type I to V?

The best prognosis (potential for continued longitudinal bone growth) is for a type I fracture. There is a progression of worsening prognosis from type I to V, with a type V fracture resulting in a cessation of physeal growth.

15. Does this mean that a type I or II fracture always has a good prognosis compared with a type III or IV fracture?

No. The Salter-Harris classification does not take into consideration the specific bone involved or location of the fracture (e.g., proximal vs. distal femur). The age of the animal and remaining growth potential of the bone involved are critical.

In general, types I and II fractures have a generally better prognosis than types III and IV fractures. The latter fracture types may have damage to a portion of the germinal cells and consequently may have cessation of growth in a portion of the physis, resulting in an angular deformity. There is an intraarticular component that may result in the subsequent development of degenerative joint disease (DJD). **Type V fractures,** because they are crushing injuries to the physis and by definition affect the germinal cells, result in cessation of growth and have the poorest prognosis.

16. What is the contribution of the blood supply to the prognosis for continued longitudinal bone growth?

Despite the proposed prognosis based on the Salter-Harris classification, damage to either the epiphyseal or the metaphyseal blood supply also affects continued growth. A traumatic event sufficient to cause a fracture through the physis also is likely to cause damage to the supplying vasculature—resulting in an irreversible injury to the germinal cells. The germinal cells undergo necrosis as a result of this interruption of the blood supply with subsequent cessation of growth. This vascular injury may occur as a result of the initial trauma or the subsequent surgical intervention to stabilize the fracture.

17. Discuss the effect of fracture location on prognosis.

The best example is the comparison of proximal (type I) and distal physeal injury (type II) of the femur. In cases with significant remaining growth, the proximal femoral physeal injury has the worse prognosis because of intracapsular vascular injury. Displacement of this physis causes an interruption of the epiphyseal blood supply. Necrosis of the germinal cell layer occurs, and growth arrest invariably results. The end result (depending on remaining growth potential) is a shortened femoral neck, coxofemoral joint laxity with subluxation, and the eventual development of degenerative joint disease (DJD). Alternatively, the distal femoral epiphysis receives its blood supply extracapsularly. The blood supply enters the epiphysis directly and may be spared when displacement of the physis occurs, and the potential for longitudinal bone growth is preserved.

18. What is the significance of patient age at the time of trauma?

A younger animal has a longer period of growth remaining and the greater potential to have a significant problem related to a short limb or an angular deformity. A puppy with a type I proximal femoral physeal fracture at 3–4 months of age has significant growth remaining, and injury causes cessation of femoral neck growth, resulting in subluxation of the femoral head and development of DJD. If the same fracture occurs by 7 months of age, 95% of femoral neck growth has occurred, and subsequent DJD problems are unlikely. When distal femoral physeal fractures occur in dogs more than 5 months of age, by that time they have achieved 80% of their longitudinal bone growth. This degree of anticipated limb shortening is not likely to result in a significant clinical dysfunction.

19. How might the age of the animal, and the relationship to its final adult size, make a difference with the prognosis?

Smaller breeds of dogs arrive at their adult height relatively sooner than larger breeds; the same physeal fracture in a chihuahua, as compared with a Great Dane, at 5 months of age has a markedly different outcome.

20. Why does limb shortening, in which only 80% of bone length is achieved, not result in a clinical problem?

Lack of functional impairment has to do with the flexed limb stance of these species. A compensatory increase in the stance angles of the adjacent joints eliminates this length discrepancy.

21. Does the specific bone in which trauma occurs make a difference regarding prognosis?

Yes. In contrast to the femur, the proximal and distal humeral physes close at approximately 10–12 and 6–7 months. The latter helps to explain why, despite a Salter-Harris type IV classification of most distal humeral fractures in young dogs, there is a good prognosis for return to function. The best example is the difference between single versus paired bones; the classic example is the radius and ulna paired bone system.

22. What is significant about the radius and ulna?

The differential rates of growth that occur at each end of the respective bones: The radius and ulna must grow longitudinally and in concert with each other. The proximal and distal radial physes account for 40% and 60% of longitudinal bone growth. The proximal and distal ulnar physes account for 10–15% and 80–85% of the longitudinal bone growth. Fractures to any of these physes that result in cessation of physeal growth in any single location result in angular limb deformities because of the constraint now present from the bone no longer keeping pace with continued growth of the remaining physes (other bone in the paired system).

23. Why is the distal ulnar physis most often affected with a type V fracture?

A shearing force to the distal radius and ulna results in compression to the distal ulnar physis because of its conical shape, causing a crushing injury, or a type V fracture. The same shearing forces to the distal radius result in a fracture through the hypertrophic zone, or a type I fracture. The end result is distal ulnar growth arrest only.

24. Does a single bone growth arrest result in angular limb deformities?

Rarely, unless the growth arrest affects only a portion of the physis.

25. Does the paired bone combination of the tibia and fibula result in angular limb deformities?

Rarely.

26. What is the overall prognosis for an animal with a physeal fracture?

In general, a **guarded** prognosis should be given for **all** fractures of a physis, regardless of the Salter-Harris classification, because there are many factors that contribute to the ultimate success or failure of treatment. If the animal has minimal growth potential remaining, the prognosis is quite good provided that accurate fracture repair is obtained.

27. What are the effects of the fixation devices on continued physeal growth?

Fixation devices that bridge the physis, such as an external skeletal fixator or a plate and screws, prevent further longitudinal bone growth. Implants that cross the physis directly (pins and screws) also can cause damage to the physis in the area of their penetration. The threads of a screw (or a threaded pin) can engage in the cartilage and prevent continued longitudinal growth. Smooth pins allow the proliferating cartilage to slide along the surface of the pin. Pins placed perpendicular to the physis have less of an effect on continued growth than pins placed obliquely. Small-diameter pins placed at an oblique angle (cross-pins) do not impede growth if an acute angle with the long axis of the bone is maintained.

BIBLIOGRAPHY

1. Brighton CT: Structure and function of the growth plate. Clin Orthop Rel Res 136:22–32, 1978.
2. Iannotti JP: Growth plate physiology and pathology. Orthop Clin North Am 21:1–17, 1990.
3. Johnson AL: Correction of radial and ulnar growth deformities resulting from premature physeal closure. In Bojrab MJ (ed): Current Techniques in Veterinary Surgery, 4th ed. Philadelphia, Lea & Febiger, 1998, pp 1094–1101.
4. Robertson WW: Newest knowledge of the growth plate. Clin Orthop Rel Res 253:270-278, 1990.
5. Salter RB, Harris WR: Injuries involving the epiphyseal plate. J Bone Joint Surg Am 45:587–622, 1963.

73. ORTHOPEDIC COMPLICATIONS

Joseph Harari, M.S., D.V.M., Dip. A.C.V.S.

1. What is a surgical complication?

A secondary condition developing during treatment of a primary disease. A complication appears unexpectedly and causes a change in existing plans, methods, or attitudes. Complications arise as a consequence of failure in following basic or established guidelines and principles.

2. What is the goal of orthopedic repairs?

A rapid return of limb functions similar to the preoperative or normal state based on early rigid internal or external fixation and preservation of periosseous soft tissues.

3. What are common complications of fracture fixation?

Abnormal limb function or disuse resulting from:

Inappropriate bone union	Neurovascular damage
Implant failure	Degenerative osteoarthritis (articular fractures)
Infection	Growth arrest (physeal fractures)
Soft tissue compromise	

4. Define inappropriate bone unions (healing).

- **Delayed unions** are due to instability, infection, avascularity, and tissue atrophy.
- **Nonunions** never achieve healing because of mechanical instability or lack of osteogenesis.
- **Malunions** produce shortened, angular, or rotational deformations.

5. What is an *elephant's foot* callus?

A radiographic diagnosis of a nonunion characterized by abundant (hypertrophic) callus associated with inadequate fracture stabilization.

6. What is a *horse's hoof* callus?

A radiographic diagnosis of a nonunion characterized by mild callus, bone resorption under a plate, and screw or plate failure associated with inefficient fracture stabilization.

7. Define a pseudarthrosis.

Formation of false joint in a delayed union or nonunion characterized by fibrous union of bone ends bathed in synovial-like (serum) fluid and surrounded by a fibrous joint capsule–like structure; motion is present at the fracture site.

8. What is the difference between oligotrophic and atrophic fracture healing?

Oligotrophic nonunions have biologic activity (vascular fibrous tissue), whereas atrophic nonunions lack tissue viability.

9. How are inappropriate unions treated?

Based on the underlying causes of the lesion:

- Implant removal or replacement—restabilization
- Autogenous cancellous bone grafting—osteogenesis
- Antibiotic therapy—systemic or sustained local delivery
- Bone débridement—resect necrotic bone, open medullary cavity
- Z-plasties—overcome contractures
- Physical therapy—restore limb function
- Arthrodesis—salvage modified limb function
- Amputation—adequate quality of life

10. Why do implants fail?

- Misapplication and inability to counteract distractive fracture site forces (compression, tension, bending, rotation).
- Normal cycling or fatigue failures of the metals over time.

11. List specific complications of plates and screws.

- Inappropriate size selection leading to breakage or stress protection.
- Inadequate load sharing by bone or ancillary implants.
- Malpositioned plate.
- Inadequate screw fixation.

12. What are specific complications of pins and wires?

Inadequate placement, number, and size of the implants.

13. What are specific complications of interlocking nails?

Nail breakage at screw hole (proximal hole, distal fragment) resulting from undersized nail or proximity to fracture site.

14. List specific complications of external fixation.

- Pin tract sepsis—excessive pin and skin motion.
- Fixator problems—configuration, pins, and clamps.
- Soft tissue impalement—neurovascular elements, muscles, and tendons.

15. List specific complications of external splintage.

- Inadequate stability or fracture reduction.
- Soft tissue compromise sores and stiff joints.
- Cast or splintage breakage.

16. Define fracture disease.

Disuse atrophy of bone, cartilage, joint capsule, ligaments, and muscles secondary to excessive immobilization after fracture repair, trauma, or external splintage. Fracture disease is most frequently associated with inadequate repair of femoral fracture (quadriceps contracture) in young dogs or humeral condyle lesions. In the former, the hind limb is held in extension, whereas in the latter, the forelimb is in a mildly flexed position.

17. How can fracture disease be avoided?

Rigid stabilization and rapid return to limb functions; temporary postoperative flexion (hind limb) or extension (forelimb) bandages to counteract muscle contractions, followed by physical therapy.

18. Which neurovascular elements are associated with orthopedic conditions?

Neurovascular Element	Orthopedic Conditions
Radial nerve	Humeral diaphysial fractures, lateral approach
Sciatic nerve	Ilial shaft, acetabular fractures; femoral pinning by greater trochanter
Median artery	Interosseous branches skewered by external fixator pins
Caudal tibial artery	Skewered by external fixator pins
Brachial artery; median, ulnar, and musculocutaneous nerves	Medial approach to humeral shaft

19. How can complications be prevented?
- Avoid "getting by" in surgery and "giving it (suspected complication) some time" as a treatment.
- Follow established and accepted perioperative protocols.
- Preoperatively, warn clients of potential complications (if they arise, they are not an unexpected problem but rather a treatable event wisely predicted by the surgeon).

BIBLIOGRAPHY

1. Martinez SA: Fracture management and bone healing. Vet Clin North Am Small Anim Pract 29:1029–1274, 1999.
2. Newton CD: Fracture repair. In Lipowitz AJ, Caywood DD (eds): Complications in Small Animal Surgery. Philadelphia, Williams & Wilkins, 1996, pp 563–599.
3. Olmstead ML: Fracture complications. Vet Clin North Am Small Anim Pract 21:641–872, 1991.

74. GROWTH DEFORMITIES

Ann L. Johnson, D.V.M., M.S., Dip. A.C.V.S.

1. Why do growth deformities most frequently affect the antebrachium?
Because of the paired bone system and the unique shape of the distal ulnar physis. Synchronous growth of the radius and ulna in the dog is essential for the development of a forelimb and requires normal functioning of the proximal and distal physes of the radius and ulna.

2. Which physis contributes the greatest percentage of bone length in the paired radius and ulnar system?
- The **radius** receives 40% of its length from the proximal physis and 60% from the distal physis.
- The **ulna** receives 85% of its length from the distal physis and 15% from the proximal physis.

3. At what age are dogs most susceptible to developing a curvature after premature physeal closure?
Although variable and based on breed, growth accelerates rapidly during the fifth to seventh months and tapers off during the ninth to tenth months. Toy-breed dogs may be finished growing by 6 months of age, whereas giant-breed dogs can continue to grow to 10 and 11 months of age.

4. What unique anatomic shape of the distal ulnar physis is responsible for its frequent involvement in growth deformities?
The **cone shape** of the distal ulnar physis prevents physeal separation during injury. Instead, forces applied to the limb cause a Salter-Harris type V crushing injury, which damages the physis and results in complete closure.

5. What are the sequela to premature closure of the distal ulnar physis?
- Shortening of the ulna
- Cranial bowing
- Valgus angulation
- External rotation
- Shortening of the radius
- Varying amounts of elbow and carpal incongruity

6. How is premature closure of the distal ulnar physis diagnosed?

Premature closure of a physis is suspected after injury to the immature forelimb, or the dog may be presented with an obvious forelimb curvature. **Radiographs** are necessary for definitive diagnosis. Craniocaudal and lateral views of the affected forelimb are made. Each radiograph should include the radius, ulna, elbow, and carpus. **Radiographs of the opposite normal limb** serve as a control for determining the normal length of the radius and ulna and the normal anatomy of the forelimb. In early cases of premature closure of the distal ulnar physis, a discrepancy in ulnar lengths may be determined before there is obvious deformity of the forelimb. Measurements of bone length and angular limb deformity should be made from the radiographs to establish a preoperative standard against which the results of treatment are compared.

7. Can curvature after a premature physeal closure be prevented by splinting or casting the limb?

No. The restraining effect of a short bone with a prematurely closed physis on the growing bone with active physes is too strong to be overcome with a splint. Surgical treatment (**ostectomy** of the affected bone) is necessary to remove the restraint on physeal growth of the paired bone and should be done as soon as possible in an immature dog with significant growth potential.

8. How is premature closure of the distal ulnar physis treated in the growing dog?

The goal of treatment is to regain unrestricted growth of the normal physes of the radius and ulna, which allows for maximal limb development and, in some cases, correction of the angular deformity. An **ulnar ostectomy** is used to release the constraint placed on the radius by the ulna and is coupled with the placement of a free autogenous fat graft to prevent premature union of the ulnar segments.

9. For show dogs, can the results of ulnar ostectomy be guaranteed?

Prognosis for normal appearance and function is guarded. Much of the outcome depends on the growth potential of the radial physes. With favorable conditions, an animal may achieve normal length of the limb and some correction of valgus angulation. Rotational deformities are not corrected. Owners must be informed of the possibility that additional surgical procedures may be necessary for complete recovery.

10. What deformities occur with premature closure of the distal radial physis?
- **Symmetric** complete closure of the distal radial physis results in a shortened but straight radius, incongruity of the elbow, and a varus angulation of the carpus.
- The limb deformity seen with **asymmetric** or partial physeal closure of the distal radius depends on the location of the closure. The most common is a caudal lateral closure of the physis, resulting in a valgus deformity of the carpus. The normal anatomy of the carpus may be disrupted.

11. How is partial premature closure of the distal radial physis treated in the growing dog?

The goal of treatment is to allow unrestricted growth of the normal portion of the distal radial physis. Tomographic examination or direct palpation by needles of the distal radial physis may help define the area of the physis that is closed and bridged with bone. The animal is treated with a **resection of the bone-bridged area of the physis** and placement of a free autogenous fat graft in the defect to prevent reestablishment of the bone bridge.

12. How is complete premature closure of the proximal or distal radial physis treated in the growing dog?

The goals of treatment are to allow unrestricted growth of the normal physes of the radius and ulna and to restore and maintain congruity of the elbow. A **radial ostectomy** and free autogenous fat graft is performed to allow continued growth of the ulna.

13. How effective are an ostectomy and fat graft if the radial and ulnar distal physes have closed and the immature dog has a significantly shortened forelimb?

An ostectomy and fat graft does not work for these patients. The preferred treatment is a **radial and ulnar osteotomy** and an external fixation, which allows **continuous distraction** of the bone ends. The circular fixator is best suited for controlled distraction to restore bone length and can be used to correct angular deformity simultaneously.

14. How is a radius curvus resulting from premature closure of the distal ulnar physis treated in the mature dog?

If the dog has not lost a significant amount of limb length, the goals of treatment are to correct angular and rotational deformities, while preserving as much length of the limb as possible during the corrective osteotomy procedure. The procedure most frequently used is the **oblique radial and ulnar osteotomy** with repositioning of the distal radial segment and **stabilization** with an external fixator. If there is significant loss of limb length, a circular fixator can be used to distract the bones after an acute corrective osteotomy. The circular fixator can also be used to correct angular deformities and lengthen the bone. Circular external fixation is a complex procedure and requires a trained surgeon along with attentive clients.

15. What is the prognosis for function and appearance after a corrective osteotomy?

Always guarded. Cosmetic appearance depends on success in restoring the normal alignment of the limb. Function is affected by any additional pathology, such as degenerative joint disease resulting from incongruent joints.

16. What techniques can be used to restore congruity of the elbow caused by premature closure of the radial or the ulnar physes?

An alternative approach, in dogs with minimal limb-length discrepancies, to treatment of incongruity of the elbow caused by premature closure of the radial physis is an **oblique ostectomy** of the proximal ulna above the interosseous ligament. A small Steinmann pin is inserted in the bone to maintain alignment of the ulna and prevent distraction by the pull of the triceps muscle. The dynamic (weight bearing and muscular contractions) shortening of the ulna allows the radial head to make contact with the capitulum of the humerus.

Treatment for elbow congruity caused by premature closure of the distal ulnar physis with minimal limb-length discrepancy or angular deformity is a **proximal ulnar osteotomy.** A small intramedullary Steinmann pin is used to maintain alignment of the ulna. The dynamic distraction of the proximal ulna caused by the pull of the triceps muscles allows the olecranon to contact the distal humerus.

17. What is pes varus?

A distal tibia deformity described in dachshunds and associated with asymmetric closure of the distal physis.

18. How is pes varus treated?

Corrective osteotomy and external skeletal fixation of the tibia.

BIBLIOGRAPHY

1. Forell EB, Schwartz PD: Use of external skeletal fixation for treatment of angular deformity secondary to premature distal ulnar physeal closure. J Am Anim Hosp Assoc 29:460–476, 1993.

2. Gilson SD, Piermattei DL, Schwartz PD: Treatment of humeroulnar subluxation with a dynamic proximal ulnar osteotomy. Vet Surg 18:114–122, 1989.
3. Johnson AL: Correction of radial and ulnar growth deformities resulting from premature physeal closure. In Bojrab (ed): Current Techniques in Small Animal Surgery, 4th ed. Philadelphia, Lea & Febiger, 1997, pp 1094–1101.
4. Johnson SG, Hulse DA: Corrective osteotomy for pes varus in the dachshund. Vet Surg 18:373–379, 1989.
5. Marcellin-Little DJ, Ferretti A, Roe SC, et al: Hinged Ilizarov external fixator for correction of antebrachial deformity. Vet Surg 27:231–245, 1998.
6. Salter RB, Harris WR: Injuries involving the epiphyseal plate. J Bone Joint Surg 45:587–622, 1963.
7. Shields Henney LH, Gambardella PC: Partial ulnar ostectomy for treatment of premature closure of the proximal and distal radial physes in the dog. J Am Anim Hosp Assoc 26:183–188, 1990.
8. Stallings JT, Lewis DD, Welch R, et al: An introduction to distraction osteogenesis and the principles of the Ilizarov method. Vet Clin Orthop Trauma 11:59–67, 1998.

75. BONE GRAFTING

Ann L. Johnson, D.V.M., M.S., Dip. A.C.V.S.

1. What is the difference between a bone autograft and allograft?
Bone transplanted from one site to another in the same animal is an **autograft.** Such grafts are histocompatible with host immune systems and do not initiate rejection responses.
Bone transplanted from one animal to another of the same species is an **allograft.** Cellular antigens of these grafts may be recognized as foreign by host immune systems and result in graft rejection.

2. Discuss the functions of a bone graft in the host site.
Bone grafts can stimulate **osteogenesis,** by providing cells capable of forming bone or by recruiting from surrounding tissues mesenchymal-type cells, which differentiate into cartilage-forming and bone-forming cells. The latter process is called **osteoinduction.** Bone grafts provide varying degrees of mechanical support, ranging from space-occupying trellises for host bone invasion to supplying weight-bearing struts within fractures. The process of vascular and osteoprogenitor cell invasion along the trellis of bone is called **osteoconduction.** All of these bone graft functions vary depending on the type of graft used.

3. What is a bone morphogenic protein (BMP)?
BMPs are found in osteoclasts and bone matrix; they are classified as growth factors involved in bone healing along with transforming growth factor-B, insulin-like growth factors I and II, acidic fibroblast growth factor, platelet-derived growth factors, fibroblast growth factor, interleukins, granulocyte colony-stimulating factors, and granulocyte-macrophage colony-stimulating factors. **BMPs induce or influence mesenchymal cell differentiation into bone-forming cells.** Demineralization of bone graft matrix allows these proteins to be active.

4. Why would a cancellous bone autograft be used?
An autogenous cancellous bone graft is used to enhance bone formation. It assists healing when optimal healing is not anticipated (cortical defects after fracture repair, adult and elderly animals with fractures, delayed unions, nonunions, corrective osteotomies, joint arthrodesis, and cystic defects), or it may be used to promote bone formation in infected fractures.
As a general rule, anytime an open fracture reduction is performed, especially in long bones, a cancellous bone autograft should be used.

5. Where is a cancellous bone autograft obtained?

Cancellous bone may be harvested from any long bone metaphysis; **proximal humerus, proximal tibia,** and **ilial wing** are most commonly used because they are accessible and contain large amounts of cancellous bone. The graft site is usually selected based on animal positioning during fracture repair.

6. Is a cancellous autograft harvested at the beginning or the end of the primary surgical procedure?

The graft is usually harvested after fracture stabilization; it may be harvested before the primary orthopedic procedure if there is concern that the donor site may be contaminated by tumor cells or bacteria at the recipient site. Alternatively a separate surgical team and instrumentation may be used to harvest the graft.

7. How do you keep cancellous autograft cells viable during the transfer?

Cancellous bone is placed directly into the recipient bed or stored in a blood-soaked sponge or blood-containing stainless steel cup. The blood clots and forms a moldable composite with the graft, which facilitates handling. To maintain viability, cancellous bone grafts are not kept in saline or treated with antibiotics. Stored grafts are secured on the instrument table to avoid disposal.

8. Why is a round access hole in the cortex of a long bone used to expose the cancellous graft?

To minimize formation of a stress riser that could contribute to fracture through the cortical defect.

9. What are the biologic steps for incorporation of the cancellous autograft into the healing fracture site?

1. **Revascularization** of cancellous bone autografts begins as early as 2 days and is usually completed within 2 weeks.

2. Transplanted osteogenic cells or differentiated mesenchymal cells become active osteoblasts, secreting **osteoid** on transplanted trabecular bone.

3. This osteoid is **mineralized** and forms new host bone in fracture sites. This new bone also incorporates the graft into host bone.

4. Eventually the necrotic cores of trabecular bone are resorbed by osteoclasts, and grafts are totally replaced by host bone.

5. Trabecular new bone is **remodeled** into cortical bone in response to the mechanical environment.

This process is usually complete within 1 year.

10. When can a metaphyseal cancellous graft site be used for a second harvest?

The donor site is initially filled with hematoma that is later replaced with fibrous connective tissue. Osteoblasts migrate to the area and deposit osteoid. Mineralization occurs, and new trabecular bone is formed within defects. This process takes approximately 12 weeks; additional cancellous bone should not be harvested from the same area before this time.

11. How frequently do complications occur with cancellous autografting?

Complications generally affect the donor site. Donor site pain is seldom clinically evident in small animals. Seroma formation or wound dehiscence may occur at donor sites. Infection or seeding of tumor to donor sites occurs rarely and can be prevented by proper sequencing of bone graft harvesting. Fractures through the donor site have been occasionally reported. Complications at the recipient site (e.g., failure of grafts to stimulate bone formation) are difficult to recognize.

12. What is the most frequent (unreported) complication of autogenous cancellous grafting?

Inadvertent loss of an unsecured, graft-ladened sponge from the surgery table (and into a kick bucket).

13. How do cancellous allografts compare with cancellous autografts?

Cancellous allografts generally perform only **osteoconductive** functions; they offer no living cells or osteoinductive properties. They do not incite the rapid healing response seen with cancellous autografts.

14. What happens to cancellous autografts when placed in an infected fracture site?

Cancellous bone autografts are recommended for treating infected fractures. For the graft to succeed, the fracture must be stabilized, and sequestered bone should be removed. In this environment, the graft is incorporated into the fracture repair. If the environment is not conducive to fracture healing, the graft is resorbed. The graft does not form a sequestrum.

15. Why would a cortical bone graft be used?

To replace missing bone. Cortical bone grafts provide excellent mechanical support but are acellular and stimulate little osteogenic response, unless the graft is demineralized and releases BMP. Demineralized bone matrix provides no structural support. Cortical allografts are used to replace large segments of cortical bone in limb salvage procedures and occasionally used to replace severely comminuted sections of middiaphyseal fractures.

16. Where are sources of cortical autografts?

Cortical autografts are harvested from areas where cortical bone can be removed without adversely affecting function (i.e., ribs, ilial wing, distal ulna, and fibula). The commonest use of a cortical autograft is transplantation of a rib to form a segmental strut for mandibular fractures. Cortical autograft harvest is done during fracture repair, and the graft is incorporated into the fracture site as a segmental graft (i.e., it is placed between fracture segments) or as a sliding onlay graft (i.e., it is placed over the fracture site). Cortical autografts are usually held in place with the implant used to stabilize the fracture.

17. How are cortical allografts harvested, prepared, and banked (stored)?

Cortical bone harvesting must be done under aseptic conditions, unless the bone is sterilized after collection. The donor animal is euthanized, and the femur, tibia, and humerus are prepared for aseptic surgery. Surgical approaches are made to the bone diaphyses, which are resected with an oscillating bone saw. The marrow canals are cleaned and flushed with saline. Sterilely harvested bones are double packaged in presterilized containers and stored at 0°C for 6–12 months. Alternatively, cleanly harvested cortical bones are double-wrapped in semipermeable packaging material and sterilized with ethylene oxide. The bones are aerated to eliminate toxic residues and stored at 0°C for 6–12 months. Cortical allografts are available commercially, and these bones are frequently freeze-dried.

18. What is the best method of stabilizing a cortical allograft?

Plate and screw fixation are needed to insure stability of host-graft interfaces for prolonged periods while fractures heal and grafts remodel. Adequate host bone must be present to allow placement of three bone screws proximal and distal to the graft.

19. What is the biology of fracture healing with a cortical allograft?

Fracture healing with cortical allografts or alloimplants consists of filling host-graft interfaces with bone, followed by graft vascularization, graft resorption, and graft replacement with host bone. Host-graft interfaces heal within 1–3 months; graft remodeling takes months to years (depending on graft length) and may never be completed. The process of remodeling can be monitored radiographically. Host-graft interfaces initially fill with cancellous-type bone. As resorption and remodeling proceed from host-graft interfaces toward the graft center, grafts change from cortical structures to porous, cancellous-type bone. Eventually the cancellous bone remodels into cortical bone.

20. When should the plate, used to secure the cortical allograft or alloimplant, be removed?
Not often. It is often difficult to determine radiographically when plate removal should be done because the amount of graft that has been remodeled may be difficult to ascertain. Because premature plate removal may predispose grafts to fracture, plate removal should not be done until definitive radiographic evidence of remodeling of the entire graft is noted. Unless complications occur, plate removal is not recommended.

21. What are complications with cortical allografts?
- Infection
- Graft rejection
- Failure of fracture repair
- Graft fracture

Graft **infection** usually results from graft or fracture site contamination and instability. This results in a large, sequestered piece of foreign material that must be debrided when fracture stabilization is performed. Cancellous bone autografts may be used to fill resultant fracture gaps. Signs of **graft rejection** (i.e., failure of graft and host bone to unite, graft resorption without replacement) are rarely noted clinically. **Plate fracture** may be observed when reduction and fixation of host-graft interfaces provides inadequate reconstruction of the bone column. **Grafts** may also **fracture** after plate removal.

22. List other novel grafting techniques described in the literature.
- Bone marrow transfer
- Fibrillar bovine collagen
- Calcium sulfate hemihydrate (plaster of Paris)
- Coralline hydroxyapatite (Coral)
- Vascularized bone transfer

CONTROVERSY

23. Is a cortical bone allograft the most appropriate treatment for a severely comminuted femoral fracture?
Using a cortical allograft to repair a severely comminuted fracture was recommended because the surgical procedure was less time-consuming than reconstructing the small multiple fragments associated with this type of fracture. Using the cortical allograft insured that the bone was reconstructed to share the load of weight bearing with the plate. The disadvantages for this procedure included the cost and labor involved with procuring bone graft and the complications that could occur with bone graft.

With the advent of biologic treatment techniques for comminuted fractures, such as closed reduction or minimally invasive surgical approaches, major segment alignment as opposed to anatomic reconstruction, and bridging plate or external fixator stabilization, cortical allografts are no longer considered an optimal treatment for comminuted fractures in dogs and cats. The biologically treated fractures heal and remodel rapidly. It is helpful to think of the multiple undisturbed fragments as massive cortical autografts and understand that the autograft is the gold standard against which all grafting procedures are compared.

BIBLIOGRAPHY

1. Fitch R, Kerwin S, Sinibaldi KR, et al: Bone autografts and allografts in dogs. Comp Cont Educ Pract Vet 19:558–575, 1997.
2. Hanson PD, Markel MD: Bone and cartilage transplantation. Vet Comp Orthop Trauma 5:163–169, 1992.
3. Johnson AL: Principles of bone grafting. Semin Vet Med Surg Small Anim 6:90–100, 1991.
4. Martinez SA, Walker T: Bone grafts. Vet Clin North Am Small Anim Pract 29:1207–1220, 1999.
5. Perry CR: Bone repair techniques, bone graft, and bone graft substitutes. Clin Orthop 360:71–86, 1999.
6. Stevenson S: Bone grafts to enhance fracture healing. Clin Orthop 355S:239–246, 1998.

76. DEVELOPMENTAL BONE DISEASES

Joseph Harari, M.S., D.V.M., Dip. A.C.V.S.

1. What are developmental disorders of bone?

Conditions unrelated to trauma, infection, or immune-mediated causes but rather associated with growth in immature animals; conditions may be present at birth (**congenital**) or have a genetic basis (**hereditary**).

2. List some common skeletal development diseases described in dogs.

In decreasing frequency based on the National Veterinary Medical Data Base System (1980–1989):
- Hip dysplasia
- Osteochondrosis
- Patella luxation
- Panosteitis

3. What is meant by term *dysplasia?*

From the Greek *dys* (abnormal) and *plassein* (to form), meaning abnormality of development.

4. List some of the less common developmental diseases in dogs.
- Craniomandibular osteopathy
- Hypertrophic osteodystrophy
- Osteochondromatosis
- Elbow dysplasia
- Retained ulnar cartilage cores

5. Define panosteitis.

A spontaneous, self-limiting, painful condition of the diaphyses and metaphyses of long bones in young, rapidly growing large or giant breeds of dogs.

6. Describe the pathophysiology of panosteitis.

Fatty degeneration of the bone marrow is followed by cellular proliferation and osteoid production. Vascular congestion secondary to osteoid synthesis leads to endosteal and periosteal reactions, subsequent bone resorption, and reestablishment of normal vascularity and adipose tissue.

7. List some pathognomonic features of panosteitis.
- Multiple limb pain.
- Pyrexia, depression, and anorexia.
- Increased intramedullary, multifocal densities identified in radiographs of long bones.

8. What does the term *pathognomonic* mean?

From the Greek, *patho* (disease) and *gnomonikos* (fit to give judgment), meaning distinct characteristics of a particular disease.

9. What are the recommended treatments for panosteitis?

Antiinflammatory analgesic (aspirin) therapy and supportive care during periods of discomfort. The disease is self-limiting with complete recovery by 1 to 2 years of age.

10. Are glucocorticosteroids or vitamin C useful in treating panosteitis?

No.

11. What is craniomandible osteopathy?

A proliferative hereditary disease of the mandible and tympanic bullae seen in young terriers exhibiting oral discomfort.

12. What is the pathophysiologic basis for the condition?

Bilateral resorption of lamellar bone and replacement by woven (immature) bone along endosteal and periosteal surfaces occurring in cyclic phases during growth.

13. How is this condition diagnosed?
- Signalment.
- Clinical signs.
- Radiographic features of bone proliferation.

14. What are the treatments for craniomandibular osteopathy?

Symptomatic therapy to alleviate discomfort, soft diet, pharyngostomy, or gastrotomy intubation to maintain normal nutritional status. The condition is self-limiting by 12 months of age (skeletal maturity).

15. Define hypertrophic osteodystrophy (HOD).

A painful, debilitating disturbance of metaphyseal bone in the long bones of young large and giant breeds of dogs.

16. Describe the pathophysiology of HOD.

An unknown cause of metaphyseal blood supply disruption leads to failure in ossification, bone necrosis, microfractures, and inflammation as well as periosteal new bone formation.

17. How is HOD recognized?
- Signalment.
- Lameness.
- Swollen metaphyseal regions of bones.
- Radiographic changes of metaphyseal lucency and circumferential periosteal new bone formation.

18. How is HOD treated?

Correction of dietary imbalances and cessation of any vitamin or mineral supplementation; analgesic and supportive fluid and nutritional treatments and padded kennels.

19. What is the prognosis for HOD?

Mildly or moderately affected animals recover from the episodic nature of the condition; severely compromised patients have a guarded prognosis—intensive care and subsequent surgery to correct limb deformation may be required.

20. Define osteochondromatosis.

Also termed *multiple cartilagenous exostoses,* this condition is characterized by multiple ossified protuberances arising from the metaphyseal cortical surfaces of long bones, vertebrae, or ribs. An unusual tracheal osteochondromatosis in Alaskan malamutes has also been reported.

21. What is the difference between dogs and cats having this condition?
- In **dogs,** the disease may be familial and the ossified nodules cease growth at skeletal maturity.
- In **cats,** the condition may be a viral-associated (sarcoma) malignant transformation.

22. How is osteochondromatosis diagnosed?

Palpation of multiple, nonpainful, firm swellings and radiography revealing multiple pedunculated or sessile excrescences arising from bone surfaces.

23. What are the treatments for osteochondromatosis?
- Surgical excision if masses produce pain or dysfunction.
- Neutering of dogs.
- Monitoring and treating for signs of FeLV in cats.

24. What is the prognosis for osteochondromatosis?
Good in dogs if the extent of the lesions are limited; in cats, it may be guarded and based on FeLV status.

25. What are retained ulnar cartilage cores?
An uncommon and variably painful lesion of the distal ulnar physes of young large and giant dogs.

26. Describe the pathophysiology of osteochondromatosis.
An unknown factor delays endochondral ossification in the distal ulnar physes, leading to ulnar growth arrest and restraint of radial development.

27. How is the condition diagnosed?
Clinical signs of angular limb deformity not associated with trauma, in young large dogs; radiography reveals radiolucent cartilage cases in the center of the physis and extending proximally into the metaphysis.

28. What are the treatments for retained ulnar cartilage cores?
- Cessation of any nutritional supplementation and feeding of a balanced diet.
- Partial ulnar ostectomy and fat grafting to reduce constraint on ulnar and radial growth.
- In mature patients, corrective radial osteotomy may be necessary to treat angular limb deformity.

29. What is the prognosis for retained ulnar cartilage cores?
Variable; based on severity of the condition.

30. What is elbow dysplasia?
Abnormal development of the elbow joint associated with:
- Traumatic physeal closures of the radius or ulna
- Hereditary-based disproportionate radial and ulnar growth in chondrodysplastic breeds
- Congenital lateral luxation in small breeds

31. List some chondrodysplastic breeds.
- Bulldog
- Pug
- Dachshund
- Beagle
- Welsh corgi
- Basset hound

32. How is disproportionate (nontraumatic) radial and ulnar growth treated?
- Neutering and cessation of breeding chondrodysplastic dogs.
- Nothing if asymptomatic.
- Corrective osteotomies of the radius and ulna to restore (if possible) congruity of the elbow joint.

33. List some corrective osteotomy procedures.
- Proximal dynamic ulnar osteotomy or ostectomy.
- Radial osteotomy or ostectomy with or without distraction.
- Distal ulnar ostectomy and fat grafting.

34. What is the prognosis after surgery?
Variable; based on the severity of the condition and success in restoring congruity to a malformed joint.

35. What is the surgical treatment for congenital elbow luxation?
Temporary pinning of the proximal ulna to the humerus to reduce the luxation and overcome aplasia of the medial collateral ligament, hypoplasia of the proximal ulna processes, and a shallow humeral trochlear notch.

36. What is the prognosis?
Variable, based on the degree of malformations and ability to reduce the luxation.

37. What is Scottish fold osteodystrophy?
Skeletal malformations of the vertebrae, fore and hind paws along with exostoses of the distal aspect of the extremities in this breed of cats. The condition is hereditable and characterized by disturbed physeal ossification and actual secondary centers entrapping soft tissue structures.

38. What are the treatments for this condition?
• Neutering.
• Breeding these cats only with straight-eared cats.
• Exostectomy.
• Arthrodesis.

39. What is the prognosis?
Variable; based on severity of osteodystrophic changes. Regrowth of exostoses can occur.

40. What is Legg-Calvé-Perthes disease?
Aseptic (or avascular) necrosis of the femoral head seen in young small breeds of dogs; may be hereditable in Manchester terriers. Named after three physicians (Arthur Legg in Boston, Jacques Calvé in France, and Georg Clemens Perthes in Germany), who independently described the condition in 1910.

41. Describe the pathophysiologic basis for the condition.
Vascular insult (unknown cause) to the proximal femoral epiphyseal and physeal bone leading to necrosis, revascularization, resorption, and remodeling with subsequent collapse of the head and neck when normally loaded.

42. List some pathognomonic clinical features of Legg-Calvé-Perthes disease.
• Unilateral or bilateral hip joint–associated lameness in young small dogs.
• Good recovery after femoral head and neck excision and physical therapy.

43. What are some confounding clinical features of Legg-Calvé-Perthes disease?
• The affected joints are dysplastic in the general sense of the term but not similar to the large dog disease.
• Patellar function needs to be evaluated in these patients.
• The debate between simultaneous or staged bilateral surgeries remains eternal.

BIBLIOGRAPHY

1. Beck JA, Simpson DJ: Surgical management of osteochondromatosis affecting the vertebrae and trachea in an Alaskan malamute. Aust Vet J 177:21–23, 1999.
2. Bojrab MJ: Disease Mechanisms in Small Animal Surgery, 2nd ed. Philadelphia, Lea & Febiger, 1993, pp 804–807, 821–833, 858–864, 892–899.

3. Harari J: Diseases of bone. In Morgan RV (ed): Handbook of Small Animal Practice, 3rd ed. Philadelphia, W.B. Saunders, 1997, pp 830–845.
4. Jacobsen LS, Kirberger RM: Canine multiple cartilaginous exostoses. J Am Anim Hosp Assoc 32:45–51, 1996.
5. Lewis DD, McCarthy RJ: Diagnosis of common developmental orthopedic conditions in canine pediatric patients. Comp Cont Educ Pract Vet 14:287–298, 1992.
6. Matthews KG, Koblik PD: Resolution of lameness associated with Scottish fold osteodystrophy following bilateral ostectomies and pantarsal arthrodesis. J Am Anim Hosp Assoc 31:280–288, 1995.
7. Munjar TA, Austin CC: Comparison of risk factors for hypertrophic osteodystrophy, craniomandibular osteopathy and canine distemper. Vet Comp Orthop Traum 11:37–43, 1998.
8. Piermattei DL, Flo GL: Handbook of Small Animal Orthopedics, 3rd ed. Philadelphia, W.B. Saunders, 1997, pp 715–730.

77. OSTEOCHONDROSIS

Joseph Harari, M.S., D.V.M., Dip. A.C.V.S.

1. Who first described osteochondrosis?

Wade Brinker, at Michigan State, may have been the first to identify osteochondrosis (humeral head lesion) retrospectively in 1939, and Wilhelm Brass in Germany was the first to report the condition in 1956.

2. Who was the first person to assimilate the various manifestations of osteochondrosis, including the pathophysiology of the condition?

Sten-Erik Olsson from Sweden in 1976.

3. What is osteochondrosis?

A multifactorial disorder of maturing cartilage cells in the epiphyses and physes of long bones in young, rapidly growing large dogs. Ischemia to the articular-epiphyseal complex leads to focal failure in endochondral ossification and retention of cartilage instead of conversion to bone. The cartilage becomes necrotic; weakens; and, after trauma, develops clefts, flaps, and sometimes loose joint bodies; synovitis and subchondral remodeling or cysts subsequently occur. An articular cartilage defect along with a degradative enzyme milieu perpetuate a degenerative osteoarthritis characterized by lameness, pain, joint effusion, capsular fibrosis, osteophytosis, and subchondral bone sclerosis.

4. List some of the inflammatory chemical mediators associated with arthritis.

- Cytokines
- Leukotrienes
- Metalloproteinase
- Prostaglandins
- Proteases
- Collagenases
- Stromelysin

5. List the causes of osteochondrosis.

- Normal trauma to weakened cartilage.
- Excessive trauma to normal cartilage.
- Hereditary predisposition.
- Rapid growth associated with high-energy dietary intake.
- Ill-defined source of vascular injury to physeal cells.

6. How common is osteochondrosis.

5.2 cases per 1000 veterinary medical teaching hospital patients; nearly 60% of the patients had a lesion involving the shoulder joint (Veterinary Medical Data Base System).

7. Where does osteochondrosis occur?

Unilaterally and bilaterally in the:
- Humeral head (caudal aspect)
- Humeral condyle (medial aspect)
- Trochlear ridges of the talus (medial more than lateral)
- Femoral condyles (lateral more than medial)

8. How is osteochondrosis diagnosed?

I. History: recurrent lameness in one or more joints not associated with trauma or systemic disease.

II. Physical examination: painful arthropathy, including swelling, crepitation, and reduced motion.

III. Diagnostic imaging:
  A. **Survey radiography**: effusion, osteochondral; defect, joint mice, osteophytes, bone sclerosis
  B. **Contrast arthrography:** cartilage and filling defects
  C. **CT**: osteochondral fragments
  D. **MRI**: cartilage and subchondral bone lesions
  E. **Scintigraphy**: arthritis

IV. Arthrocentesis: nearly normal, nonseptic, non–immune-mediated

V. Arthroscopy: atraumatic, confirmatory for diagnosis and treatment

9. Discuss treatment options for osteochondrosis.

Arthroscopy or arthrotomy is performed for resecting diseased cartilage, and subchondral bone curettage is performed to stimulate fibroplasia and retrieval of loose osteochondral fragments. Antiarthritic medications, such as aspirin, glucocorticosteroids, carprofen, etogesic, polysulfated glycosaminoglycans, hyaluronan, glucosamine, and chondroitin sulfate, are also used.

10. What are the surgical approaches for treating osteochondrosis of the humeral head?

Craniolateral with tenotomy of the infraspinatus muscle, **caudolateral** with dissection between the acromial and scapular parts of deltoideus (with or without teres minor tenotomy), and **caudal** approach between deltoideus and triceps muscles. All usually require technical assistance for limb manipulations to examine humeral head lesions.

11. What is osteochondritis dissecans?

The combination of an articular cartilage cleft and flap (dissecting lesion) and synovitis. From the Latin *dissec,* to separate.

12. What is a joint mouse?

A loosened cartilage flap ossified via nourishment from synovial fluid and either free-floating within the joint or attached to the synovium. Joint crepitation during palpation or ambulation, associated with these fragments is said, by some clinicians, to resemble a **squeaking** noise.

13. What is an important clinical consequence of osteochondrosis?

Bicipital tenosynovitis secondary to migration of cartilaginous or osseous fragments from the shoulder joint into the biceps tendon sheath.

14. How is bicipital tenosynovitis diagnosed?

Not easily at times, because of subtleness of signs: lameness and pain during palpation of the intertubercular groove and tendon. Survey and contrast radiography may reveal fragments, filling defects, and synovial irregularities. Ultrasonography of the tendon and sheath may reveal abnormal changes; arthroscopy provides direct visualization of the structures.

15. How is bicipital tenosynovitis treated?

- Rest and local glucocorticosteroid (prednisolone acetate) injection for early inflammatory lesions.
- Resection of the tendon from the supraglenoid tubercle and transfixation (**tenodesis**) to the medial aspect of the greater tubercle with a bone screw and spiked washer or suturing techniques.

16. What is the prognosis for bicipital tenosynovitis?

Prognosis is good after surgery and fair with medical treatment.

17. With removal of cartilage lesions on the humeral head for treatment of osteochondrosis, should the edges of the defect be perpendicular or beveled?

Cartilage defects fill more completely with fibrocartilage after curettage or forage if the edges remain perpendicular to the joint surface.

18. What is the success rate for surgical treatment of osteochondrosis in the shoulder joint?

Excellent, after a convalescence of 1–2 months.

19. What is the commonest complication of the surgery?

Seroma from excessive patient activity and inadequate hemostasis or tissue apposition during closure.

20. What lesions are associated with osteochondrosis of the elbow joint?

Osteochondrosis of the medial aspect of the humeral condyle is frequently identified in joints with ununited anconeal process and fragmented medial coronoid process.

21. What is the prognosis after cartilage resection and bone curettage for osteochondrosis of the elbow joint?

Good if degenerative osteoarthritis has not developed in the joint; however, large clinical studies evaluating treatment for this singular lesion (and not for ununited anconeal process and fragmented medial coronoid process) are lacking.

22. What is ununited medial epicondyle?

An equivocally painful ossicle located within the origins of the flexor tendons in young dogs (Labrador retrievers) without a history of trauma; suspected to be either an osteochondrosis lesion or ectopic calcification. Treatment is via surgical excision.

23. What is the prognosis for osteochondrosis of the stifle joint?

Most authors report a guarded prognosis for large lesions in young dogs; small lesions or easily retrieved joint fragments have a better prognosis, although large case numbers are not evident.

24. What breeds of dogs are most frequently affected with osteochondrosis of the hock joint?

- Rottweilers
- Labrador retrievers

25. What is the prognosis after surgical treatment for tibiotarsal osteochondrosis?

Convalescence usually requires 1 month; residual lameness may be common. Pericapsular fibrosis secondary to arthritis and instability and periodic antiarthritic treatments may be features during recovery.

26. List the five recommended surgical approaches to the hock joint for treatment of osteochondrosis.
1. **Plantaromedial**   4. Dorsolateral
2. Caudal   5. Plantarolateral
3. Dorsomedial

27. Which dietary components are related to development of osteochondrosis?
Excessive feedings with high-energy, fat-containing and calcium-containing food.

28. What are some useful recommendations to reduce the effect of improper nutrition on the development of osteochondrosis?
- Limit food intake based on calculated energy requirements.
- Dietary fat content should be 8–12%.
- Dietary calcium content should be 1–1.5%.
- Avoid vitamin or mineral supplementation.

29. How is the resting energy requirement (RER) calculated?
RER (kcal/dog) = (30 × wt in kg) + 70

CONTROVERSIES

30. Which is the best surgical approach for treatment of humeral head osteochondrosis?
Probably arthroscopy. Studies have revealed greater surgical exposure with the craniolateral versus caudolateral approach, although weight bearing on the affected limb and joint range of motion may be less. Craniodorsal retraction of infraspinatus and teres minor muscles gives better exposure than separating the muscles. The caudal approach gives excellent exposure to the caudal cul-de-sac for removal of joint fragments, although major neurovascular elements (caudal circumflex humeral artery and vein, axillary nerve) must be identified and preserved. Although surgeons debate the merits of each approach, arthroscopists are rewarded with better visualization of the joint and reduced postoperative morbidity.

31. Is surgery beneficial for dogs with osteochondrosis of the tarsal joint?
Probably, but not absolutely, if the patient is young, has minimal degenerative changes in the joint, undergoes a minimally invasive or arthroscopic procedure for a small lesion or free-floating fragment in a relatively stable joint. Progressive postoperative arthritic changes, as evaluated by radiographs, may be a consistent feature, although not synonymous with clinical evidence of lameness.

BIBLIOGRAPHY
1. Harari J: Osteochondrosis. Vet Clin North Am Small Anim Pract 28:1–195, 1998.
2. Nixon AJ: Cartilage resurfacing techniques: Methods to prevent osteoarthritis. Annual Meeting of American College of Veterinary Surgeons Proceedings, San Francisco, Oct 1998, p 204.
3. Olsson SE: Pathology, morphology and clinical signs of osteochondrosis. In Bojrab MJ (ed): Disease Mechanisms in Small Animal Surgery, 2nd ed. Philadelphia, Lea & Febiger, 1993, pp 777–796.
4. Piermattei DL, Flo GL: Handbook of Small Animal Orthopedics and Fracture Repair, 3rd ed. Philadelphia, W.B. Saunders, 1997, pp 192–197, 300–317.
5. Read RA: Osteochondrosis and elbow arthrosis in young dogs. Waltham Focus 3:2–10, 1993.
6. Schenck RC, Goodnight JM: Osteochondritis dissecans. J Bone Joint Surg Am 78:439–454, 1996.
7. Stobie D, Wallace LJ: Chronic bicipital tenosynovitis in dogs. J Am Vet Med Assoc 207:201–207, 1995.

78. ELBOW DYSPLASIA

Mary K. Quinn, D.V.M.

1. What is elbow dysplasia?

A group of developmental diseases of the cubital joint, which are thought to be forms of osteochondrosis. These conditions include:

- **ununited anconeal process (UAP)**
- **Osteochondrosis** of the humeral condyle
- **fragmented medial coronoid process**
- Ununited medial epicondyle (included by some authors)

2. What are the typical signalment and clinical signs of affected patients?

- Young, large-breed, rapidly growing dogs with unilateral or bilateral forelimb lameness.
- Signs may be acute or gradual in onset.
- Affected animals may **warm out** of the lameness or may be worse after exercise because of secondary degenerative joint disease.

3. Discuss congenital lateral luxation of the elbow.

Congenital lateral luxation of the elbow in toy breeds is considered by some to be a true elbow dysplasia. The disease is occasionally seen in small breeds of dogs. A proposed cause is aplasia of the medial collateral ligament resulting in underdevelopment of the coronoid and anconeal process as well as a shallow trochlear notch. There is usually no trauma to the physis, and the exact cause is unknown.

4. What is UAP?

Failure of the ossification center of the anconeal process to fuse with the olecranon. Normally the fusion is complete by **5 months** of age. This disease is seen primarily in large-breed dogs, with the German shepherd, basset hound, and St. Bernard being overrepresented. Instability or detachment of the process leads to inflammation and eventual osteoarthritis.

5. Discuss the causes of UAP.

There is a positive association with growth plate trauma caused by rapid or long periods of growth. The disease is heritable in the German shepherd. There is evidence to suggest UAP is a manifestation of osteochondrosis or a failure of endochondral ossification. Some dogs have been found to have an elliptic semilunar notch, which forms a poor articulation with the humerus. The end result is increased pressure against the anconeal process, which separates the anconeal growth plate or prevents proper fusion.

6. What are the clinical signs of UAP?

- Usually clinical signs are not apparent before 5–8 months of age.
- There is decreased range of motion at the elbow joint limiting the swing phase of the gait.
- Often the dog stands with the paw externally rotated.
- Crepitus may be present in older animals.

7. How is UAP diagnosed?

Both elbows should be **radiographed** (lateral-to-medial view) with the joint in acute flexion to facilitate visualization of the anconeal process. Osteoarthritis may be apparent in chronic conditions. Fusion of the process does not occur before 5 months of age.

8. List treatment options for UAP.
- Surgical **excision** following lateral arthrotomy
- Proximal **ulnar osteotomy** to promote fusion
- Lag screw **fixation** in young animals

9. Which ridge of the humeral trochlea is most commonly affected with osteochondrosis?
Medial aspect of the humeral condyle.

10. Which breeds of dogs and ages are most commonly affected with osteochondrosis?
Retrievers, Bernese mountain dogs, and rottweilers between 5–8 months of age.

11. What are the typical clinical signs?
- Forelimb lameness and a stiff gait, which can worsen with exercise or after rest.
- Joint swelling may be palpated between the lateral epicondyle of the humerus and the olecranon.
- Pain may be elicited over the medial collateral ligament or by stressing the ligament (flexing the carpus 90° and rotating the foot laterally).

12. How is osteochondrosis diagnosed?
A triangular subchondral defect on the medial aspect of the humeral condyle may be evident on the craniocaudal **radiographic** projection. Roughening of the medial epicondylar surface may be an early sign. One may see only evidence of degenerative joint disease in chronic cases.

13. List the treatment options for osteochrondrosis.
- Exploration of the joint, removal of any remaining cartilage flap, and curettage to clean the edges of the lesion
- **Muscle separating technique** between the pronator teres and the flexor carpi radialis muscles
- **Longitudinal myotomy** of the flexor carpi radialis
- Epicondylar **osteotomy**
- **Arthroscopy,** which provides access for diagnosis and treatment with minimal morbidity

14. What is FCP?
Fragmented medial coronoid process of the ulna. The breeds affected, clinical signs, and etiopathology are similar to osteochondrosis. Rottweilers are unique in that, often, the coronoid is still attached, but a fissure is present instead of a fragment.

15. What is a kissing lesion?
A cartilage abrasion of the medial aspect of the humeral condyle caused by the loose coronoid process rubbing against the humerus. Typically the lesion is approximately 2 mm wide and extends practically the entire length of the articular surface. In younger dogs, the lesion may be narrower than osteochondrosis. In older dogs, the two lesions appear similar.

16. What are the radiographic signs?
- Craniocaudal, lateral, and flexed lateral views should be obtained to rule out UAP, osteochondrosis, and ununited medial epicondyle.
- Typically the actual fragment **cannot** be visualized with survey radiographs.
- Occasionally, blunting of the coronoid process and a small vertical line may be present.
- Often excessive osteoarthritis makes identification of the coronoid process difficult.
- Early in the disease process, osteophytes on the anconeal process may be evident.
- On the craniocaudal view, osteophytes may also appear medially on the coronoid process and the humeral condyle.
- Although radiographic signs may be suggestive of FCP, definitive diagnosis often requires **arthrotomy** or **arthroscopy.**

17. Discuss alternative imaging modalities.

A **CT scan** may show the separated coronoid or the fissured coronoid in affected Rottweilers. The technique should be used judiciously because overinterpretation occurs if loose osteophytes are present.

MRI has also been evaluated for usefulness in diagnosis of FCP. Compared with radiography, MRI was useful for detection of nondisplaced fragmented or fissured coronoid processes. The images correlated well with surgical findings.

18. Describe the surgical treatment for FCP.

Removal of all loose pieces of bone is the surgical objective. The approach to the joint is the same as previously mentioned for osteochondrosis. Sharp adduction and internal rotation of the antebrachium improves exposure. Placing a fulcrum on the lateral aspect of the elbow is also helpful. Either the fragmented process is loose and readily apparent, or it may require breakage at the fissure line. The operation can be performed bilaterally in young dogs, even if unilaterally lame. Older arthritic dogs probably benefit from surgery of the lame limb only because the prophylactic benefit has already been lost.

19. What is the prognosis for FCP?

The prognosis for function is good if the FCP is removed before degenerative joint disease is severe. Radiographically the arthritis is known to progress, but most dogs improve postoperatively. By 3 months postoperatively, most dogs recover maximal clinical function. Surgical removal of loose elbow fragments has been shown to resolve lameness even in older dogs with severe radiographic evidence of osteoarthritis.

20. What is ununited medial epicondyle?

Detached ossified bodies located at either the medial joint line or caudally just distal to the medial humeral epicondyle, believed to be a form of osteochondrosis in which fragments of cartilage avulse with the tendon. Over time, the cartilage changes to bone and enlarges. Lameness results when bone fragments rub against the humerus or ulna. In the mature dog, the fragments are just outside the articular surface and cause little irritation. Surgical removal of the fragments is usually helpful if there is no other coexisting elbow condition. Some clinicians believe this condition to be the result of two types of calcification within the flexor tendons at their attachment to the medial epicondyle. One, which can be unilateral or bilateral, is associated with elbow incongruity. The second form is a result of traumatic separation of the epicondyle with the attached flexor tendons.

21. Discuss the role of elbow incongruity.

Wind found that developmental incongruity of the trochlear notch of the ulna was associated with the development of UAP, osteochondrosis, and FCP. In affected animals, a slightly elliptic trochlear notch with a decreased arc of curvature develops. This arc is too small for the humeral trochlea, which causes major points of contact in the area of the anconeal process and medial coronoid process. The result is increased weight bearing forces and constant micromotion resulting in UAP and FCP. Osteochondrosis results from interference of endochondral ossification caused by excessive pressure generated by the abnormal height of the medial coronoid process.

22. What is the role of elbow arthroscopy?

Arthroscopy of the elbow joint allows systematic inspection of the medial and lateral humeral condyles, medial and lateral coronoid processes, caudad and middle parts of the head of the radius and the olecranon. Evolution of equipment and techniques has made arthroscopy an acceptable, and often desirable, alternative to standard imaging or arthrotomy for the diagnosis and treatment of many lesions of the elbow.

BIBLIOGRAPHY

1. Boulay JP: Fragmented medial coronoid process of the ulna in the dog. Vet Clin North Am 28:51–74, 1998.

2. Brinker WO, Piermattei DL, Flo GL: Handbook of Small Animal Orthopedics and Fracture Repair, 3rd ed. Philadelphia, WB Saunders, 1997, pp 293–317.
3. Flo GL: Surgical removal of fragmented coronoid processes and fractured anconeal process in an older dog with evidence of severe degenerative joint disease. J Am Vet Med Assoc 213:1780–1782, 1998.
4. Fox SM, Brubridge HM, Bray JC, et al: Ununited anconeal process: Lag-screw fixation. J Am Anim Hosp Assoc 32:52–56, 1996.
5. Kippenes H, Johnston G: Diagnosis imaging of osteochondrosis. Vet Clin North Am 28:137–160, 1998.
6. Roy RG, Wallace LJ, Johnston GR: A retrospective long-term evaluation of ununited anconeal process excision on the canine elbow. Vet Comp Orthop Traumatol 7:94–97, 1994.
7. Sjorstrom L: Ununited anconeal process in the dog. Vet Clin North Am 28:75–86, 1998.
8. Snaps FR, Balligand MH, Saunders JH, et al: Comparison of radiography, magnetic resonance imaging and surgical findings in dogs with elbow dysplasia. Am J Vet Res 58:1367–1370, 1997.
9. Wind AP: Elbow incongruity and developmental elbow diseases in the dog: Parts 1 and 2. J Am Anim Hosp Assoc 22:711–724, 725–730, 1986.
10. Van Bree JH, Van Ryssen B: Diagnostic and surgical arthroscopy in osteochondrosis lesions. Vet Clin North Am 28:161–189, 1998.
11. Zontine WJ, Weitkamp RA, Lippincott CL: Redefined type of elbow dysplasia involving calcified flexor tendons attached to the medial humeral epicondyle in three dogs. J Am Vet Med Assoc 194:1082–1085, 1989.

79. HIP DYSPLASIA

Ron McLaughlin, D.V.M., D.V.Sc., Dip. A.C.V.S.

1. What is hip dysplasia?

A skeletal developmental defect that occurs commonly in dogs and rarely in cats. It is characterized by hip joint laxity early in life leading to joint degeneration. It occurs most often in large, rapidly growing breeds of dogs and usually affects both hip joints.

2. What is the cause of hip dysplasia?

A combination of genetic (polygenic) and environmental factors that lead to laxity of the immature hip joint. The joint laxity leads to subluxation and poor congruence between the femoral head and the acetabulum. The resultant abnormal forces across the joint interfere with normal development and cause overload of articular cartilage. With time, degeneration (capsular fibrosis, articular erosion, subchondral bone sclerosis, osteophytosis) of the joint occurs.

3. List some environmental factors that affect the development and progression of canine hip dysplasia?

- Rapid weight gain in growing animals
- A high plane of nutrition (excessive caloric intake)
- Reduced pelvic muscle mass
- A mismatch between skeletal and muscular developments

4. List the clinical signs in a dog with hip dysplasia.

Decreased activity	Narrow stance
Difficulty rising	Hip pain
Reluctance to run or climb stairs	Atrophy of thigh muscles
Intermittent, hind limb lameness	Hypertrophy of shoulder muscles
Bunny hopping	Crepitus and decreased hip joint motion
Swaying gait	

5. How is hip dysplasia diagnosed?
- A tentative diagnosis is based on **signalment, history, clinical signs,** and **physical examination** findings.
- In most cases, hip joint laxity (**positive Ortolani sign** or **Bardens test**) is palpable.
- Joint looseness may not be present in chronic cases because of periarticular fibrosis.
- A definitive diagnosis requires radiographic identification of hip joint laxity or secondary morphometric and degenerative changes within the joint.

6. What are the Ortolani sign and Bardens test?
- **Ortolani sign:** Dorsal coxofemoral luxation followed by abduction of the femur results in a **click** as the femoral head is reseated in the acetabulum. (**Ortolani** was an Italian pediatrician who identified a palpable and audible click while examining a 5-month-old infant in Ferrara, Italy in 1935.)
- **Bardens test:** Elevation of the femoral shaft produces lateral displacement of the greater trochanter. (**Bardens** and **Hardwick,** Indiana veterinarians, described lateral displacement of the femur in dogs in 1968.)

7. What are the typical radiographic findings of hip dysplasia?
Joint subluxation
- Incongruity between the femoral head and acetabulum
Degenerative joint disease
- Flattening of the femoral head
- Thickening of the femoral neck
- Shallow acetabulum
- Irregular acetabular margin
- Enthesiophyte formation at the joint margins
- Sclerosis of the subchondral bone
- Increased density of the periarticular soft tissues

Hip dysplasia usually affects both hips, and one side may appear radiographically to be more severely affected than the other.

8. The Orthopedic Foundation for Animals (OFA) has a registry program to evaluate pelvic radiographs and grade hip conformation. What is the radiographic positioning method recommended by the OFA?

Dogs are usually heavily sedated and radiographed in dorsal recumbency with the pelvis symmetric. Both hips are fully extended (hip-extended position), the femurs are parallel, and the stifles are rotated internally to place the patellae on the midline.

9. How are pelvic radiographs evaluated?

Radiographs are evaluated for **hip joint congruity** and **evidence of degenerative disease** and given a score:
- **Normal** (excellent, good, fair)
- **Borderline dysplastic**
- **Dysplastic** (mild, moderate, severe)

10. PennHip is another registry program to evaluate hip radiographs and grade hip conformation. What is the radiographic positioning method advocated by PennHip?

Distraction/compression radiographic views are obtained with the dog under heavy sedation or general anesthesia and in dorsal recumbency. The hind limbs are in a neutral position (hips not extended) to maximize joint laxity and prevent **winding up** of the joint capsule. The first view is a compression view with the femoral heads fully seated into the acetabula. The second view is a distraction view obtained by placing a custom-made device between the legs at the level of the ventral pelvis to create maximal lateral displacement of the femoral heads. The relative amount of femoral head displacement (joint laxity) is quantified to obtain a **distraction Index** (DI).

11. How is the DI used in radiographic evalution?

The DI ranges from **0 to 1** and is calculated by dividing the distance that the geometric center of the femoral head moves laterally from the center of the acetabulum by the radius of the femoral head.

- A DI of 0 indicates a fully congruent joint.
- A DI of 1 indicates a complete luxation with little or no acetabular coverage of the femoral head.

12. Does the estrus cycle have an effect on coxofemoral joint laxity as evaluated by the OFA and PennHip techniques?

No.

13. What other radiographic views for evaluating hip dysplasia have been described?

- Dorsolateral hip testing using radiography and CT of patients in sternal recumbency and a **kneeling** position.
- Pelvic stress radiography with dogs in dorsal recumbency, femurs angled at 60°, and manually **pushed** craniodorsally.

14. List the treatment options available for dogs with hip dysplasia.

1. **Immature dog with joint laxity and no degenerative joint disease:**
   - Triple pelvic osteotomy to correct forces on the joint and minimize progression of osteoarthritis
   - Medical management
2. **Immature dog with joint laxity and degenerative joint disease:**
   - Medical management
   - Femoral head and neck excision or total hip replacement if unresponsive to medical treatment
3. **Mature dog with degenerative joint disease:**
   - Medical management
   - Total hip replacement or femoral head and neck excision

15. List the factors that must be considered when selecting treatment for a dog with hip dysplasia.

Dog's age, size, and activity	Femoral head shape
Degree of laxity	Clinician's preferences
Degree of osteoarthritis	Home environment
Quality and depth of acetabulum	Medical and surgical costs

16. What is included in the medical treatment of hip dysplasia?

- Controlled activity
- Weight loss
- Physical therapy
- Antiinflammatory and analgesic medications
- Disease-modifying osteoarthritic agents

17. What is a TPO?

A corrective surgical procedure that reorients the acetabulum (following three osteotomies—pubic, ischial, and iliac) to establish congruity between the femoral head and acetabulum. It increases acetabular coverage of the femoral head to eliminate subluxation and improve joint stability. The rotated acetabulum is stabilized with an angled bone plate and screws.

18. What are the indications for performing a TPO to treat hip dysplasia?

Young dogs (6–12 months old) with radiographic evidence of joint laxity, minimal or no degenerative joint disease, and clinical signs of hip dysplasia are considered candidates for TPO. To be successful, the procedure must be performed early in the disease process, before osteoarthritic changes develop and while the remodeling capability exists to allow development of a more congruent joint. Early correction of the abnormal biomechanical forces acting on the joint may minimize the progression of osteoarthrosis and may allow development of a more normal joint as the dog matures.

19. List complications that have been described after TPO surgery.

Excessive narrowing of pelvic canal	Implant failures
Temporary constipation	Persistent joint incongruity
Sciatic nerve injury	Wound infection

20. When is a total hip replacement used to treat hip dysplasia?

Total hip arthroplasty is the replacement of the femoral and acetabular components of the coxofemoral joint with prosthetic implants. In dogs with hip dysplasia, total hip arthroplasty is generally reserved for dogs with severe degenerative joint disease unresponsive to medical therapies. A cemented modular system composed of a polyethylene acetabular cap, a cobalt-chrome femoral head, a titanium femoral stem, and polymethyl methacrylate cement is frequently used.

21. List the complications of total hip replacement surgery.

Infection	Implant loosening
Luxation	Sciatic nerve injury
Persistent lameness	Femoral fracture

22. When is a femoral head and neck excision arthroplasty used to treat hip dysplasia?

This is a salvage procedure used when significant degenerative joint disease is present and hip pain cannot be controlled medically or when total hip replacement is cost prohibitive. The goal is to eliminate hip pain by removing the femoral head and neck and initiating the development of a fibrous pseudarthrosis that permits ambulation. The procedure can be performed in dogs of all sizes; however, results are usually better in smaller, lighter dogs (<20 kg).

23. What is a biceps sling?

Partial resection of the biceps femoris muscle used as an interpositional pad between the remaining proximal femur and acetabulum during femoral head and neck excision.

24. What is a femoral neck–lengthening procedure?

A surgical procedure that involves creating a longitudinal split in the proximal femur. Wedges are inserted to increase the distance from the greater trochanter to the femoral head, effectively **lengthening** the femoral neck and reducing subluxation. The use of the procedure is controversial.

CONTROVERSIES

25. Discuss the controversy between the OFA system and the PennHip systems for the radiographic diagnosis of hip dysplasia.

The OFA system has been the standard for many years. A scientific study comparing radiographic techniques found the distraction method used in PennHip to be 2.5 times more sensitive in identifying joint laxity. Because of the hip-extended positioning method, the OFA system is accurate in detection of hip dysplasia once secondary changes occur but is less accurate in detecting joint laxity alone. The grading system used by OFA is subjective, and the repeatability of the scores has been questioned. One report found an examiner variability of 48–75% using the OFA scoring system. The PennHip system is better able to show joint laxity, and this looseness, as measured by the DI, is strongly correlated with the future development of osteoarthritis in some breeds.

26. Do polysulfated glycosaminoglycans (PSGAG) help dogs with hip dysplasia?

Given to puppies susceptible to hip dysplasia, PSGAG improved radiographic, laboratory, and necropsy evaluations. Given to adult dogs with hip dysplasia, PSGAG failed to improve significantly (statistically) orthopedic scores compared with controls. Nonsteroidal antiinflammatory drugs, such as carprofen and etodolac, have been documented to improve limb function clinically in dogs with degenerative disease of the hip joint.

27. Is a TPO indicated for a young patient with palpable laxity and no clinical signs?

Some surgeons prefer to operate only on symptomatic patients, whereas others believe the complications of surgery are outweighed by the benefits, especially in breeds predisposed to dysplasia and subsequent degenerative changes. Others downplay the efficacy of TPO surgery and prefer total hip replacement (or femoral head excisions) later in life for the animal. An absolute correct and scientifically valid decision may be elusive; clinical and professional preferences (or prejudices) may be important influences.

28. Can femoral head and neck excision arthroplasty be used successfully in large dogs?

Successful recovery from femoral head and neck excision surgery depends on the evaluator. Although few clinicians would argue about reduced weight bearing and range-of-motion characteristics compared with a normal hip or a total hip replacement patient, functional postoperative pain-free limb usage has been described by owners and authors in large, active dogs that have been stimulated to use the limbs early during convalescence.

29. Are there other surgical procedures that have been used in the past to treat hip dysplasia?

Several, once common, procedures are not currently recommended, including **pectineal myotomy, BOP shelf arthroplasty,** and **intertrochanteric osteotomy.**

- **Pectineal myotomy** (or myectomy) may temporarily alleviate muscular or pericapsular pain, although it has little effect on the progression of joint disease.
- The **BOP shelf arthroplasty** procedure failed to promote a new dorsal acetabular shelf of bone to reduce subluxation (autogenous iliac bone transfer may be more realistic).
- **Intertrochanteric osteotomy,** used to improve coxofemoral biomechanics by varization, normoversion, and medialization of the femoral head and neck, has not prevented progressive degenerative joint disease in affected patients.

BIBLIOGRAPHY

1. Adams WM, Dueland RT: Early detection of canine hip dysplasia: Comparison of two palpation and five radiographic methods. J Am Anim Hosp Assoc 34:339–346, 1998.
2. Bardens J, Hardwick H: New observations on the diagnosis and causes of hip dysplasia. VM/SAC 63:238–245, 1968.
3. Cook JL, Tomlinson JL: Pathophysiology, diagnosis and treatment of canine hip dysplasia. Comp Cont Educ Pract Vet 18:853–865, 1996.
4. Corley EA: Role of the Orthopedic Foundation for Animals in the control of canine hip dysplasia. Vet Clin North Am 22:579–593, 1992.
5. Evers P, Kramek BA: Clinical and radiographic evaluation of intertrochanteric osteotomy in dogs. Vet Surg 26:217–222, 1997.
6. Farese JP, Todhunter RJ: Dorsolateral subluxation of hip joints in dogs measured in a weight-bearing position with radiography and computed tomography. Vet Surg 27:393–405, 1998.
7. Flückiger MA, Friedrich GA: A radiographic stress technique for evaluation of coxofemoral joint laxity in dogs. Vet Surg 28:1–9, 1999.
8. Johnson AL, Smith CW: Triple pelvic osteotomy, effect of limb function and degenerative joint disease. J Am Anim Hosp Assoc 34:260–264, 1998.
9. Lust G: An overview of the pathogenesis of canine hip dysplasia. J Am Vet Med Assoc 210:1443–1450, 1997.
10. Oakes MG, Lewiss DD: Evaluation of shelf arthroplasty as a treatment for hip dysplasia in dogs. J Am Vet Med Assoc 208:1838–1845, 1996.

11. Ortolani M: Congenital hip dysplasia in the light of early diagnosis. Clin Orthop 119:6–10, 1976.
12. Rasmussen LM, Kramek BA: Preoperative variables affecting outcome of triple pelvic osteotomy. J Am Vet Med Assoc 213:80–85, 1998.
13. Smith GK: Advances in diagnosing canine hip dysplasia. J Am Vet Med Assoc 210:1451–1462, 1997.

80. TRAUMATIC JOINT LUXATIONS

Ron McLaughlin, D.V.M., D.V.Sc., Dip. A.C.V.S.

1. Why is a complete physical examination so important in a patient suspected of having a traumatic joint luxation?
Concurrent injuries are common in patients receiving sufficient trauma to luxate a joint.

2. List possible concurrent injuries.
- Fractures
- Diaphragmatic hernias
- Abdominal hernias
- Bladder ruptures
- Pulmonary contusions
- Neurologic deficits
- Traumatic myocarditis
- Ligamentous injuries

3. Which is the most commonly luxated joint in dogs?
The coxofemoral joint.

4. What causes coxofemoral luxation?
Trauma, although severe hip dysplasia can also lead to complete luxation of the joint.

5. In a coxofemoral luxation, the femoral head is displaced in which direction?
Most hip luxations are **craniodorsal** (approximately 75%). This is due, in part, to the pull of the gluteal muscles on the greater trochanter. The remainder of hip luxations are ventral or caudad.

6. List the clinical signs of a coxofemoral luxation.
- Severe lameness (often non–weight bearing)
- External rotation of the limb (stifle outward, hock inward)
- Asymmetry of the hips
- Apparent shortening of the luxated limb

7. What is the examination technique for palpating the hip joint to identify a coxofemoral luxation?
The **thumb displacement test.** The clinician's thumb is positioned in the palpable depression between greater trochanter and ischial tuberosity. As the limb is externally rotated, the greater trochanter moves caudally, and the clinician's thumb is displaced from the depression if the hip joint is reduced. When the hip is luxated, the femoral head slides cranially along the ilium when the limb is externally rotated and the clinician's thumb is not displaced.

8. Why is it important to radiograph the hips when a coxofemoral luxation is suspected?
To confirm and characterize (craniodorsal, ventral, or caudad) the luxation. Radiographs also

allow the clinician to evaluate the pelvis for acetabular or femoral head fractures, and concurrent hip disease.

9. How soon after injury should the coxofemoral luxation be reduced?

As soon as possible to minimize destruction of cartilage and to decrease muscle spasticity and fibrosis. It is important that the patient is stable and able to undergo anesthesia safely before reduction is attempted. Closed reduction is usually successful if performed in the first several days after luxation.

10. Describe the technique for closed reduction of a craniodorsal coxofemoral luxation.

General anesthesia (or sedation and an epidural) is usually required. The patient is placed in lateral recumbency (with the luxated limb up), and an assistant stabilizes the pelvis using a towel or strap positioned between the patient's hind limbs. The clinician performing the reduction grasps the hind limb at the hock and stifle. The limb is externally rotated and pulled distally. The limb is then internally rotated and abducted to reduce the joint. Once the joint is reduced, firm medial pressure is applied to the trochanter as the limb is manipulated through a full range of motion. This process removes blood clots, joint capsule, and other soft tissues from the acetabulum. The stability of the joint is also assessed during this manipulation. Joint reduction is confirmed by palpation and radiography.

11. Once a closed reduction is achieved, how is the joint stabilized to prevent reluxation?

Application of an Ehmer sling.

12. How does an Ehmer sling work to stabilize the joint and prevent reluxation?

Not well. The sling is designed to prevent weight bearing and positions the femoral head deeply within the acetabulum by holding the limb in an internally rotated and abducted position. Ehmer slings are able to prevent reluxation in only about 50% of cases.

13. List the potential complications of using an Ehmer sling after closed reduction.

- Reluxation of the coxofemoral joint before, during, or after an Ehmer sling is applied.
- Gradual loosening of the sling, which can also lead to reluxation of the joint several days later.
- Swelling of foot and soft tissue injuries caused by the tape.

14. What is one contraindication for performing closed reduction for a coxofemoral luxation?

Articular fractures of the femoral head or acetabulum.

15. List the indications for open reduction and stabilization of a coxofemoral luxation.

Articular fractures	Chronic luxation
Unsuccessful closed reduction	Joint examination
Joint reluxation	Internal fixation

16. What surgical approaches are commonly used for open reduction of a coxofemoral luxation?

A **craniolateral approach** to the hip is used most commonly. A trochanteric osteotomy can be used to increase exposure. When reattaching the greater trochanter, it may be positioned caudodistally to increase the medial pull of the gluteal muscles and abduct and internally rotate the femur, increasing joint stability.

17. What is the extracapsular suture method for stabilizing a coxofemoral luxation?

Occasionally, after the femoral head is reduced, the joint capsule can be sutured. In many cases, the joint capsule is damaged and cannot be sutured completely. In these cases, two screws (with washers) are placed in the dorsal acetabular rim (at approximately the 10 o'clock and 1 o'clock positions). Suture (nonabsorbable) material is woven from the femoral neck to the screws, creating a **web** over the joint and preventing reluxation.

18. What is the trochanteric rotation suture method for stabilizing a coxofemoral luxation?

Placement of nonabsorbable suture between the greater trochanter and ventral wing of the ilium to internally rotate the proximal femur and seat the head into the acetabulum.

19. What is the Devita pin method of stabilizing a coxofemoral luxation?

Placing an intramedullary pin from ventral to the ischium, over the femoral neck and embedding it into the ilium. The pin provides dorsal acetabular support to prevent reluxation.

20. List potential complications of the Devita pin technique.
- Pin migration
- Injury to the sciatic nerve during pin placement
- Damage to the femoral head
- Reluxation

21. Describe the toggle pin technique for stabilizing coxofemoral luxations.

A hole is drilled through the femoral neck and head, and another hole is drilled through the medial acetabular wall. A nonabsorbable suture is passed through the hole in the femoral neck and anchored to a small, metal clip. The metal clip (made by bending a Kirschner wire) is then inserted through the acetabular hole to anchor the suture. The suture (tied laterally below the greater trochanter) effectively replaces the ligament of the head of the femur and provides stability.

22. How does triple pelvic osteotomy help stabilize a luxated (reduced) hip joint?

It allows the acetabulum to be reoriented to enhance the dorsal coverage of the femoral head. It would be useful only when stabilizing craniodorsal hip luxations.

23. What options are available if both closed and open techniques are unsuccessful in stabilizing a coxofemoral luxation?

Femoral head and neck excision arthroplasty or total hip replacement may be used. Transarticular pinning has been infrequently described in the literature, although joint disease and patient size are limiting factors.

24. Are shoulder luxations congenital or caused by trauma in dogs?

Both. Shoulder luxations are relatively uncommon in the dog, but when they do occur, they are usually a result of trauma. Lateral luxations are more prevalent in large-breed dogs. Small dogs, particularly toy poodles and shelties, can have medial shoulder luxation with no evidence of trauma.

25. Are all congenital shoulder luxations reducible?

No. If diagnosed early, the joint may be surgically reconstructed and stabilized. Some congenital luxations are irreducible because of malformations of the glenoid and humeral head. Severe erosion of the glenoid may be present in cases of chronic luxation. Excision of the glenoid or arthrodesis of the scapulohumeral joint may be required in such cases.

26. What are the common clinical signs of a traumatic shoulder luxation?

Dogs are often non–weight bearing and hold the limb flexed at the elbow. Palpation reveals the relative malpositioning of the acromial process and the greater tubercle of the humerus.

27. After closed reduction of a traumatic shoulder luxation, what type of external coaptation may be used to provide stability?
- A Velpeau sling is preferred for stabilizing medial luxations (it distracts the humeral head laterally).
- A non–weight-bearing sling or Spica splint is preferred for stabilizing lateral luxations.

28. What surgical techniques are used to provide stability after open reduction of a shoulder luxation?
Once the joint is reduced, the joint capsule and surrounding soft tissue are imbricated. The tendon of the biceps brachii can be transposed to provide support. For medial luxations, the tendon in transposed medially; for lateral luxations, the tendon is transposed laterally.

29. What are the clinical signs of a traumatic elbow luxations?
- Acute non–weight-bearing lameness
- Pain
- Soft tissue swelling
- Reduced range-of-motion at the elbow joint
The limb is carried with the elbow flexed and adducted, while the foot and antebrachium are abducted.

30. Are elbow luxations more often medial or lateral?
Almost always lateral because of the restrictive size and shape of the medial humeral epicondyle. Because the elbow is an inherently stable joint, luxation often includes rupture (midsubstance tears or avulsion injuries) of the collateral ligaments and possibly concurrent fractures. Radiography of the joint is imperative.

31. Can closed reduction of an elbow luxation be successful?
Yes. Closed reduction is successful in most cases if performed within the first few days after luxation. A limb bandage helps reduce soft tissue swelling and assists in the reduction; patients with early closed reduction have a better prognosis than patients with chronic injuries undergoing open reduction.

32. Describe the technique for closed reduction of an elbow luxation.
General anesthesia is required, and muscle relaxants may help. Reduction can be achieved by applying medial pressure to the radial head and the olecranon with elbow maximally flexed. Alternatively the elbow is flexed, and the antebrachium is abducted. The ulna is then rotated to engage the anconeal process within the condylar ridge of the humerus. The limb is then extended and internally rotated to reduce the radiohumeral joint. Flexion of the elbow should complete the reduction.

33. How is joint stability assessed after closed reduction?
Careful palpation of the elbow after reduction is important to evaluate the collateral ligaments. The elbow and carpus are flexed to 90°, and the paw is rotated medially and laterally. If the collateral ligaments are intact, the paw rotates laterally to approximately 45° and medially to approximately 70°. If the lateral collateral ligament is damaged, the paw rotates medially to 140°. If the medial collateral ligament is torn, the paw rotates laterally to approximately 90°. Physical comparison to the contralateral normal elbows is helpful along with posttreatment radiographs.

34. List the indications of open reduction of an elbow luxation.
- Joint fractures
- Unstable joint
- Unsuccessful reduction
- Visualization of joint structures

35. What treatments are used for open reduction?
- Collateral and annular ligament repairs
- Temporary transarticular fixation
- Postoperative coaptation

36. In which breeds of dog does congenital elbow luxation occur?
- Pekingese
- Yorkshire terriers
- Boston terriers
- Shelties
- Dachshunds
- Bassets

37. What are the clinical signs of congenital elbow luxation?
Clinical signs occur as early as 3–6 weeks of age and are characterized by **lateral luxation** and **flexion of the elbow** with the antebrachium pronated.

38. List the surgical techniques available for repairing damaged collateral ligaments in tarsocrural luxations.
1. Direct suturing of the ligament using a locking loop suture pattern and nonabsorbable suture material.
2. Prosthetic ligament replacement using screws and washers and nonabsorbable suture.
3. Replacement of the long and the short components of the collateral ligament (preferred technique).

BIBLIOGRAPHY

1. Evers P, Johnston GR: Long-term results of treatment of traumatic coxofemoral joint dislocation in dogs. J Am Vet Med Assoc 210:59–64, 1997.
2. Fox SM: Coxofemoral luxations in dogs. Comp Cont Educ Pract Vet 13:381–388, 1991.
3. Hunt C, Henry WB: Transarticular pinning for repair of hip dislocation in the dog. J Am Vet Med Assoc 187:828–833, 1985.
4. Milton JL, Horne RD: Congenital elbow luxation in the dog. J Am Vet Med Assoc 175:572–582, 1979.
5. Murphy ST, Lewis DD: Traumatic coxofemoral luxation in dysplastic dogs managed with a triple pelvic osteotomy. Vet Comp Orthop Traumatol 10:136–140, 1997.
6. O'Brien MG, Boudrieau RJ: Traumatic luxation of the elbow joint in dogs. J Am Vet Med Assoc 201:1760–1765, 1992.
7. Piermattei DL, Flo GL: Orthopedic conditions of the fore and hind limbs. In Handbook of Small Animal Orthopedics and Fracture Treatment, 3rd ed. Philadelphia, W.B. Saunders, 1997.
8. Vasseur PB: Clinical results of surgical correction of shoulder luxation in dogs. J Am Vet Med Assoc 182:503–505, 1983.

81. PATELLAR LUXATIONS

C. W. *Smith*, D.V.M., M.S., Dip. A.C.V.S.

1. What is patellar luxation?
Displacement of the patella from the trochlear sulcus; also known as **patellar ectopia.**

2. What types of patellar luxations occur?
- Patellar luxations can be **medial** or **lateral.**

- **Medial luxation** is commoner than lateral luxation in all breeds and sizes (75–80% of all cases).
- **Large dogs** have a higher percentage of lateral luxations than small and toy breeds.
- **Bilateral involvement** occurs in 20–25% of the cases.

3. **Why does the trochlear groove fail to develop in animals with early patellar luxations?**

Articular cartilage is the growth plate for the epiphysis and responds to increases and decreases of pressures. Increased pressure retards growth, and decreased pressure accelerates growth. Without the patella in the trochlear groove, there is no pressure to retard cartilage growth, and no groove develops. Continued pressure of the patella in the trochlear groove is responsible for development of the normal depth of the trochlear groove.

4. **What is the cause of patellar luxation?**

Patellar luxations can be **congenital** or **traumatic.** Most are congenital and related to changes and influences of the hip joint, quadriceps mechanism, and pelvic limb conformation.

5. **Describe the clinical signs of animals with patellar luxations.**

Clinical signs vary with the degree of luxation. Some animals are asymptomatic. Animals with grades 1 and 2 patellar luxations have intermittent weight-bearing lameness characterized by carrying the leg in a flexed position. Reduction of the luxation may occur when the animal extends the leg. Animals with grades 3 and 4 luxations exhibit a crouching position because of the inability to extend the hind limbs. Pain may be evident in some patients when chondromalacia of the patella and femoral condyle is present.

6. **List other musculoskeletal abnormalities that occur with medial patellar luxations.**

Coxa vara
Decreased femoral neck anteversion
Medial displacement of the quadriceps muscle group
Lateral torsion and bowing of the distal femur
Femoral epiphysis dysplasia
Rotational instability of the stifle joint
Tibial deformities

7. **What is coxa vara and valga?**

- **Varus**—decreased (<135°) angle of inclination (angle between femoral neck and shaft in a ventrodorsal projection).
- **Valgus**—increased (>145°) angle of inclination.

8. **What is femoral neck anteversion and retroversion?**

- **Anteversion**—cranial displacement of the femoral neck relative to the femoral condyles.
- **Retroversion**—caudal displacement of the femoral neck relative to the condyles.

9. **What is the association between hip dysplasia and lateral patellar luxations?**

Hip dysplasia, coxa valga, and lateral patellar luxation have **not** been consistently associated or documented as concurrent or causative conditions.

10. **Why are torsional and angular deformities associated with medial patellar luxations?**

Torsional and angular deformities are caused by abnormal pressures exerted on the growth plates because of the displacement of the quadriceps muscle group. Increased pressure on the medial side of the femoral growth plate slows growth, whereas decreased pressure on the lateral side accelerates growth. This leads to lateral bowing of the distal femur. Tibial deformation occurs with the same types of forces acting on the proximal and distal tibial growth plates. Medial displacement of the tibial tuberosity, medial bowing of the proximal tibia, and lateral torsion of the distal tibia occur.

11. What is the grading system used to characterize the degree of luxation and deformity in patellar luxations?

The **Putnam classification** (University of Guelph, Ontario, 1968):

Grade 1. The patella can be luxated manually with the leg in extension but returns to the trochlea when released. There is minimal or no deviation of the tibial tubercle and minimal to slight rotation of the tibia. Animals exhibit intermittent patellar luxations and occasionally carry the leg in flexion.

Grade 2. The patella can be manually reduced but reluxates when released. There is slight medial deviation of the tibial tubercle and 30° medial tibial rotation. Animals exhibit frequent patellar luxations.

Grade 3. The patella is constantly luxated and may be reduced manually but reluxates when released. There is moderate deviation of the tibial tubercle and 30–60° of tibial rotation. The trochlea is shallow. The animal uses the leg held in a semiflexed position.

Grade 4: The patella is fixed in the luxated position and cannot be reduced. There is severe deviation of the tibial tubercle and 60–90° of tibial rotation. The trochlea is shallow or nonexistent. The animal's use of the leg is poor, and the leg is held in a flexed position.

12. How are patients with congenital medial patella luxation classified based on clinical signs?

Brinker's classification:

- Neonates and puppies with early abnormalities (grades 3, 4)
- Young to mature animals with intermittent problems (grades 2, 3)
- Older animals with acute injuries or joint degeneration (grades 1, 2)

13. Discuss characteristics of patellar luxations in the cat.

Congenital and traumatic forms of patellar luxations occur, but only 2% are due to trauma. Medial luxations are commoner than lateral luxations. Devon Rex and Abyssinian cats appear to be predisposed to medial patellar luxation. Angular and torsional deformities are not common in the cat. Diagnosis is most frequently made in young cats <1 year of age. Affected cats usually are weight bearing; moderate-to-severe luxations require surgical correction and have a good prognosis after treatments.

14. How frequently does ruptured cruciate ligament occur in small, old dogs with chronic medial patellar luxations?

15–20%

15. Why would patellar luxation predispose a dog to cruciate ligament failure?

- Loss of quadriceps muscles in reducing cranial drawer motion
- Abnormal stifle joint development causing stress of ligaments
- Concomitant degeneration of CrCL with age

16. What are the treatment principles used for the surgical correction of patellar luxations?

- **Realign the quadriceps mechanism:** tibial tubercle transplantation
- **Trochleoplasty:** to increase depth of the trochlea
- **Soft tissue support:** repair and reinforcement

17. List three trochleoplasty techniques.

1. **Trochlear sulcoplasty**—cartilage and subchondral bone resections.
2. **Trochlear wedge recession**—osteochondral wedge placed in a deeper groove.
3. **Trochlear chondroplasty**—in young dogs, cartilage flap and subchondral curettage.

18. What are advantages of preserving cartilage with a chondroplasty or wedge recession procedure?

Maintenance of trochlear-patellar articular cartilage contact, resulting in quicker return of limb function compared with sulcoplasty.

19. List soft tissue reconstruction techniques that are used to help stabilize the patella.
- Overlap tightening of the lateral or medial retinaculum
- Fascia lata overlap
- Patellar and tibial antirotation suture ligament
- Desmotomy of medial or lateral retinaculum
- Quadriceps release

20. What is the commonest cause of failure for the surgical treatment of patellar luxations?
When the surgeon tries to overcome skeletal malformations by soft tissue reconstructive techniques. All grades 2 and higher need realignment of the quadriceps mechanism.

21. Is congenital patellar luxation hereditary?
Medial patellar luxation in toy and small breeds of dogs is believed to be hereditary.

22. What is the commonest error made in trochleoplasty proedures?
The resected trochlear groove is not wide enough to allow the patella to ride deeper.

23. In small dogs with medial patellar luxation, does surgery reduce the progression of osteoarthritis?
No. In studies of dogs with bilateral lesion, progressive osteoarthritis was noted in treated and control groups. Increasing age at surgery was the only factor to correlate positively with the severity of joint degeneration.

24. What is genu valgum?
Lateral patellar luxation in large breeds characterized by hip dysplasia (increased angle of inclination and anteversion of the femoral neck) and externally rotated (knock-knee) limbs.

25. How is lateral patellar luxation treated?
Based on the grade or severity of the deformity and clinical signs. Soft tissue and orthopedic procedures are similar to treatments for medial patellar luxation except performed on opposite sides of the joint (lateral relief, medial imbrication, medial tuberosity transposition).

26. What is the association between medial patellar luxation and hip dysplasia in cats?
Weak at best because the conditions can develop alone or in combination, and cats are frequently asymptomatic.

BIBLIOGRAPHY

1. Hayes AG, Boudrieau RJ, Hungerford LL: Frequency and distribution of medial and lateral patellar luxation in dogs: 124 cases (1982–1992). J Am Vet Med Assoc 205:716–720, 1994.
2. Hulse DA, Johnson AL: Management of joint diseases. In Fossum TW (ed): Small Animal Surgery. St. Louis, Mosby, 1997, pp 976–985.
3. Piermattei DL, Flo GL: Brinker, Piermattei, and Flo's Handbook of Small Animal Orthopedics and Fracture Repair, 3rd ed. Philadelphia, W.B. Saunders, 1997, pp 516–534.
4. Remedios AM, Basker A: Medial patellar luxation in 16 large dogs. Vet Surg 21:5–9, 1992.
5. Roy R, Wallace L: Retrospective evaluation of stifle osteoarthritis in dogs with bilateral medial patellar luxation and unilateral repair. Vet Surg 21:475–479, 1992.
6. Smith GS, Langenbach A: Evaluation of the association between medial patellar luxation and hip dysplasia in cats. J Am Vet Med Assoc 215:40–45, 1999.

82. CRUCIATE LIGAMENT INJURIES AND TREATMENTS

Robert M. Radasch, D.V.M., M.S., Dip. A.C.V.S.

1. What are the origin and insertion points of the cranial cruciate ligament (CrCL)?
- Origin—medial surface of the lateral femoral condyle.
- Insertion—craniomedial surface of the tibial plateau beneath the intermeniscal ligament.

2. Is the CrCL one solid ligamentous structure?
No. It is divided into a small craniomedial and large caudolateral bands, which spiral around each other as the CrCL courses distally and medially.

3. What is the function of the CrCL?
To prevent craniocaudal movement of the tibia relative to the femur. It also limits excessive internal rotation of the tibia and, with the caudal cruciate ligament, provides a limited degree of varus-valgus support to the stifle joint during flexion.

4. Do the two distinct CrCL bands have any clinical importance?
Yes. Each band has a different function depending on the stifle joint flexion or extension. Animals can rupture one band (**partial CrCL tear**), while the other remains intact.

5. What is the function of each CrCL band?
The craniomedial band is taut during all phases of flexion and extension, whereas the caudolateral band is taut only in extension and becomes lax during flexion. The **craniomedial band** is the primary check against craniocaudal drawer motion.

6. With partial CrCL injuries, does one band tear more commonly than another?
Yes. The smaller craniomedial band ruptures more frequently than the caudolateral band. This results in subtle drawer motion in flexion but not in extension.

7. Why does the CrCL rupture?
- **Excessive internal rotation of the tibia** causes the CrCL to become twisted, subjecting the ligament to injury from the caudomedial edge of the lateral femoral condyle.
- **Hyperextension of the stifle** causes the roof of the femoral intercondylar notch to sever the CrCL.
- **Biomechanical loss of structural and material strength** of the ligament as a result of aging predisposes the CrCL to rupture from nontraumatic causes.
- **Conformational (breed dependent) abnormalities** result in straight standing stifle angles, and the roof of the intercondylar notch gradually cuts away or causes tearing of the craniomedial band of the ligament.
- **Anticollagen antibodies and immune complexes** may weaken the ligament.

8. List the three most common clinical presentations associated with CrCL injury.
1. **Acute tear**—sudden non–weight-bearing or partial weight-bearing lameness, which may improve slightly over 3–6 weeks.
2. **Partial tear**—a cyclical, recurrent mild weight-bearing lameness that resolves with rest or antiinflammatory drugs. Eventually the CrCL completely tears, and a non–weight-bearing lameness occurs. These animals often have significant degenerative joint disease of the stifle by the time the CrCL completely tears.

3. **Chronic tear**—acute exacerbation (severe lameness) of a chronic problem (mild lameness) and degenerative joint disease.

9. Do all dogs and cats with CrCL tears require surgery?

No. Dogs weighing less <10 kg and cats often have adequate clinical function without surgery. Some surgeons believe conservative nonsurgical treatment in small dogs and cats may provide a good short-term clinical outcome but may predispose these patients to more severe progressive degenerative joint disease in the long-term compared with an animal in which surgery was performed. Concomitant or subsequent (unstable stifle) meniscal injury may require surgery.

10. List typical physical examination findings for an animal with an acute CrCL rupture.

Cranial drawer motion, increased internal tibial rotation
Joint effusion
Possible meniscal click
Pain elected on flexion and extension of joint

11. What tests can be performed clinically to identify stifle joint laxity and diagnose a CrCL tear?

Positive cranial-drawer test (stifle palpation)
Positive tibial-compression test (stifle and hock palpation)

12. List typical physical examintion findings for an animal with a partial CrCL tear.

- Subtle drawer motion, with the joint in flexion, if the craniomedial band of the CrCL has torn. If the caudolateral band has torn or there is an incomplete interstitial tear of the CrCL, no instability is detected regardless of joint position.
- Crepitation on flexion and extension of the stifle.
- Pain on hyperextension of the joint.
- Medial joint **buttress:** periarticular joint fibrosis and osteophyte formation near the medial collateral ligament.
- Joint effusion.

13. How often can cranial drawer motion (either in flexion or extension) be detected in patients with a partial CrCL tear?

In a study of 25 patients with partial CrCL tears, only 50% of the patients had abnormal cranial drawer motion.

14. List typical physical examination findings for a chronic CrCL tear.

Crepitation on flexion and extension of stifle
Thigh musculature atrophy
Partial or intermittent lameness
Possible meniscal click
Possible anterior drawer motion
Periarticular joint capsule fibrosis (medial buttress)

15. Can an animal have a complete CrCL tear and no anterior drawer motion?

Sure. Severe degenerative joint disease and periarticular joint fibrosis can make detection of anterior drawer difficult. Some animals in which the caudal pole of the medial meniscus is folded cranially do not have drawer motion because the torn meniscus acts as a wedge in the joint, preventing drawer motion.

16. Is cranial drawer motion normal in immature patients?

Yes. Often young animals (<1 year old) have increased joint laxity (**puppy drawer**) with 3–5 mm of drawer present and an intact CrCL. A distinct end point is palpated as the tibia is moved cranially.

17. Do animals with bilateral CrCL tears have unusual clinical signs?
They appear as neurologic patients. The animal will not stand (crouched stance) unless forced to walk (**on eggshells**).

18. Is it common for a dog with CrCL reconstruction to injure the contralateral ligament?
Yes. Approximately 30–40% of dogs rupture the opposite CrCL within 12–18 months. This percentage increases (60%) if there is radiographic evidence of degenerative joint disease.

19. What is the signalment for an animal at a higher than average risk for a contralateral CrCL tear?
  Large, active animals
  Rottweiler breed
  Middle-aged to older, spayed, female patients
  Overweight patients

20. In patients with an intermittent, non–weight-bearing lameness, pain on flexion and extension of the joint, and no drawer motion, are there any noninvasive, beneficial diagnostic tests?
Yes. These tests support, but cannot always confirm, CrCL injury. A definitive diagnosis usually requires **joint exploration** (or **arthroscopy**).
  • Synovial fluid analysis (increased joint fluid quantity and elevation in total WBC count)
  • Radiography (osteophytes along the femoral trochlear ridge, the tibial plateau and fabella, joint effusion, displacement of fat pad)
  • Nuclear scintigraphy (joint inflammation)
  • MRI (anatomic defects)

21. List epidemiologic parameters that place a dog at a high risk for CrCL rupture.
  Age (peak prevalence in dogs 7–10 years old or <4 years old)
  Large breed (rottweilers, Newfoundlands, retrievers, mastiffs, akitas)
  Neutered dogs (hospital population)
  Weight (>22 kg)

22. What percentage of dogs develop progressive osteoarthritis after a CrCL rupture has been surgically reconstructed?
Nearly 100%.

23. What are the two general categories of CrCL reconstruction techniques?
  1. Extracapsular (outside of the joint)
  2. Intracapsular

24. List some commonly performed extracapsular techniques.
  • **Lateral (with or without medial) retinacular stabilization:** Large, monofilament non-absorbable sutures are placed from around the lateral (with or without medial) fabella through a hole in the proximal tibial crest.
  • **Imbrication technique:** Multiple imbrication sutures (Lembert or mattress pattern) are placed along the lateral or medial joint capsule and fascia to stabilize the joint (often combined with retinacular sutures).
  • **Fibular head transposition:** The fibular head and lateral collateral ligament are advanced cranially resulting in tension in the lateral collateral ligament and elimination of drawer motion.
  • **Tibial plateau leveling osteotomy** (TPLO): A cylindrical osteotomy of the proximal tibia is performed, and the tibial plateau is rotated, leveled, and stabilized with a bone plate to eliminate cranial tibial thrust.

25. List some commonly performed intracapsular techniques.
- **Over the top procedure:** An autogenous graft of tissue is passed through the stifle joint, over the top of the lateral femoral condyle to mimic biomechanically the function of the CrCL. The graft is usually harvested from the patellar ligament and may contain a small wedge of patella and a portion of the quadriceps tendon or fascia lata.
- **Under and over technique:** A 1–2 cm strip of fascia lata (with or without patellar tendon) is harvested and left attached to the proximal tibia, is passed under the intermeniscal ligament and through the joint, and is secured over the lateral femoral condyle.
- **Paatsama technique:** A 1–2 cm wide strip of fascia lata is harvested and left attached to the proximal tibia. The graft is then passed through bone tunnels created in both the proximal tibia and distal femur, which are placed at the anatomic origin and insertion points of the CrCL.
- **Arthroscopic placement of an artificial synthetic CrCL:** This has been performed in a limited number of clinical cases yielding impressive results.

26. What is a notchplasty?
A technique, often performed in humans, in which a stenotic intercondylar fossa of the femur is enlarged.

27. What structures are in the intercondylar fossa (ICF)?
CrCl
Caudal cruciate ligaments
Fat

28. Why would a notchplasty be performed?
- Because veterinary surgeons would try anything to improve the results of CrCL reconstructions.
- If there is stenosis of the ICF resulting from degenerative changes caused by a CrCL tear, placement of a ligament substitute in an orthotopic position may be difficult. Enlargement of the ICF permits better positioning and reduces trauma of the graft.
- There is some speculation that certain breeds or individual animals may have congenital ICF stenosis. If this is true, a prophylactic notchplasty might reduce the potential for CrCL rupture in these patients.

29. When using an extracapsular fabellotibial suture technique, does the type of knot used to secure the monofilament suture matter?
Yes. Experimentally a square knot is superior to a surgeon's or a sliding, half-hitch knot.

30. Does placing a clamp across the first throw of a square knot used to secure the fabellotibial suture significantly weaken it?
Probably not, assuming adequate material was chosen in the first place. A study showed clamping the square knot had no adverse effects on the material properties of nylon polybutester, polypropylene, and nylon fishing line. This technique increased the stiffness of 27-kg leader fishing line.

31. Does the sterilization technique alter the strength of monofilament fishing lines commonly used to perform extracapsular repairs?
Depends on the material. Both steam sterilization and ethylene oxide have minimal effects on, and are suitable for, nylon leader line. Steam sterilization and ethylene oxide weakened standard nylon fishing line; ethylene oxide resulted in less weakening of the nylon.

32. How many throws should be placed when using monofilament fishing line to perform an extracapsular repair?
Five; no significant improvement in strength is gained by using more throws.

33. Monofilament fishing line has become a popular material to perform extracapsular repairs. Is one type of fishing line better?
Yes. Monofilament nylon leader line has been found to be stiffer and resists higher loads than the standard nylon fishing line.

34. When performing a fabellotibial extracapsular reconstruction, what is the weakest part of the repair?
Assuming adequate size monofilament suture is used, the weakest point is where the monofilament suture passes around the fabella through the femoral-fabella ligaments. Often the monofilament suture can **saw** through the soft tissue, resulting in recurrence of anterior drawer motion.

35. A crimp clamp system has become available for monofilament loop fixation when performing a fabellotibial extracapsular repair. Is this technique biomechanically superior to tied knots?
Possibly. The crimp clamp system was found to be superior (experimentally) to knotted loops in all single load and cycled parameters tested, which include load to failure, initial loop tension, loop elongation, mode of failure, and point of failure. This assumes the weak link of the repair is the knot or crimp and not the anchor point of the suture around the fabella.

36. Which type of suture has been associated with pericapsular infections and draining tracts?
Large, braided (multifilament) suture.

37. List the commonest complications associated with fibular head transportation (FHT).
- Iatrogenic fracture of the fibular head and neck
- Tearing or elongation of the lateral collateral ligament
- Postoperative seroma formation over the proximal lateral tibia
- Meniscal pathology and cranial drawer motion (experimentally)

38. What nerve is in the vicinity of the surgical approach for FHT?
The peroneal nerve passes caudally and below the fibular head.

39. What are the signs of inadvertent peroneal nerve injury?
- Overextension of the tarsus
- Knuckling of the digits
- Sensory loss over the dorsal aspect of the paw or the lateral aspect of the limb

40. When performing an autograph replacement for CrCL reconstruction, does harvest location of the graft affect its strength?
Yes. A graft based on the lateral one third of the patellar tendon and fascia lata was found to be superior to other harvested grafts. Grafts taken from the central and lateral portions of the patellar tendon are biomechanically superior. Lateral grafts failed sequentially (versus abruptly as in central or medial grafts), which may allow recoverability of function if traumatically overloaded. The lateral graft is also wider and more accessible than a central graft.

41. When an autograft is harvested from dogs, is it as strong as the normal CrCL?
No. The CrCL can withstand approximately 3.5–9.5 times more load before failure and is 3–6 times stiffer than grafts taken from the central, middle, or lateral one third of the patellar tendon. This is in contrast to human studies, which have shown that some autogenous grafts are stronger than the intact CrCL; this exemplifies why one cannot always extrapolate veterinary information from human data.

42. After an autograft is harvested, is its blood supply damaged?
Yes. After the graft is harvested, it is completely avascular and requires 5–6 months for the

revascularization process. During this time, the graft undergoes ischemic necrosis, which compromises its material properties, making it susceptible to failure.

43. After an autograft revascularizes, will it ever be as strong as a normal CrCL?
No. Even after 26 weeks, the graft reaches its maximum strength, which is only 28% that of a normal CrCL.

44. Can an extracapsular and intracapsular repair be combined?
Some surgeons advocate an extracapsular lateral retinacular stabilization technique in combination with an intracapsular autograft. They speculate that the extracapsular repair would support the stifle during the graft's revascularization period, minimizing graft failure.

45. After performing a TPLO, will the stifle be palpably stable?
No. Cranial drawer motion will always be present. With this technique, cranial tibial thrust is eliminated by leveling the tibial plateau, but no replacement of the CrCL is performed.

46. What is a meniscal release?
A technique in which the caudal meniscotibial ligament of the medial meniscus is transected to allow the caudal pole of the medial meniscus to move independently of the tibia.

47. What is considered an excessive tibial plateau slope?
Anything >26°.

48. Are there situations in which a TPLO should not be considered?
Yes. If the dog's CrCL is normal or the measured tibial plateau slope requires >12 mm of rotation (using a 24-mm biradial saw blade) to level it. Performing a TPLO with rotations >12 mm of the tibial plateau isolates the tibial tubercle and may predispose it to fracture from the pull of the quadriceps tendon.

49. If a dog has a tibial plateau slope requiring >12 mm of rotation, is there anything else that can be done?
Yes: combining a TPLO with a cranial closing wedge osteotomy of the cranial surface of the tibia.

50. List potential complications associated with a TPLO.
- Plate breakage
- Screw breakage or loosening
- Tibial tubercle fracture
- Implant infection
- Seroma
- Malalignment of the osteotomy
- Nonunion
- Overrotation of the tibial plateau, resulting in subsequent damage to the caudal cruciate ligament

51. How effective has the TPLO procedure been?
Retrospective evaluation of 394 patients having a TPLO performed for either a complete or partial CrCL tear found normal function and activity returned for an excellent results in 73% of the cases, good function in 21%, fair result in 3%, and poor results in 2%. These evaluations were performed 1–8 years postoperatively. There is not a controlled study (yet) that compares the TPLO to other intracapsular and extracapsular procedures. Surgeons report the TPLO procedure has provided earlier return to function (often 2–4 weeks postoperatively) and better long-term results in dogs weighing >60 lb, compared with other techniques.

52. List critical factors in recovery from CrCL injury and surgery.
- Active postoperative physical therapy and rehabilitation
- Reduction of patient obesity
- Use of nonsteroidal antiinflammatory drugs to reduce discomfort
- Medial meniscus structure and function
- Possibly, cartilage-enhancing drugs

53. What lifestyle changes may be beneficial in recovering animals?
- Swimming activities to strengthen parapatellar support structures, maintain joint motions, and avoid concussive effects on damaged cartilage.
- Avoidance of leaps out of pick-up trucks and decks or marathons on concrete surfaces.

54. What are the origin and insertion points of the caudal cruciate ligament?
- **Origin**—intercondyloid fossa of the craniolateral (inside) surface of the medial femoral condyle.
- **Insertion**—popliteal notch of the tibia.

55. What is the function of the caudad cruciate ligament?
To prevent caudal translation of the tibia during flexion. It acts in concert with the CrCL to provide rotational support in flexion and varus-valgus stability during extension.

56. How often do isolated ruptures of caudal cruciate ligament occur?
Rarely.

57. Why is isolated rupture rare?
- The caudal cruciate ligament is positioned in the joint such that loads sufficient to cause ligament damage are directed toward the CrCL.
- The caudal cruciate ligament is stronger than the CrCL.
- The direction of force needed to cause a caudal cruciate ligament tear is seldom clinically encountered.

58. What type of injury causes an isolated caudal cruciate ligament tear?
A cranial-to-caudal blow directed against the proximal tibia, most often a result of an automobile injury or the result of falling on the limb with the stifle flexed.

59. What physical examination findings are common with a dog presented with an isolated caudal cruciate ligament tear?
- Subtle caudal drawer motion (if palpation begins correctly with the joint in a neutral position)
- Mild intermittent, non–weight-bearing lameness

60. Do all isolated tears of the caudal cruciate ligament need to be repaired?
No. Retrospective clinical and experimental studies found the prognosis to be good regardless how or if the patient was treated. Long-term prospective studies for efficacy of caudal cruciate ligament repairs have not been performed. Some surgeons recommend surgical reconstruction for large-breed dogs and athletic animals.

61. List surgical options that are currently available to reconstruct a torn caudal cruciate ligament.
- **Suture stabilization**—large monofilament sutures placed from the caudomedial corner of the tibia and fibular head to the proximal patellar tendon. Imbrication of the caudal and lateral joint capsule is also performed.

- **Caudal redirection of the medial collateral ligament** using a bone screw and spiked washer to eliminate caudal drawer motion.
- **Tenodesis**, or entrapment, of the popliteal tendon on the caudolateral aspect of the joint with a bone screw and spiked washer placed into the caudal tibia.

62. What is the terrible triad injury?
Combination of (1) CrCL, (2) caudal cruciate ligament, and (3) medial collateral ligament tears. Damage to the joint capsule, menisci, and lateral collateral ligament often occurs. This type of injury is often the result of an automobile injury or being kicked by a large animal. **Total stifle joint derangement, stifle joint luxation,** and **multiple ligamentous stifle joint injuries** are terms used to describe the combination of lesions.

63. List treatment options for traumatic stifle derangement.
- Resection or suturing (peripheral) of torn menisci
- Repair of collateral ligament instabilities
- Repair of cruciate ligament instabilities
- Repair of capsular and retinacular tears
- External splintage (2–4 weeks) followed by physical therapy
- Stifle joint arthrodesis or hind limb amputation in severe, irreparable cases

64. How are medial or lateral collateral ligament injuries repaired?
- Suturing of interstitial tears
- Reattachment of origin and insertion fragments with implants
- Replacement with figure-8 nonabsorbable suture

65. What is the prognosis for treatment of traumatic stifle joint derangement?
Good to fair based on the severity of the injury and ability to repair individual lesions. Limb function is regained, although stifle joint range of motion is reduced by 30–40°.

CONTROVERIES

66. Is one form of CrCL reconstruction more successful than another?
One of the most frequently (and intensely) debated questions at surgery meetings during the past 10 years. Multiple studies have failed to prove (objectively) that one technique is superior to another; in general, success rates of 80–90% have been described for everything.

67. Do many dogs with CrCL rupture have concurrent immune-mediated synovitis?
Possibly. The debate is whether the lymphoplasmacytic synovitis is an immune-mediated arthropathy, causing weakening of the CrCL and eventual rupture, or if the chronic instability and joint degeneration with a CrCL tear lead to the lymphoplasmacytic synovitis.

68. When and why would a meniscal release incision be performed?
It should be performed during TPLO in animals with an intact caudal pole of the medial meniscus. Because a TPLO does not prevent cranial drawer, if an intact medial meniscus is left in place, the patient may develop a subsequent tear.

BIBLIOGRAPHY

1. Anderson CC, Tomlinson JT: Biomechanical evaluation of a crimp clamp system for loop fixation of monofilament nylon leader material used for stabilization of the canine stifle joint. Vet Surg 27:533–539, 1998.
2. Caporn TM, Roe SC: Biomechanical evaluation of the suitability of monofilament nylon fishing and leader line for extra-articular stabilization of the canine cruciate-deficient stifle. Vet Comp Orthop Traumatol 9:126–133, 1996.
3. Chauvet AE, Johnson AL: Evaluation of fibular head transposition, lateral fabellar suture, and conserva-

tive treatment of cranial cruciate ligament rupture in large dogs. J Am Anim Hosp Assoc 32:247–254, 1996.

4. Duval JM, Budsberg SC: Breed, sex, and body weight as risk factors for rupture of the CrCL in dogs. J Am Vet Med Assoc 215:811–814, 1999.

5. Dupuis J, Harari J: Cruciate ligament and meniscal injuries in dogs. Comp Cont Educ Pract Vet 15:215–233, 1993.

6. Galloway RH, Lester SJ: Histopathological evaluation of canine stifle joint synovial membrane collected during repair of cranial cruciate ligament rupture. J Am Anim Hosp Assoc 31:289–294, 1995.

7. Huber D, Egger EL: The effect of knotting method on the structural properties of large diameter nonabsorbable monofilament sutures. Vet Surg 23:260–267, 1999.

8. Moore KW, Read RA: Rupture of the cranial cruciate ligament in dogs—parts I and II. Comp Cont Educ Pract Vet 18:223–234, 381–391, 1996.

9. Nwadike BS, Roe SC: Mechanical comparison of suture material and knot type used for fabello-tibial sutures. Vet Comp Orthop Traumatol 11:47–52, 1998.

10. Piermattei DL, Flo GL: The stifle joint. In: Handbook of Small Animal Orthopedics and Fracture Repair, 3rd ed. Philadelphia, W.B. Saunders, 1997, pp 516–580.

11. Slocum B, Devine T: Tibial plateau leveling osteotomy for repair of cranial cruciate ligament rupture in the canine. Vet Clin North Am Small Anim Pract 23:777–795, 1993.

12. Vasseur PB: Stifle joint. In Slatter D (ed): Textbook of Small Animal Surgery, 2nd ed. Philadelphia, W.B. Saunders, 1993, pp 1817–1865.

13. Whitehair JG, Vasseur PB, Willits NH: Epidemiology of cranial cruciate ligament rupture in dogs. J Am Vet Med Assoc 203:1016–1019, 1993.

83. MENISCECTOMY

Elizabeth J. Laing, D.V.M., D.V.Sc., Dip. A.C.V.S.

1. What is a meniscus?
A plate of fibrocartilage that divides a joint cavity into two parts.

2. List three functions of a meniscus.
1. Aids in joint lubrication by spreading synovial fluid during movement
2. Absorbs shock and transmits load across articular surfaces
3. Increases stifle joint stability

3. How many menisci are in the dog?
Six. Two in each stifle (medial and lateral) and one in each temporomandibular joint.

4. What causes a meniscal injury?
In most cases, meniscus injuries occur concurrent with or secondary to cranial cruciate ligament (CrCL) injury.

5. Is this a common problem?
Among dogs and cats with stifle injuries, yes. Reported incidence ranges from 10% in small dogs and cats with acute CrCL instability to >90% in large or obese dogs with chronic instability.

6. Which meniscus is more commonly injured?
The **medial meniscus,** specifically the caudal portion.

7. Why?
The medial meniscus is more firmly attached to the tibia by the joint capsule and medial collateral ligament. In patients with CrCL instability, increased cranial drawer motion and internal

stifle rotation places the femoral condyle in contact with the caudal horn of the medial meniscus. The increased pressure on the caudal meniscal rim causes longitudinal shearing and compression injuries. The lateral meniscus is more mobile and less prone to injury.

8. **List the various types of meniscal injuries.**
   - **Longitudinal** or **bucket-handle tears** of the medial meniscus are the commonest.
   - **Compression** or **crushing** of the caudal horn of the medial meniscus; these injuries may progress to longitudinal tears if left untreated.
   - **Peripheral detachments** usually occur after severe stifle trauma and usually have concurrent cruciate and collateral ligament tears and joint capsule disruption.
   - Miscellaneous other injuries:
        Axial fringe tears
        Transverse tears
        Discoid menisci
        Calcified menisci

9. **Is the type of injury important?**
   Yes and no.
   - For the novice surgeon, knowing the common sites of injury increases the chance of recognizing and subsequently treating these injuries at surgery.
   - For the patient, the type of tear has little bearing on prognosis.

10. **What physical findings are suggestive of a meniscal injury?**
   Meniscal injuries should be suspected in **every** animal presenting with CrCL instability, especially those with a persistent lameness that does not improve with time, rest, and antiinflammatory medication. The amount of drawer motion can sometimes decrease after a meniscal tear if the torn portion becomes wedged between the cranial femoral condyle and the tibia. Gently pushing caudally on the tibial tubercle to replace the meniscus may allow better evaluation of drawer motion in these cases.

11. **What is a meniscal click?**
   An audible or palpable snap produced when the torn piece of meniscus slips between the tibia and femoral condyle during stifle flexion or drawer motion.

12. **Is a meniscal click pathognomonic for a meniscal injury?**
   No. Just as a meniscal tear may be seen but not heard, a stifle click may not necessarily indicate a torn meniscus. Other causes include crepitus from osteophytes or surgical sutures, cruciate ligament tags rubbing between articular surfaces, and luxation of the long digital extensor tendon.

13. **What diagnostic (other than arthrotomy) tools may be useful?**
   - Diagnostic arthroscopy
   - Contrast arthrography
   - MRI
   Unless calcified, menisci are not visible on survey radiographs.

14. **What is the recommended treatment for a meniscal injury?**
   Surgery: a partial or complete **meniscectomy.**

15. **What surgical approach is most useful?**
   It depends on the surgeon's preference. A **medial** parapatellar arthrotomy provides the best view and access to the medial meniscus. Others prefer a **lateral** approach, presumably because they like the challenge or familiarity with the approach (including CrCL repair). In either case, visualization is enhanced with the patient in dorsal recumbency, the affected leg extended caudally, and the surgeon standing at the end of the table.

16. How can visualization of the medial meniscus be enhanced?
- Cranial displacement of the tibia by an assistant
- Wedging a curved hemostat or Hohmann retractor gently into the popliteal fossa to force the tibia forward
- Vertical and horizontal placements of Gelpi retractors across the joint tables
- Use of a headlamp and small probes
- Arthroscopy

17. How much of the meniscus should be removed?
All of the torn portion and maybe more. Although most surgeons agree that meniscectomy is the treatment of choice for meniscal injury, the relative merits of partial and total meniscectomy are often debated.

18. When should one consider performing a primary meniscal repair?
Direct suturing of meniscal injures is reserved for acute peripheral capsular tears without irreparable meniscal damage. Chronic or severe tears, especially if confined to the avascular portion of the meniscus, do not heal well and are better treated with meniscectomy.

19. What structures can be damaged during a meniscectomy?
- Articular cartilage
- Caudal cruciate ligament
- Medial collateral ligament (when working medially)
- Long digital extensor tendon (when working laterally)

20. What is the prognosis after a meniscectomy?
The more meniscal tissue removed, the greater the risk of subsequent articular cartilage degeneration and secondary osteoarthritis. This should not dissuade the surgeon from the procedure, however, because considerable relief of pain and lameness can be achieved by removing a severely damaged meniscus.

CONTROVERSIES

21. Is there any benefit in removing the entire meniscus when just a portion of it is torn?
Yes, at least in theory. Total meniscectomy removes any potential pathology, such as compression injury, in the intact portion of the meniscus that may have otherwise been overlooked at surgery. Also, by incising along the outer vascularized meniscal rim, this procedure may facilitate future meniscal regeneration. Finally, it is often technically easier for the novice surgeon to remove the entire portion rather than just the caudal horn.

22. What is the disadvantage of total meniscectomy?
The patient loses the spacer function of the meniscus, resulting in increased contact stress to the articular surfaces and potentially exacerbating the development of degenerative joint disease. Total meniscectomy has experimentally been shown to produce more degenerative articular cartilage changes than partial meniscectomy.

23. What is vascular access channeling?
A technique to enhance meniscal regeneration after partial meniscectomy. The meniscus is incised from the synovial attachment to the inner edge, theoretically allowing active pluripotential cells arising from the synovium to reach the damaged inner section of the meniscus and achieve healing. In experimental cases, menisci undergoing this procedure had increased regeneration when compared with menisci undergoing partial excision alone. It has not been evaluated in the clinical setting.

24. What is a meniscal release?

The caudal horn of the medial meniscus is incised at or near its lateral attachment on the intercondyloid eminence, to allow the caudal horn more freedom of movement during stifle motion and avoid the crushing effect of the femoral condyle. It is recommended for intact menisci in conjunction with **tibial plateau leveling osteotomy,** to minimize postsurgical meniscal damage after CrCL repair. Although of theoretic interest, its use has not been evaluated in conjunction with other methods of stabilization, and its long-term effects are unknown.

BIBLIOGRAPHY

1. Arnoczky SP: Pathomechanics of cruciate ligament and meniscal injuries. In Bojrab MJ (ed): Disease Mechanisms in Small Animal Surgery. Philadelphia, Lea & Febiger, 1993, pp 764–776.
2. Dupuis J, Harari J: Cruciate ligament and meniscal injuries in dogs. Comp Cont Educ Pract Vet 15:215–232, 1993.
3. Flo GL: Meniscectomy. Vet Clin North Am: Small Anim Pract 23:831–844, 1993.
4. Hulse DA, Shires PK: The meniscus: Anatomy, function, and treatment. Comp Cont Educ Pract Vet 5:765–774, 1983.
5. Slocum B, Devine Slocum TD: Meniscal release. In Bojrab MJ (ed): Current Technique in Small Animal Surgery, 4th ed. Baltimore, Williams & Wilkins, 1998, pp 1197–1199.

84. TENDON INJURIES

Ron McLaughlin, D.V.M., D.V.Sc., Dip. A.C.V.S.

1. Is there such a disease as biceps bursitis in the dog?

No. Anatomically, there is no bursa associated with the biceps tendon as it traverses the shoulder joint. It is common for the tendon and its enveloping synovial sheath to become inflamed (**bicipital tenosynovitis**).

2. What causes bicipital tenosynovitis?

Inflammation of the biceps tendon and its synovial sheath may result from a strain injury to biceps, direct trauma to the tendon, or irritation from an osteochondrosis-related joint mouse. Adhesions between the tendon and the sheath may eventually limit shoulder joint motion.

3. What are the typical signalment and clinical signs of a dog with bicipital tenosynovitis?

Signalment
- Medium to large breed
- Middle-aged
- Hunting and active dogs

Clinical signs
- The onset of clinical signs is usually gradual.
- Initially, the lameness is mild, intermittent, and associated with exercise.
- The dogs willingly bear weight on the limb but are reluctant to flex and extend the shoulder joint (pain is induced as the tendon slides through the groove).
- Eventually the shoulder muscles atrophy.
- Pain can be elicited by applying digital pressure to the tendon region and manipulating the shoulder joint.

4. How is bicipital enosynovitis diagnosed?

- Relevant history
- Clinical signs

- Radiography
- Ultrasonography

Radiographs may rule out other causes of shoulder lameness and, in more chronic cases, reveal calcification of the tendon and osteophytes on the intertubercular groove. Ultrasonographic evaluation may reveal irregularities in the tendon body, tendon ruptures, synovial hyperplasia, and joint mice.

Synovial fluid analysis, nuclear scintigraphy, and contrast arthrography are rarely used but may help confirm a diagnosis of bicipital tenosynovitis.

5. Discuss treatment of bicipital tenosynovitis.

Results are better if the disease is treated early before degenerative joint or groove disease develops. The initial treatment is rest (6 weeks) and nonsteroidal antiinflammatory drugs. Intraarticular or local prednisolone acetate injections (20–40 mg) are often successful (about 70%) if used before severe pathologic changes occur and if adhesions or joint mice are not present. Tenodesis (surgical transposition of the origin of the biceps tendon) is indicated when response to medical treatment is unsatisfactory or when adhesions or joint mice restrict joint motion. The tendon is removed from the intertubercular groove and reattached to the humerus using a screw and spiked washer. Approximately 50–60% of dogs regain full use of the limb and a normal gait after surgery. The remainder are often intermittently lame as a result of chronic degenerative joint disease.

6. What is infraspinatus contracture?

An uncommon cause of lameness in hunting dogs resulting from acute trauma causing partial rupture and scarring of the infraspinatus muscle and tendon.

7. What are the clinical signs associated with infraspinatus contracture?

- Dogs generally develop an acute lameness while hunting.
- The initial lameness resolves but is replaced in 3–4 weeks by a chronic lameness characterized by an inability to internally rotate (pronate) the shoulder joint.
- Attempts to pronate the shoulder during examination cause the scapula to lift away from the body wall.
- The dogs are not painful during palpation, and the elbow is adducted while the paw is abducted.
- The limb is circumducted during ambulation.
- The condition can affect both forelimbs.

8. What is the treatment for infraspinatus contracture?

Tenotomy and excision of the insertion of the muscle on the proximal humerus. A craniolateral approach to the shoulder joint is used. The dog's gait should return to normal almost immediately after surgery.

9. Can mineralization of the supraspinatus tendon cause lameness in dogs?

Maybe. Mineralization of the supraspinatus tendon has been reported as an incidental finding and a cause of lameness in large dogs. The mineralization is evident radiographically near the greater tubercle of the humerus. Overuse or repetitive trauma may lead to degeneration of the tendon and dystrophic calcification, similar to calcifying tendonopathies seen in humans.

10. How is mineralization of the supraspinatus tendon differentiated from mineralization associated with bicipital tenosynovitis?

Dogs with mineralization of the supraspinatus tendon are typically not painful when flexing the shoulder joint. A tangential radiograph of the intertubercular groove is helpful to distinguish the location of the calcification.

11. What structures comprise the common calcaneal tendon (Achilles tendon)?
- Gastrocnemius tendon (largest component)
- Superficial digital flexor (SDF) tendon
- Common tendon of the biceps femoris, semitendinosus, and gracilis muscles

12. What clinical signs are associated with avulsion of the gastrocnemius tendon from its insertion on the calcaneus?
- Dogs are usually lame immediately after the injury and have a painful swelling proximal to the calcaneus.
- A defect in the tendon may be palpable or demonstrated ultrasonographically.
- With time, weight bearing resumes, and a characteristic stance develops: The stifle is extended, the hock is moderately flexed, and the digits are flexed.

13. What causes the gastrocnemius tendon to avulse?
Degeneration of the tendon-bone junction is postulated as the cause in older, overweight females. Although an uncommon clinical entity in cats, traumatic rupture of the tendon has been reported.

14. Why do the digits flex during weight-bearing after avulsion of the gastrocnemius tendon?
Because of the added weight applied to the intact SDF tendon (as is passes over the calcaneus).

15. What are the origin and insertion of the SDF tendon?
The SDF tendon originates on the lateral fabella of the stifle joint, courses distally along with the gastrocnemius muscle, and crosses over the proximal end of the calcaneus before inserting on the digits.

16. Luxation of the superficial digital flexor tendon is a cause of lameness reported most commonly in what breeds of dogs?
- Shelties
- Collies

17. What is the commonest luxation of the SDF tendon?
The SDF tendon is held in place by a medial and lateral retinacula as it passes over the tip of the calcaneus. The medial attachment is smaller and weaker and more likely to rupture, allowing the tendon to luxate laterally.

18. What morphologic differences in the proximal calcaneus may predispose dogs to luxation of the SDF tendon?
In many Sheltie and collie dogs with SDF luxation, the calcaneus is slender, the calcaneal groove is shallow, and the tip of the calcaneus is slanted distolaterally.

19. What are the clinical signs associated with luxation of the SDF tendon?
- A mild, intermittent lameness and swelling near the tip of the calcaneus.
- A popping sensation that may be palpated over the calcaneus as the tendon luxates and reduces.

20. Discuss the recommended treatment for luxation of the SDF tendon.
Stabilization of the tendon using external coaptation is usually unrewarding. Surgical stabilization is indicated and consists of replacing the tendon in the calcaneal groove and imbricating the torn retinaculum. Polypropylene mesh has been used for surgical failure and revisions of imbrication.

21. What are clinical signs of deep digital flexor tendon injuries?
Penetrating wounds to the palmar or plantar aspects of the distal limb producing variable lameness and hyperextension of the digits.

22. List the basic principles of tendon surgery.
* Atraumatic and aseptic techniques
* Strict hemostasis
* Anatomic, end-to-end anastomosis with monofilament, nonabsorbable suture using patterns designed specifically for tendon repair

23. List some suture patterns that are used for tendon repairs.
Mason-Allen
Krackow
Modified Kessler (locking loop)
Three-loop pulley horizontal mattress
Modified Bunnell-Mayer

24. How do tendons heal?
Via extrinsic and intrinsic (epitenon) mechanisms characterized by inflammation, phagocytosis, fibroplasia, and collagen deposition. Passive motion and controlled mobilization beginning 3 weeks after injury are ideal for reducing adhesions and increasing tensile strength. Realistically, in veterinary patients, external splintage and immobilization are used for 6 weeks after injury or surgery.

BIBLIOGRAPHY

1. Bloomberg MS: Tendon, muscle and ligament injuries and surgery. In Olmstead ML (ed): Small Animal Orthopedics. St. Louis, Mosby, 1995, pp 473–499.
2. Guerin S, Burbridge H: Achilles tenorrhaphy with a modified surgical technique and cranial half cast. Vet Comp Orthop Traumatol 11:205–210, 1998.
3. Houlton JEF, Dyce J: The use of polypropylene mesh for revision of failed repair of SDF in dogs. Vet Comp Orthop Traumatol 6:129–130, 1993.
4. Mauterer JV, Prata RG, Carberry CA, et al: Displacement of the tendon of the superficial digital flexor muscle in dogs: 10 cases (1983–1991). J Am Vet Med Assoc 8:1162–1165, 1993.
5. Mughannam A, Reinke J: Avulsion of the gastrocnemius tendon in three cats. J Am Anim Hosp Assoc 30:550–556, 1994.
6. Piermattei DL, Flo GL: Diagnosis and treatment of orthopedic conditions of the fore and hindlimbs. In Handbook of Small Animal Orthopedics and Fracture Treatment, 3rd ed. Philadelphia, W.B. Saunders, 1997.
7. Reinke JD, Mughannam AJ: Lateral luxation of the superficial digital flexor tendon in 12 dogs. J Am Anim Hosp Assoc 29:303–309, 1993.
8. Reinke JD, Mughannam AJ, Owners JM: Avulsion of the gastrocnemius tendon in 11 dogs. J Am Anim Hosp Assoc 29:410–418, 1993.
9. Stobie D, Wallace LJ: Chronic bicipital tenosynovitis in dogs. J Am Vet Med Assoc 207:201–207, 1995.
10. Williams N, Payne JT: Deep digital flexor tendon injuries. Comp Cont Educ Pract Vet 19:853–861, 1997.

85. TRAUMATIC MYOPATHIES

Randall B. Fitch, D.V.M., M.S., Dip. A.C.V.S.

1. What is the prevalence of muscle injuries in the dog?
The true prevalence in dogs is unknown but probably underestimated. Skeletal muscle constitutes approximately 50% of the total body mass in the dog, but only 5% of referred muscu-

loskeletal cases. The low frequency in dogs and cats may be due to failures in reporting and diagnosing injuries, especially when they accompany more apparent or severe injuries.

2. List the major mechanisms of muscle injury.
- Contusion
- Laceration
- Rupture
- Strain
- Compartment syndrome
- Ischemia
- Denervation

3. How does muscle heal?
By the same mechanisms as all tissues:
- Inflammation
- Débridement
- Repair and remodeling

The type and severity of injury determine whether the muscle heals by **regeneration of functional myofibrils** or **scar formation.** The extracellular matrix that surrounds and organizes muscle fibers also provides a scaffolding for regenerating myofibers and the building blocks (mucopolysaccharides, proteoglycans, and collagen) required for repair. The orientation and structure maintained by the extracellular matrix is essential for muscle contraction.

4. Is fibrosis beneficial or detrimental in the healing of muscle?
Although fibrous scar tissue provides tensile strength and plays a part in normal muscle healing, excessive scar tissue impedes muscle fiber regeneration and interferes with muscle contraction. Healing by scar tissue may decrease by 50% the muscle's functional ability to produce tension. Resection of devascularized or fibrotic muscle may be required to regain functional characteristics of the muscle. Apposition and immobilization of tissue edges minimize scar tissue formation and allow penetration of regenerating muscle fibers.

5. What type of suture patterns should be used in muscle?
Ideally, none. The holding strength of muscle is poor, and muscle, being a dynamic organ, is ill-suited for any suture penetrating the contractile components. When it is possible, the surgeon should take advantage of surrounding tendons and aponeuroses for suture purchase. Sutures can be placed in muscle sheaths using a mattress pattern or tension-relieving sutures (e.g., near-far-far-near suture pattern) with absorbable, monofilament suture, which may require bolstering with stents or fascia lata. Multiple sutures may be preplaced so that the repair can be progressively tightened to overcome natural muscle contraction.

6. When should physical therapy be initiated after muscle repair?
Mobility across the healing muscle should not begin until the remodeling stage of healing is reached. Premature mobilization of muscle after injury or surgery increases granulation and scar tissue production, resulting in poor penetration by regenerating muscle fibers and disruption of the repair. Prolonged immobilization results in irregular orientation of muscle fibers, decreased tensile strength, and excessive scar contraction. Controlled motion and stress during later stages of healing are required to promote functional parallel orientation of regenerating muscle. For optimal function, complete **immobilization** is recommended for the first 3 weeks after repair or injury. The immobilization period is followed by **controlled mobilization** (restricted activity with cage confinement or soft support bandage, controlled leash walks, and passive range of motion) for an additional 3–6 weeks, then a gradual return to normal activity over several weeks.

7. What is a muscle strain injury?
Injury during athletic activities from overstretch and overuse resulting in disruption of muscle fibers, most commonly near the muscle-tendon junction. These injuries are characterized by inflammation, followed by healing with marked fibrosis.

- Grade I muscle strains (the least severe) involve tearing of a few muscle fibers with pain and local spasm.
- Higher grades indicate increased structural damage, pain, and hemorrhage, with grade IV being complete muscle rupture.

8. Does muscle strain injury affect muscle function?

Strength of muscle contraction is greatly affected by strain injury, but recovery appears to be rapid. Muscle disruption and minor hemorrhage are present immediately after injury. Inflammation becomes pronounced in the days following, and by 1 week, the inflammation is replaced by fibrous tissue. Some muscle fibers regenerate, but normal histology is not restored, and scar tissue persists. Healing of muscle by fibrous scar tissue predisposes it to reinjury and possible muscle contracture.

9. If damaged muscle is predisposed to trauma, what preventive measures can be taken to avoid reinjury?

Although stretching is considered by many to prevent muscle strain injury, evidence for this is lacking. Stretching may be difficult to initiate in pets. Muscle is viscoelastic; **warm-up** exercise or simply warming up the temperature of the muscle has a protective effect in muscle injury.

10. Which is the most commonly injured region of muscle?

Musculotendinous junction.

11. What muscle strain injuries have been reported in the dog?

FORELIMB	HIND LIMB
Rhomboideus	Iliopsoas
Serratus ventralis	Tensor fascia lata
Biceps	Sartorius
Pectorals	Pectineus
Triceps	Gracilis
Flexor carpi ulnaris muscles	Achilles mechanism

12. How are muscle strain injuries diagnosed?

- Mature, athletic dogs are most commonly affected and present with varying degrees of lameness, focal swelling, subcutaneous hemorrhage, palpable muscle displacement, and pain.
- Muscle strain injury should not be treated as an exclusionary diagnosis.
- Further confirmation can be provided through direct specific palpation (shaving the region can be enlightening in some cases), specific stressing of the muscle in question, sonographic imaging, and MRI.

13. How is muscle strain injury treated?

- Ice packs during the first 24 hours posttrauma
- Warm compresses after 24 hours
- Compressive wraps
- Antiinflammatory medications
- Analgesic medications
- Muscle relaxants
- Rest
- Controlled physical therapy
- Surgery

Although acute, minor injuries appear to respond well to nonaggressive treatment, chronic and severe muscle injuries may not. Severe muscle strains may require a more aggressive approach involving surgical débridement, repair, or tenomyectomy.

14. What is muscle contracture?
Muscle is replaced by a noncompliant, nonfunctional fibrous tissue that restricts normal motion, often adhering to the adjacent joint and interfering with normal limb action. The commonest muscle contractures in the dog include the infraspinatus, quadriceps, gracilis, supraspinatus, and semitendinosus muscles.

15. Discuss treatment of muscle contractures.
Based on the location of the lesion.
Infraspinatus contracture results in tethering of normal shoulder motion producing an unusual limb action characterized by circumduction of the leg. Treatment is by infraspinatus tenotomy, which releases the infraspinatus tendon pull and restores a nearly normal gait.
Quadriceps muscle contracture occurs primarily in young, active dogs after fractures of the distal femur with voluntary or enforced immobilization of the limb, resulting in fibrous ankylosis of the stifle joint. Initially, many of these changes are reversible, but they become permanent after several weeks. The prognosis for advanced quadriceps contracture is poor even with treatment and commonly results in a nonfunctional leg. Treatment should be directed toward prophylaxis (90°–90° flexion splint for 3–5 days) and early recognition of this condition. Rigid fracture stabilization and early return to function are critical to preventing the lesion. Resection of fibrotic tissues, restabilization of femoral fractures, and active physical therapy may help chronic conditions.
Gracilis muscle contracture occurs in active, middle-aged German shepherd dogs. Affected dogs are able to maintain normal activity and exercise freely but have a characteristic **jerky** gait. Surgery (resection of affected muscle) initially alleviates the lameness, but recurrence has been reported several months after surgery. Both conservatively and surgically treated dogs remained active and healthy with no progression of the disorder, although the abnormal gait remained unchanged.
Fibrotic myopathy of the semitendinosus muscle also is reported in the German shepherd dog, resulting in restrictive fibrotic bands in the muscle producing a characteristic gait abnormality with hyperflexion of the stifle joints. Surgical resection of these fibrous bands produces only temporary relief with recurrence usually within 6 months.

16. Discuss myositis ossificans.
Myositis ossificans results in mineralization within muscle possibly producing discomfort and lameness. It has been described in several locations in the dog, including muscles of the caudal hip region, shoulder, quadriceps, and cervical musculature. Large, middle-aged, active dogs are most commonly affected. Lameness is believed to result from mechanical interference caused by the mineralized mass; the size and location of the mineralization plays an important role in the severity of lameness. Surgical excision of the mass is curative; local injections of antiinflammatory medications, including steroids, is usually unrewarding.

17. What is compartment syndrome?
Pressure-induced injury to muscle resulting from swelling or hemorrhage within a confined osteofascial space. Elevated interstitial pressure impairs microvascular perfusion and produces neuromuscular injury with pain, swelling, and eventual necrosis of muscle. Three general mechanisms exist for increasing the compartmental pressure:
1. Hemorrhage or injection into the compartment
2. Postischemic tissue swelling within the compartment
3. External pressure from a bandage or cast

18. What are the clinical symptoms and locations of compartment syndrome in the dog?

Symptoms	Locations
• Nonresolving swelling	• Craniolateral crus
• Pain	• Caudal crus
• Tense muscle	• Caudal antebrachium
	• Quadriceps (cranial femur)

19. How is compartment syndrome diagnosed?

By measuring **compartmental pressure** using a pressure catheter (Wick catheter, Slit catheter, transducer-type catheter, and hypodermic needle connected to a three-way stopcock and manometer). Normal intrafascial pressure is − 2 to +8 mm Hg. Pressures exceeding 30 mm Hg are clinically significant and result in necrosis of skeletal muscle if the duration is >8 hours.

20. Are there common muscle injuries that occur in humans that may be undiagnosed in the dog?

Yes. An example is **delayed-onset muscle soreness** (DOMS). In this common condition, muscle pain occurs 24–72 hours after vigorous exercise. Muscle weakness may persist for several days after resolution of soreness.

BIBLIOGRAPHY

1. Bloomberg M: Muscles and tendons. In Slatter D (ed): Textbook of Small Animal Surgery. Philadelphia, WB Saunders, 1993, pp 1996–2020.
2. de Haan JJ, Beale BS: Compartment syndrome in the dog: Case report and literature review. J Am Anim Hosp Assoc 29:134–140, 1993.
3. Kriegleder H: Mineralization of the supraspinatus tendon: Clinical observations in seven dogs. Vet Comp Orthop Trauma 8:91–97, 1995.
4. Layton CE, Ferguson HR: Lameness associated with coxofemoral soft tissue masses in six dogs. Vet Surg 16:21–24, 1987.
5. Leighton RL: Quadriceps contracture. In BMJ (ed): Disease Mechanisms in Small Animal Surgery. Philadelphia, Lea & Febiger, 1993, pp 1076–1078.
6. Lewis D: Gracilis or semitendinosus myopathy in 18 dogs. J Am Anim Hosp Assoc 33:177–188, 1997.

86. ARTHRODESIS

Trevor N. Bebchuk, D.V.M.

1. What is the difference between arthrodesis, fusion, and ankylosis?

Arthrodesis is surgical fixation of a joint designed to accomplish fusion of the joint surfaces by promoting the proliferation of bone cells. **Fusion** of a joint is the end result of arthrodesis, but it may occur naturally after severe joint disruption (comminuted intraarticular fractures). Arthrodesis should be distinguished from **ankylosis,** which is the immobility or consolidation of a joint because of disease or injury and is usually a result of periarticular contracture and fibrosis.

2. For which joints has arthrodesis been described?

- Carpus
- Tarsus
- Metacarpophalangeal
- Metatarsophalangeal
- Stifle
- Elbow
- Shoulder joints of the appendicular skeleton
- Intervertebral joints

3. What is the purpose of bone graft in arthrodesis?

The bone graft hastens the rate of bone fusion (**cancellous graft**) and, in some instances, provides structural support (**cortical graft**).

4. What are the different properties of cancellous and cortical bone graft?

CANCELLOUS BONE GRAFT	CORTICAL BONE GRAFT
Osteoconductive properties	Osteoconductive properties
Osteoinductive properties	Structural support
Osteogenic properties	

5. Which type of bone graft is used most often in arthrodeses?
Cancellous bone graft; cortical grafts have been used as inlay grafts for additional structural support.

6. What sites can be used for harvest of cancellous bone graft?
- Proximal lateral humerus
- Proximal medial tibia
- Iliac crest.

In the mature animal, the proximal humerus provides the most accessible and greatest quantity of graft. In young animals, the flared metaphyses of most long bones contain good cancellous bone with high osteogenic potential.

7. How should bone graft be treated during harvest and transfer?
The graft should be collected before application and placed in a sterile metal bowl immersed with the patient's blood. It must be protected from dehydration, and graft chips should be <2–3 mm in diameter to maximize graft nutrition by diffusion. Graft should be placed loosely at the site on viable bone and healthy soft tissues closed over the wound.

8. List the means of stabilization for arthrodesis.
- Dynamic compression plate
- Specialty bone plates such as T-plates and 2.7/3.5 hybrid dynamic compression plates
- Transarticular lag screws
- Cross pins
- Pins and tension band wire
- External skeletal fixators

9. Is rigid internal fixation alone adequate for successful arthrodesis?
No. In many situations, the fixation is placed on the compression side rather than the tension side of an arthrodesis. A region that normally has motion and is now fixed is less mechanically stable than a bone with proper rigid internal fixation. Fixation, regardless of its stiffness, is in a mechanically compromised position. For these reasons, it is advisable to use supplemental support, such as a cast, splint, or non–weight-bearing sling, in most arthrodeses.

10. What are the major considerations for selecting a method of arthrodesis?
- Amount of motion at the joint
- Stability of the fixation

For a joint with a large amount of normal mobility, more rigid fixation is required than for a less mobile joint.

11. Is it important to remove the articular cartilage when performing an arthrodesis?
Yes. The cartilage should be removed to leave congruent bone surfaces of subchondral cancellous bone to facilitate fusion. Any areas of cartilage not removed can lead to delayed fusion. Drilling (or forage) into subchondral bone (medullary cavity) also aids in osteogenesis.

12. Which planes must be evaluated during an arthrodesis?
- Flexion = extension
- Varus = valgus
- Axial or rotational alignment

13. List the basic principles of successful arthrodesis.
- Complete removal of all articular cartilage
- Autogenous cancellous bone grafting
- Rigid internal fixation
- Supplemental external fixation
- Functional angle of fusion

14. What adjustments may need to be made to normal stifle angle when performing stifle arthrodesis?
During stifle arthrodesis, femoral and tibial osteotomies (to remove the articular cartilage and provide congruency for stabilization) cause limb shortening. Leg length can be recovered by stabilizing the joint in an angle 5°–10° greater (more extension) than the normal (contralateral) standing stifle angle.

15. Which types of injures are appropriately treated by arthrodesis?
In general, the procedure is indicated for conditions that result in pain, instability, and loss of joint function for which no reconstructive option is available.
- Acute severe joint derangements involving loss of bone or ligamentous structures such that joint integrity cannot be reestablished.
- Chronic joint instability not amenable to reconstructive surgery.
- Painful intraarticular or periarticular malunion or nonunion.
- Painful degenerative joint disease not amenable to medical therapy.
- Severe growth deformities and congenital luxations.
- Peripheral nerve injury that results in loss of function of a distal joint.

16. List contraindications for arthrodesis.
- Fulminating infection
- Previously fused, contralateral joints (elbow and stifle)

17. Discuss complications and morbidity associated with arthrodesis.
Delayed union, malalignment, and implant complications. **Limb disuse** is the major manifestation of morbidity. The more distal the joint, the less likelihood of morbidity after arthrodesis because distal joints are less mobile than proximal joints. Other sources of morbidity include implant breakage, loosening, and osteomyelitis.

18. How does a bone plate affect the bone proximal and distal to an arthrodesis?
Stress risers at the plate ends proximal and distal to the arthrodesis can lead to fractures. This is a risk in the metacarpals and metatarsals after pancarpal or pantarsal arthrodesis because the bones are small and the plates are larger than normal to accommodate the radius or tibia. Increasing the length of the metacarpal bone covered by the plate may decrease the risk of fractures.

19. How long does it generally take an arthrodesis to achieve joint fusion?
8–20 weeks before fusion is radiographically evident. The range is based on:
- Type of injury
- Patient age
- Quality and quantity of graft material
- Type of fixation

20. What are the appropriate angles of arthrodesis for the shoulder, elbow, carpus, and tarsus?
In all joints, this angle should be (measured with a goniometer) equal to the opposite limb in a standing position. If this is not possible, the following guidelines (canine) may be used:
- Elbow — 130°–140°
- Carpus — 170°
- Shoulder — 105°–110°
- Tarsus 135°–145°

21. Is the functional outcome after successful arthrodesis acceptable?
- Arthrodesis of the carpus and tarsus provides a functional, pain-free limb with mild gait abnormalities.
- Arthrodesis of the elbow, shoulder, and stifle results in a more obvious gait disturbance; most dogs use the leg with pain-free function at slower gaits and when standing.
- Amputation may be an option in some dogs.

BIBLIOGRAPHY

1. Cofone MA, Smith GK, Lenehan TM: Unilateral and bilateral stifle arthrodesis in eight dogs. Vet Surg 21:299–303, 1992.
2. Decamp CE, Martinez SA, Johnston SA: Pantarsal arthrodesis in dogs and a cat: 11 cases (1983–1991). J Am Vet Med Assoc 203:1705–1707, 1993.
3. de Haan JJ, Roe SC, Lewis DD: Elbow arthrodesis in twelve dogs. Vet Comp Orthop Trauma 9:115–118, 1996.
4. Li A, Gibson N, Carmichael S: Thirteen pancarpal arthrodeses using 2.7/3.5 mm hybrid dynamic compression plates. Vet Comp Orthop Trauma 12:102–107, 1999.
5. Piermattei DL, Flo GL: Principles of joint surgery. In Piermattei DL, Flo GL (eds): Brinker, Piermattei and Flo's Handbook of Small Animal Orthopedics and Fracture Repair. Philadelphia, WB Saunders, 1997, pp 201–220.
6. Whitelock RG, Dyce J, Houlton JEF: Metacarpal fractures associated with pancarpal arthrodesis in dogs. Vet Surg 28:25–30, 1999.

87. OSTEOMYELITIS

Joseph Harari, M.S., D.V.M., Dip. A.C.V.S.

1. What is osteomyelitis?
Inflammation of the periosteum, cortex, and medullary cavity of bone; most frequently associated with bacterial infections, although nonsuppurative osteomyelitides associated with skeletal mycotic infections or reactions to metal implants have been described.

2. Name the causes of osteomyelitis.
Trauma or operative procedures (most common)
Contiguous extension from soft tissue structures
Hematogenous spread from distant focus (diskospondylitis)

3. What are the pathophysiologic events of septic osteomyelitis?
- Bacterial colonization, replication
- Vascular stasis, tissue ischemia
- Capillary permeability, neutrophilic infiltration, and engulfment of bacteria
- Neutrophil lysis, enzymes release, tissue destruction

- Focal abscessation (Brodie's abscess) if adequate host defenses or periosseous invasion and inflammation leading to bone destruction

4. What is a sequestrum?
Dead bone involved as a nidus for inflammation or infection.

5. What is an involucrum?
Zone of sclerotic bone surrounding inflammatory or septic bone disease.

6. List clinical signs of osteomyelitis.
Focal pain, swelling, discharge at wound site
Limb dysfunction
Leukocytosis, nonregenerative anemia
Pyrexia (infrequent)

7. List radiographic signs of osteomyelitis.

Soft tissue swelling	Delayed healing
Irregular periosteal reactions	Cortical lysis
Implant failure	Increased medullary density

8. When do radiographic changes become evident?
At a minimum, 10–14 days after injury or surgery.

9. How is osteomyelitis diagnosed?
Clinical history of trauma or surgery
Clinical signs
Radiographic changes
Cytologic and microbiologic evaluations of wounds
Nuclear scintigraphy (increased uptake)

10. Which aerobic bacteria have been associated with osteomyelitis?

Staphylococcus (most common)	*Pseudomonas*
Escherichia coli	*Corynebacterium*
β-hemolytic *Streptococcus*	*Pasteurella*
Proteus	*Klebsiella*

11. Which anaerobic bacteria have been associated with osteomyelitis?
Bacteroides
Peptostreptococcus
Clostridium
Fusobacterium
Actinomyces

12. List characteristics of anaerobic infections.
Polymicrobial Gram staining results
Persistent exudative lesions
Failure in antibiotic treatment or aerobic bacterial isolation

13. Why are anaerobic infections of osteomyelitis difficult to identify?
- True low rates of incidence
- Sampling, transport, or isolation errors
- Difficulty in performing antimicrobial sensitivity patterns
- Overlooked in polymicrobial infections involving more common aerobes

14. What are important considerations for antibiotic therapy of osteomyelitis?
1. What are the likely causative organisms?
2. What is the susceptibility of these microbes?
3. Will drug therapy provide effective local concentration?
4. What are untoward effects of the drug therapy?

15. List characteristics of mycotic infections.
Geographic distribution
Hematogenous dissemination after spore inhalation
Multicentric lesions
Possible underlying immunodeficiency

16. Which mycotic agents have been identified with osteomyelitis?
Coccidioides immitis
Blastomyces dermatitidis
Histoplasma capsulatum
Cryptococcus neoformans

17. What are cryptic infections?
Chronic, recurrent, or dormant bacterial proliferation associated with plates or screws and often not producing overt clinical signs. Causative agents produce a peribacterial mucopolysaccharide film (glycocalyx) promoting adherence to implants and covering the microbes as a barrier to cellular and humeral defense mechanisms and antimicrobial therapy.

18. What is bacterial slime?
The glycocalyx or biofilm composed of matrix and serum proteins, ions, cellular debris, and carbohydrate.

19. How is osteomyelitis treated?
- Débridement of necrotic bone and soft tissues
- Lavage with isotonic solutions
- Open wound drainage, closure via second intention
- Removal of failed implant and fracture restabilization
- Cancellous bone grafting
- Appropriate antimicrobial therapy

20. Name the benefits of using autogenous cancellous grafts in the treatment of osteomyelitis.
- To fill in osteomyelitic bone cavity
- To substitute for resected nonviable bone
- To promote healing of a motion-associated, septic nonunion

21. List some commonly used antibiotics.
- Amoxicillin-clavulanate
- Cefazolin
- Ciprofloxacin or enrofloxacin
- Clindamycin
- Cloxacillin
- Metronidazole
- Potentiated sulfas

22. What are the spectra of activity of commonly used antimicrobial drugs?

DRUG	GRAM-POSITIVE AEROBES	GRAM-NEGATIVE AEROBES	ANAEROBES
Amoxicillin-clavulanate	+ +	+	+ +
Cefazolin	+	+	+
Clindamycin	+ +	−	+ +
Cloxacillin	+ +	−	+
Enrofloxacin	+	−	+ +
Potentiated sulfas	+	+	+

23. How long should bacterial infections be treated?
Minimum of 2–4 weeks; continued even after cessation of overt clinical or radiographic signs.

24. What is the Papineau technique for treatment of chronic osteomyelitis?
• Open drainage after débridement (saucerization)
• Delayed internal fixation and autogenous, cancellous bone grafting
• Second intention wound healing or secondary closure

25. What are some novel approaches to treatment of osteomyelitis?
• High local wound concentration delivery via gentamicin-impregnated polymethyl methacrylate beads.
• Local, biodegradable (polylactic acid polymers, collagen) implants containing ampicillin, gentamicin, or cephazolin
• Regional or intravascular perfusion via pumps or direct injections

26. How can osteomyelitis be avoided?
• Aseptic and biologic surgical techniques
• Appropriate prophylactic or therapeutic antimicrobial therapy
• Early detection and aggressive intervention to prevent bone necrosis and implant failures

BIBLIOGRAPHY

1. Dernell WS: Treatment of severe orthopedic infections. Vet Clin North Am Small Anim Pract 29:1261–1274, 1999.
2. Johnson KA: Osteomyelitis in dogs and cats. J Am Vet Med Assoc 205:1882–1887, 1994.
3. Muir P, Johnson KA: Anaerobic bacteria isolated from osteomyelitis in dogs and cats. Vet Surg 21:463–466, 1992.
4. Radasch RM: Osteomyelitis: In Harari J (ed): Surgical Complications and Wound Healing. Philadelphia, WB Saunders, 1993, pp 223–253.
5. Tobias KM: Schneider RK: Use of antimicrobial-impregnated polymethyl methacrylate. J Am Vet Med Assoc 208:841–845, 1996.

88. OSTEOARTHRITIS

Spencer A. Johnston, V.M.D., Dip. A.C.V.S.

1. What is osteoarthritis (OA)?
The gross and histopathologic, biochemical, and biomechanical alterations (including deterioration) in articular cartilage and periarticular tissues leading to decreased joint function. Clinically, it is characterized by joint pain, tenderness, limitation of movement, crepitus, occasional effusion, and variable degrees of local inflammation. The term *degenerative joint disease* is often used synonymously with OA.

2. Describe the alterations in articular cartilage.
Articular cartilage is composed primarily of chondrocytes and cartilage matrix and is a smooth surface that serves to distribute load over the surface of the joint and provide nearly frictionless movement between the ends of the bones. The cartilage matrix contains mainly collagen, proteoglycans, and water. Collagen provides tensile strength, and proteoglycans contribute compressive strength to this tissue. The earliest changes of osteoarthritis are characterized by **disruption** and **loss** of the **collagen fibrils** and **proteoglycans.** This eventually leads to gross changes ranging from fibrillation and fissures to complete loss of surface cartilage, exposing un-

derlying bone. As these changes occur, cartilage loses its ability to distribute forces over the surface of the joint, and there is decreased smooth joint motion.

3. Discuss causes of OA.

OA usually occurs secondary to some type of injury to the cartilage. This injury may occur as the result of direct **trauma** to the cartilage, such as a fracture involving the articular surface. Alternatively, cartilage trauma may result from **abnormal biomechanics** associated with the loss of ligamentous support, such as cruciate ligament rupture. OA may also result from **abnormal cartilage development** whereby chondrocytes in the abnormal cartilage are injured by normal forces, as in the case of osteochondritis dissecans.

In nearly all instances, some type of injury or abnormality of the chondrocyte initiates the release of prostaglandin E_2 and proteoglycan and collagen fragments. The synovial membrane is stimulated by these substances to produce inflammatory products, such as cytokines (interleukin-1, interleukin-6, and tumor necrosis factor-α) and more prostaglandins. The cytokines stimulate the anabolic and catabolic function of the chondrocytes, so that there is increased production of collagen, proteoglycans, and metalloproteinases (which break down collagen and proteoglycans). If this cycle of increased anabolic and catabolic function continues, the anabolic capacity is eventually exhausted, and catabolic processes prevail, leading to deterioration of the articular cartilage and periarticular fibrosis.

4. Do joints wear out as the result of overuse?

Not really. Articular cartilage has limited ability to repair itself after injury. It is a metabolically active tissue that responds to stresses. Although aging changes occur in articular cartilage, there is evidence to suggest that a high level of activity does not cause OA unless that activity places a supraphysiologic force on the joint.

5. Will a dog with an acetabular fracture, cruciate ligament rupture, or hip dysplasia develop OA?

Yes.
- With **articular fractures,** an injury to the cartilage is sustained, initiating a complex series of biochemical changes that result in further damage to the joint.
- With **cruciate ligament rupture,** the articular cartilage experiences abnormal forces that initiate the same change.
- Although genetic factors have a large role in the development of **hip dysplasia,** the clinical manifestations of hip dysplasia in the mature dog are due to the osteoarthritic changes that result from this complex condition.

6. Do all patients suffering an injury to cartilage develop severe OA?

No. Articular cartilage has a variety of control mechanisms to limit cartilage destruction. These products include tissue inhibitors of metalloproteinase (TIMP) and various growth factors (insulin-like growth factor) to promote cartilage repair. If normal biomechanical function can be restored (anatomic alignment and reduction of an articular fracture), further cartilage injury may be reduced or avoided. If other factors can be modified to reduce stress placed on an injured joint, it is less likely that further chondrocyte injury will occur. OA can range from being mild (not requiring treatment) to severe instances requiring joint replacement or fusion.

7. If OA is a disease of articular cartilage and articular cartilage is aneural, why do patients experience pain with this condition?

Although OA is defined primarily by changes in the articular cartilage, it is not the only tissue affected. In addition to articular cartilage, there are changes in the synovial membrane, joint capsule, and subchondral bone. The **joint capsule** has a rich supply of **nociceptors** (pain receptors), and the subchondral bone also contains nociceptors, although to a lesser degree. Stimulation of these nociceptors owing to biochemical changes that occur within the joint as well as owing to alterations in biomechanics and stresses placed on the periarticular tissues results in pain associated with movement, leading to the discomfort typically associated with OA. Pain does not come from the articular cartilage itself but is a consequence of the cascade of changes associated with damage to this normally smooth, nearly frictionless surface.

8. Which is worse — loss of motion or pain associated with OA?

Pain is usually considered to be the major complaint associated with OA. Loss of function, typified by decreased range of motion, can usually be accommodated unless an individual is performing at a high athletic level. For the typical pet, pain relief is the primary goal.

9. What is the best way to treat OA?

Specific recommendations vary in each case.

- Therapy common to all patients with OA includes modification of exercise patterns to include regular periods of exercise that does not place excessive strain on the affected joint (instead of irregular periods of highly strenuous exercise) and weight loss, if appropriate.
- The next level includes treatment with nonsteroidal antiinflammatory drugs (NSAIDs).
- The last level involves surgery to replace or eliminate the joint.

10. Why exercise a painful joint that has altered biomechanics?

One of the ways that the joints are spared excessive loads is through the support of the muscles, ligaments, and tendons surrounding the joint. If a joint is not used, these tissues atrophy, which results in less support for the already abnormal joint. This causes the already abnormal cartilage to experience more force, contributing to further damage to the articular surface and resulting in more pain. Moderation of exercise, so that pericapsular muscle mass is maintained (without causing excessive loads on the articular cartilage) is considered beneficial.

11. How much exercise is appropriate?

Common sense needs to prevail here. Some patients are good about limiting their activity, whereas others run and jump until they cannot use the limb anymore. For patients that exercise hard and suffer pain and stiffness, the owners must try to limit the amount of strenuous activity through leash restriction or controlled duration and type of activities (especially on hard surfaces).

12. Does obesity cause OA?

Obesity alone is unlikely to cause OA. Obesity causes increased stress on joints. If these joints are abnormal to begin with, either because of previous injury or because of congenital predisposition (hip dysplasia), obesity exacerbates the changes and clinical signs associated with OA. Often the clinical signs of OA can be substantially alleviated by weight reduction.

13. How do NSAIDs work?

By inhibiting prostaglandin production, decreasing the low level of peripheral inflammation present in OA. NSAIDs also provide analgesia by inhibiting prostaglandin production in the central nervous system.

14. Do NSAIDs cure OA?

No. NSAIDs are useful for treating the pain associated with OA and increasing the patient's levels of comfort and function.

15. Discuss the role of COX-2 inhibitors.

Cyclooxygenase (COX) is the major enzyme responsible for the conversion of arachidonic acid (produced as the result of cell membrane damage) to prostaglandins. Prostaglandins, specifically prostaglandin E_2, increase the sensitivity of nociceptors to stimuli and are important mediators of pain in the osteoarthritic joint. Other prostaglandins produced as the result of cyclooxygenase activity include prostaglandin E_1, prostacyclin, and thromboxane, among others. These prostaglandins have important physiologic functions.

In the early 1990s, two forms of cyclooxygenase were discovered and named **COX-1** and **COX-2**. COX-1 is thought to be responsible for the production of prostaglandins associated with **normal physiologic function** and is found in such tissues as the stomach, kidney, endothelium, and platelets. COX-2 was thought to be induced as the result of **inflammation** and responsible for producing prostaglandins such as prostaglandin E_2. It was hypothesized that if COX-2 could be inhibited without inhibiting COX-1, many of the side effects associated with NSAID use could be avoided.

Although the entire story regarding the use of NSAIDs is not as straightforward as the description of COX-1 and COX-2 would lead one to believe, there is early evidence to suggest that COX-2-specific inhibitors do decrease the number of serious side effects (especially related to the gastrointestinal system) associated with NSAID use in humans. There is no evidence to suggest that they are any more effective for the palliation of painful symptoms associated with OA or that they can halt or reverse the progression of OA.

16. What NSAIDs are approved for use in dogs?
- Phenylbutazone
- Meclofenamic acid
- Carprofen
- Etodolac

Of these, only **carprofen** and **etodolac** have undergone study in trials specifically designed to test their efficacy in dogs with OA.

Aspirin has been used for many years in dogs, but is not approved by the U.S. FDA for this purpose.

17. Which NSAID is the most effective for alleviating the painful symptoms of OA?
There have not been any studies in veterinary medicine comparing NSAIDs for efficacy in treating OA. There is evidence from human studies to suggest that a specific NSAID may be more effective for a single individual. It is reasonable to believe that if one NSAID is not effective for a particular patient, that patient may respond to a different NSAID. A lack of response does not mean that all NSAIDs would be ineffective for that patient.

18. What side effects are associated with NSAIDs?
The major side effect is usually GI bleeding, ranging from mild to severe and life-threatening. Although consistent difference among NSAIDs has not been noted with respect to efficacy, there is a well-recognized difference among NSAIDs with respect to ability to cause GI bleeding. Other GI effects include vomiting and diarrhea.

19. What about hepatotoxicity?
Carprofen has been reported to cause hepatotoxicity in a small percentage of dogs that receive it. This condition is characterized by hepatocellular necrosis. Hepatotoxicity, regardless of the NSAID involved, seems to be an idiosyncratic reaction and is perhaps due to unusual metabolism of the drug in certain patients whereby toxic metabolites of the drug result from hepatic metabolism. An alternative hypothesis is that hepatotoxicity is due to an immune-mediated phenomenon. Most patients that develop hepatotoxicity recover from the condition if the drug is discontinued and they receive supportive care.

20. What about nephrotoxicity?
NSAIDs work by inhibiting prostaglandins, and prostaglandins are important for vasodilation in the kidney. In animals that are normovolemic, there is little prostaglandin activity in the kidney and the effect of NSAID administration seems to be negligible. There is little evidence to suggest that long-term administration of NSAIDs to healthy animals results in renal failure. NSAIDs should be used cautiously in patients that have preexisting renal disease or are hypovolemic.

21. What are the treatments for OA in cats?
- Environmental modifications to reduce leaping and climbing
- Weight reduction if obese patient
- Aspirin
- Possibly butorphanol or corticosteroids
- Possibly oral nutritional supplements (glucosamine and chondroitin sulfate)

CONTROVERSIES

22. Are glucosamine and chondroitin sulfate efficacious?
Maybe. Glucosamine and chondroitin sulfate are marketed as nutritional supplements and have **not** undergone the scientific scrutiny of pharmaceuticals such as NSAIDs. As a result, convincing evidence of their efficacy is not necessary for them to be sold.

There is a growing body of evidence that indicates glucosamine and chondroitin sulfate can modulate the metabolism of chondrocytes *in vitro*. This modulation often includes an increase in proteoglycan synthesis or a decrease in metalloproteinase production, or both. There is a paucity of well-controlled, double-blind studies indicating the effectiveness of these products clinically. Some evidence (studies in humans) is beginning to emerge that the products may be effective for treating symptoms associated with low grades of OA, but it is not yet clear that the products modulate the actual progression of OA.

23. What are the most effective dose and formulation of glucosamine and chondroitin sulfate?
Because the nutritional supplementation industry is not strictly controlled, there are many different formulations available. The actual content of glucosamine or chondroitin sulfate in these products may vary. Scientific dose-efficacy studies have not been performed to determine the most effective dose for many of these products.

24. Discuss the role of polysulfated glycosaminoglycans (PSGAGs)?
Although there is *in vitro* information suggesting that PSGAGs may be effective in stimulating proteoglycan production, increasing hyaluronan production, and decreasing degradative enzyme activity in isolated chondrocytes or cartilage explants, results of various studies have been inconsistent. A beneficial effect has been reported in the cruciate ligament transection model (acute injury) of canine OA. Although there are many anecdotal reports regarding efficacy of this product, there are no published studies involving a large number of clinically affected dogs that confirm the efficacy of this product. A study by Lust et al. showed a protective effect of PSGAGs when given to puppies genetically predisposed to hip dysplasia.

25. Do glucosamine, chondroitin sulfate, or PSGAGs cause any harm?
Although minor alterations in clotting profiles have been reported, they do not have a major clinical impact, unless another disease process, which also affects clotting, is present. Minor gastrointestinal upset has been anecdotally reported for **glucosamine** and **chondroitin sulfate** in a small percentage of canine patients and a larger percentage of human patients.

BIBLIOGRAPHY

1. Budsberg SC, Johnston SA, Schwarz PD: Efficacy of etodolac for the treatment of osteoarthritis of the hip joints in dogs. J Am Vet Med Assoc 214:206–210, 1999.
2. Johnston SA: Osteoarthritis. Vet Clin North Am Small Anim Pract 27:699–953, 1997.
3. Johnston SA, Fox SM: Mechanisms of action of anti-inflammatory medications used for the treatment of osteoarthritis. J Am Vet Med Assoc 210:1486–1492, 1997.
4. Kealy KD, Lawler DF, Ballam JM: Five-year longitudinal study on limited food consumption and development of osteoarthritis in coxofemoral joints of dogs. J Am Vet Med Assoc 210:222–225, 1997.

5. Lust G, Williams AJ, Burton-Wurster N: Effects of intramuscular administration of glycosaminoglycan polysulfates on signs of incipient hip dysplasia in growing pups. Am J Vet Res 53:1836–1843, 1992.
6. MacPhail C, Lappin MR, Meyer DJ: Hepatocellular toxicosis associated with administration of carprofen in 21 dogs. J Am Vet Med Assoc 212:1895–1901, 1998.
7. Reimer ME, Johnston SA, Leib MS: The gastroduodenal effects of buffered aspirin, carprofen, and etodolac in healthy dogs. J Vet Intern Med 13:472–477, 1999.
8. Vasseur PB, Johnson AL, Budsberg SC: Randomized, controlled trial of the efficacy of carprofen, a nonsteroidal anti-inflammatory drug, in the treatment of osteoarthritis in dogs. J Am Vet Med Assoc 206:807–811, 1995.

IV. Neurosurgery

89. INTERVERTEBRAL DISK DISEASE

Ron McLaughlin, D.V.M., D.V.Sc., Dip. A.C.V.S.

1. What is the name of the outer, fibrous portion of the intervertebral disk?
Annulus fibrosus.

2. What is the name of the central, gelatinous portion of the intervertebral disk?
Nucleus pulposus.

3. What is Hansen type I disk degeneration?
Occurs primarily in chondrodystrophic breeds of dogs. **Chondroid metaplasia** (more collagen, less proteoglycans, less water) of the nucleus pulposus and weakening of the annulus fibrosus begin at 2–9 months of age. As the disease progresses, routine spinal movement can result in prolapse of the nucleus pulposus through the degenerative annulus. The herniated disk material causes signs of acute, compressive myelopathy. Dogs often show clinical signs of acute disk herniation at 3–6 years of age.

4. What is Hansen type II disk degeneration?
Occurs in nonchondrodystrophic dogs, including large breeds. **Fibroid metaplasia** occurs within the disk and leads to protrusion or bulging of the disk. The result is a chronic, slowly progressive myelopathy in older dogs (5–12 years of age).

5. What causes the neurologic dysfunction associated with disk herniation?
- Dynamic force of the herniated disk material injuring the spinal cord.
- Physical displacement of the spinal cord by disk material in the epidural space (mass effect).
- Hypoxic changes caused by pressure on the vascular system within the cord.
- Ischemia and edema within the cord.
- Increased pressure caused by cord swelling within the confines of the dura and vertebral canal.
- Inflammatory response to the herniated disk material.

6. What are the goals of the neurologic examination?
Determination of the location and severity of the spinal lesion.

7. What is the difference between paresis and paralysis (plegia)?
- **Paresis** is a partial deficit in motor function.
- **Plegia** indicates complete loss of voluntary movement.
Some authors use **plegia (paralysis)** to indicate voluntary motor and sensory (deep pain) losses.

8. What is a useful grading system for neurologic signs?
Increasing severity with higher number:
- Grade 1—spinal pain.
- Grade 2—mild ataxia (proprioception deficits).
- Grade 3—severe ataxia, no weight bearing.

- Grade 4—no voluntary motor function.
- Grade 5—no motor function or deep pain perception.

9. What is meant by the term upper motor neuron (UMN) disease?

UMNs are the motor systems in the brain that control the lower motor neurons and are responsible for initiation and maintenance of movement and tone in the extensor muscles of the body. The primary clinical sign of UMN disease is paresis or paralysis caudal to the injury, along with exaggerated reflexes (hyperreflexia) and increased extensor tone. UMN disease of the hind limbs indicates a lesion cranial to L4 and is commonly seen with thoracolumbar disk herniation. UMN disease to the forelimbs suggests a lesion cranial to T3. Atrophy after UMN injury is mild and gradual and a result of disuse.

10. What is meant by the term lower motor neuron (LMN) disease?

LMNs are the efferent neurons connecting the central nervous system to the muscles. They are located in the gray matter of all spinal cord segments where their axons form peripheral spinal nerves. LMN disease is characterized by paralysis, decreased muscle tone, and decreased reflexes (hyporeflexia or areflexia). Muscle atrophy occurs quickly after LMN injury. LMN disease can occur after disk herniation affecting the brachial or pelvic intumescence.

11. What are clinical signs in a dog with thoracolumbar disk herniation?

- The forelimbs and cranial nerves are normal.
- The hind limbs show signs of upper motor neuron disease. Depending on the severity and chronicity of the herniation, the hind limbs may be paretic or paralyzed. If ambulatory, the patient is often ataxic and has hyperreflexic femoral and patellar reflexes.
- Other signs might include focal hyperpathia along the spine, bowel or bladder dysfunction, reluctance to jump or climb stairs, crying in pain, and an arched back (kyphosis).

12. What clinical signs might be seen in a dog with cervical disk herniation?

- The cranial nerves are normal.
- Dogs have neck pain, are reluctant to move their head or neck, cry out in pain, and have few neurologic deficits.
- Neurologic signs, if present, are usually consistent with UMN disease (including paresis, ataxia, and hyperreflexia affecting the hind limbs, forelimbs, or both).
- Paralysis of the limbs is uncommon after cervical disk herniation but can occur.

13. What is a root signature?

In some cases, dogs present for forelimb lameness (hold limb in flexion) or associated with neck pain. This is called a **root signature** and is caused by compression or irritation of the nerve roots (C6-T2 cord segments between C4-5 to T1-2 vertebrae) innervating the forelimb.

14. What are the differential diagnoses for interverebral disk disease?

- Fibrocartilaginous emboli
- Spinal trauma (fracture or luxation)
- Primary or metastatic neoplasia of the spinal cord or vertebrae
- Myelomalacia
- Myelitis
- Meningitis
- Diskospondylitis
- Endocrine neuropathies
- Degenerative myelopathy
- Vertebral anomalies and spinal dysraphism
- Demyelinating diseases
- Peripheral neuropathies

15. What are the most common sites for cervical disk herniation?
C2-3 and decreasing caudally.

16. What are the most common sites for thoracolumbar disk herniation?
T11-12 to L1-2 (75%).

17. Why does thoracolumbar disk herniation occur infrequently cranial to T10?
An intercapital ligament courses dorsally over the disks from T2 to T10 and helps prevent herniation of disk material into the epidural space.

18. List the typical survey radiographic findings of intervertebral disk herniation.
- Narrowing or wedging of an intervertebral disk space
- Change in shape of the intervertebral foramen at the site of the herniation
- Narrowing of the space between facets
- Mineralized disk material visible in the spinal canal

19. How accurate are survey radiographs?
Evaluation of these films may **fail** to determine accurately the site of herniation in 30–40% of patients.

20. What are the typical myelographic signs of intervertebral disk herniation?
- Extradural compression, including loss or deviation of the contrast column over the disk space.
- Spinal cord may appear widened on the orthogonal radiographic view.

21. How accurate is myelography?
Evaluation correctly identifies the site in 85–95% of patients.

22. What other imaging modalities may be helpful in diagnosing disk herniation?
MRI and **CT** are beneficial but available only in a limited number of hospitals.

23. How does one evaluate a patient for conscious deep pain sensation?
The clinician firmly pinches the patient's digits with a forceps and assesses the response. Conscious perception of pain is indicated by the patient crying out, or attempting to bite, attempting to get away; in some cases, the response may be limited to dilation of the pupils. Withdrawing the foot without conscious recognition of pain is a **reflex** and suggests only loss of deep pain sensation.

24. What is progressive myelomalacia?
Also called **hematomyelia** or **progressive, hemorrhagic myelomalacia.** Although the exact cause is uncertain, it is likely the result of severe ischemia caused by trauma, hemorrhage, vasospasm, and hypoxia within the damaged spinal cord. Massive catecholamine release may be an important factor in the development of myelomalacia. The ischemic cord quickly undergoes necrosis and complete nervous tissue destruction. The autocatalytic process causes ascending and descending necrosis of motor neurons and sensory fibers. Clinical signs include LMN dysfunction and ascending analgesia soon after spinal trauma. The prognosis is grave, and patients usually die of respiratory failure within days of injury.

25. When is medical therapy indicated for treatment of disk herniation?
In patients with pain alone (no neurologic deficits) or with a first episode of mild ataxia. Medical treatment is also recommended in patients when the prognosis is grave with or without surgery, such as those with a loss of deep pain recognition for >48 hours or those with myelomalacia.

26. What is the appropriate medical therapy for disk herniation?
- The most important part of medical therapy is **strict confinement.**
- **Analgesics** and **anti-inflammatory medications** are often given but may have minimal effect on the disease.
- For paralyzed patients, care should include prevention of decubital ulcers, proper bladder care, and physical therapy.

27. What surgical procedures are used for treatment of disk herniation?
Disk herniation is generally treated by **decompressive surgery.** Cervical disk herniations can be decompressed by performing a ventral slot procedure. Thoracolumbar herniations are usually decompressed by performing a hemilaminectomy or foraminotomy procedure. The herniated disk material is removed from the epidural space.

28. What are the advantages of a hemilaminectomy compared with a dorsal laminectomy?
- Allows complete removal of the herniated disk material
- Less invasive
- Less traumatic to the cord
- Less likely to result in a postoperative scarring that can compress the spinal cord

29. What is a laminectomy membrane?
Constrictive fibrosis between epaxial musculature and the spinal cord and dura mater after decompressive surgery.

30. How is a laminectomy membrane avoided?
- Retaining lateral facets and lamina during dorsal laminectomy
- Placement of absorbable gelatin sponge or fat in bone defects
- Meticulous closure of overlying muscles and fascia

31. What is the prognosis after surgery?
Variability in clinical signs, treatments, and postoperative follow-up evaluations make it difficult to provide definitive, scientifically valid statements. In general, dogs with deep pain before surgery recover 65–95% of the time, usually within 6 weeks. Recovery rates for dogs with loss of deep pain sensation before surgery are 25–75%.

32. What are indications of recovery?
Reverse order of preoperative signs:
- Deep pain perception
- Voluntary motor function
- Ataxia—proprioception deficits
- Weight bearing, ambulation

33. How common are recurrences after disk surgery?
After decompressive thoracolumbar disk surgery, recurrent neurologic signs occur in 35–42% of the patients. Reoperations were described in 6% of dogs, primarily Dachshunds.

34. When is a durotomy indicated?
Many surgeons believe a durotomy is rarely, if ever, helpful. Some surgeons perform a durotomy in patients with severe neurologic deficits, a grave prognosis, and when the spinal cord appears to be severely injured. Although a durotomy is unlikely to be helpful in these circumstances, gross visualization of myelomalacia assists in providing a true prognosis to the owner.

35. What is meant by the term UMN bladder?
Injury to the spinal cord between the brain stem and L7 (cranial to the innervation to the bladder) can result in detrusor areflexia and sphincter hypertonus (UMN bladder). The bladder be-

comes distended and is difficult to express manually. Permanent damage to the detrusor muscle can occur if the condition is not treated properly.

36. What is the appropriate therapy after surgery for a disk herniation?
- In paralyzed patients, frequent bladder expression or closed urinary collection systems are used to keep the bladder decompressed and to minimize the development of cystitis.
- Physical therapy is used to prevent decubital ulcers and minimize muscle atrophy.
- Analgesics are indicated for the first several days after surgery.
- Steroid therapy is controversial and is likely to have minimal effect >24 hours after surgery.
- Complications of steroid use (primarily gastrointestinal complications) are common and may preclude the use of steroids for more than the initial perioperative period.

37. List other (nonsurgical) treatments for disk disease.
- **Chemonucleolysis:**—percutaneous, fluoroscopically guided, intradiskal injection of collagenase.
- **Thermal ablation:**—fluoroscopically guided YAG laser.
- **Acupuncture:**—for mildly affected patients.

CONTROVERSIES

38. When are corticosteroids used for treatment of disk herniation?
Most studies indicate corticosteroids are helpful only in controlling spinal disease if administere before spinal injury, which is difficult to do in a clinical situation. Most clinicians use steroid therapy in disk cases. Methylprednisolone sodium succinate (30 mg/kg) is administered intravenously and followed by a continuous infusion (5 mg/kg/hr for 24 hours). Others prefer to administer two subsequent doses of 15 mg/kg every 8 hours rather than an infusion. Steroid administration >24 hours after injury is unlikely to have therapeutic effect.

39. When is surgery indicated for treatment of disk herniation?
Many dogs respond, at least initially, to medical treatment. Surgery is likely to yield better results than medical treatment in patients with multiple episodes of ataxia and paresis, those with moderate or severe neurologic deficits, and those that have not responded or have worsened with medical therapy. Dogs with acute loss of deep pain sensation (<24 hours) are more likely to improve after surgery than with medical therapy. Whenever surgery is considered, early surgical decompression is the key to success.

40. When is intervertebral disk fenestration indicated?
The procedure involves opening the annulus fibrosus and removing the nucleus pulposus to reduce the incidence of future disk rupture. To date, no studies have definitively shown that the incidence of future herniation is significantly reduced or the likelihood of future herniation is sufficiently high to warrant this surgical procedure. Many surgeons perform a disk fenestration procedure on the surrounding disks after decompressive surgery at the herniated site, particularly in the cervical region. Many surgeons that do not believe fenestration is warranted complete the procedure in the cervical region (because it is easy to perform) but do not fenestrate disks in the thoracolumbar region, where it is more difficult.

BIBLIOGRAPHY

1. Dhupa S, Glickman N: Reoperative neurosurgery in dogs with thoracolumbar disc disease. Vet Surg 28:421–428, 1999.
2. Jerram RM, Dewey CW: Acute thoracolumbar disk extrusion in dogs: Parts I, II. Comp Cont Educ Pract Vet 21:922–930, 1037–1046, 1999.
3. Oliver JE, Lorenz MD: Pelvic limb paresis, paralysis, or ataxia. In Oliver JE, Lorenz MD (eds): Handbook of Veterinary Neurology, 2nd ed. Philadelphia, WB Saunders, 1993, pp 128–169.

4. Schultz KS, Walker M, Moon M: Correlation of clinical, radiographic, and surgical localization of inter-vertebral disc extrusion in small-breed dogs: A prospective study of 50 cases. Vet Surg 27:105–111, 1998.
5. Wheeler SJ, Sharp NJ: Small Animal Spinal Disorders: Diagnosis and Surgery. London, Mosby-Wolfe, 1994, pp 68–108.

90. VERTEBRAL FRACTURES AND LUXATIONS

Otto I. Lanz, D.V.M., Dip. A.C.V.S.

1. What are the initial evaluations of a dog with suspected vertebral column fracture?
1. Life-threatening injuries should be dealt with accordingly.
2. The next priority is immobilization of the spine to prevent further displacement of an unstable spinal fracture-luxation. The animal should be placed onto a flat board and taped in lateral recumbency.
3. A neurologic examination should be performed to localize and determine the severity of the lesion. Palpation of the spine and assessment of spinal cord reflexes, pain perception, and cranial nerves should be performed.

2. What medications should be administered if a spinal injury is suspected?
Once the neurologic assessment has been made, opioids can be administered as an analgesic. **Methylprednisolone sodium succinate** or **prednisolone sodium** succinate is the treatment of choice. The protocol is 30 mg/kg IV bolus, followed by a 15 mg/kg bolus 2 hours later. Additional 15 mg/kg IV bolus doses are continued every 6 hours for 24 hours. Starting treatment >8 hours after spinal trauma is detrimental by causing inhibition of neuronal sprouting and neuronal glucose uptake. **Cimetidine** and **misoprostol** have been used for treatment of gastric ulceration.

3. What diagnostic tests should be performed?
- Radiographs
  Lateral and horizontal beam (ventrodorsal projection) radiographs of the suspected fracture
  Thoracic radiographs to rule out pulmonary contusions, diaphragmatic hernia, and pneumothorax.
- A complete blood count
- Serum chemistry analysis
- Urinalysis

4. Discuss the three-compartment theory.
The canine vertebrae are divided into three regions defined by anatomic structures:
1. The **dorsal** compartment contains the articular facets, laminae, pedicles, spinous processes, and supporting ligamentous structures.
2. The **middle** compartment contains the dorsal longitudinal ligament, the dorsal annulus, and the dorsal vertebral body.
3. The **ventral** compartment contains the remainder of the vertebral body, the lateral and ventral aspects of the annulus, nucleus pulposus, and the ventral longitudinal ligament.
Radiographs are assessed to evaluate which of the three compartments are damaged. When two or three compartments are fractured or displaced, the fracture is considered **unstable**. If only one compartment is involved, the fracture is considered **stable**.

5. When is myelography performed for spinal fractures?

- Myelography is usually not performed if the spinal fracture can be treated conservatively or if there is a substantially displaced fracture-luxation that obviously requires surgery.
- Myelography should be performed in animals with marked neurologic deficits and normal or equivocally abnormal radiographs. In these cases, myelography can identify persistent spinal cord compression resulting from an extruded disk, which may need surgical decompression.
- Myelography can also detect occult spinal lesions (20% of animals with spinal trauma) and spinal cord transection in animals with no deep pain.

6. What are the advantages of performing preoperative CT and MRI scans in animals with spinal fractures?

CT

- Visualizes osseous abnormalities, such as vertebral fractures
- Accurately identifies fracture stability by determining which compartments are involved
- Helps surgeon plan surgery and determine which means of fixation will be used through three-dimensional reconstruction of the vertebral fracture

MRI

- Offers superior soft tissue definition, which is helpful when evaluating the spinal cord.

7. Where do most spinal fracture-luxations occur?

In the junction of a mobile and immovable (static/kinetic) vertebral segment. In dogs and cats, these areas include:

- Lumbosacral junction
- Thoracolumbar junction
- Cervicothoracic junction
- Atlantoaxial junction
- Atlanto-occipital junction

8. What are the primary forces responsible for causing vertebral fracture-luxations?

The forces responsible are bending (**extension, flexion**), torsion (**rotation**), and compression (**axial loading**). Flexion injuries of the spine are the most common type of injury and usually cause the most severe neurologic dysfunction.

9. List the elements of nonsurgical management.

- Strict cage rest for 4–6 weeks
- Back braces or body casts
- Cessation of steroids, use of analgesics
- Serial neurologic examinations (deterioration warrants reevaluation, with or without surgery or euthanasia)

10. List the indications for surgical intervention of spinal fracture-luxations.

- Substantial neurologic deficits
- Evidence of spinal cord compression based on radiographs, myelogram, or CT scans.
- Stable fracture that is responding poorly to conservative therapy
- Deteriorating neurologic status after conservative management
- Vertebral instability (two or three affected compartments) demonstrable on radiographs or CT scans.

11. What factors must be considered when selecting a surgical technique for stabilization of vertebral fracture-luxations?

- Location of the lesion
- Presence of a compressive lesion within the canal

- Size of the animal
- Equipment available
- Experience of the surgeon

12. List surgical techniques for stabilization of vertebral fractures-luxations.

Pins and polymethyl methacrylate   Pins and wires

Vertebral body plating   External fixators

Spinous processes plating

13. What are the advantages of using pins and polymethyl methacrylate?

- Relative ease of application
- Versatility for most regions of the spine
- Affords good stabilization
- Is stronger than dorsal fixation
- No special instrumentation needed
- Relatively inexpensive materials

14. What is the optimal number and configuration of pins when using pins and polymethyl methacrylate?

An **eight-pin configuration** with the pins angled away from the fracture site. The pins in the cranial two vertebral bodies are directed in a caudoventral direction, and the pins in the caudal two vertebral bodies are directed in a cranioventral direction. Pins are placed on both sides of the vertebral body.

15. Can a four pin configuration be used?

If a four-pin configuration is used, the pins should be angled toward the fracture site. The pins in the cranial vertebral body are angled caudoventrally and the pins in the caudal vertebral body are angled cranioventrally.

16. List the advantages and disadvantages of spinous process plating.

Advantages

- Inherent stability provided by the articular facets; supraspinous and interspinous ligaments preserved.
- Can be combined with other techniques (vertebral body plating or pins and methyl methacrylate).

Disadvantages

- Plate slippage and fracturing of the spinous processes in the postoperative period.
- Spinous processes must be large and the bone compact to support the plate.
- A minimum of two spinous processes on each side of the fracture-luxation must be engaged with the plate and the plate placed close to the base of the spinous process.

17. How many cortices should be engaged when using a vertebral body plate for stabilization of spinal fracture-luxations?

At least four cortices engaged cranial and caudal to the fracture-luxation. Stabilization of two adjacent vertebral bodies is recommended; however, if a midbody vertebral fracture is encountered, three vertebral bodies should be spanned with the vertebral body plate.

18. Describe the anatomic landmarks for placing pins or screws in a vertebral body.

- When placing screws or pins from a dorsolateral approach to the thoracic spine, the tubercle of the ribs and the base of the accessory processes are used as landmarks.
- In the lumbar vertebrae, the accessory processes and transverse processes are used as landmarks. Pins and screws placed in the thoracic vertebrae or lumbar vertebrae should be directed at a 45° angle relative to the spinous processes.

- When ventral stabilization of the cervical spine is performed, screws or pins are directed in a dorsolateral direction at a 30°–35° angle from the ventral midline of the vertebral body.

19. What kind of joint is the atlantoaxial joint?

A diarthrodial joint that lacks the support of an intervertebral disk. This joint depends entirely on the fibrous joint capsule and surrounding ligaments for stability.

20. What causes atlantoaxial instability?

A congenital or developmental problem resulting in instability of the atlantoaxial joint. Instability may result from fracture, absence, hypoplasia, or malformation of the odontoid process, resulting in a nonfunctional attachment of the ligamentous structures supporting the atlas and axis. Rupture or laxity of the alar, apical, transverse, or dorsal atlantoaxial ligaments may also result in laxity between the atlas and axis.

21. What is the usual signalment and history of an animal presented for atlantoaxial instability?

Atlantoaxial instability occurs primarily in toy-breed dogs <1 year of age. Dogs that are presented with clinical signs of atlantoaxial instability at an older age have instability since birth, but recent trauma causes a significant amount of instability leading to spinal cord compression.

The history of an animal with atlantoaxial instability is one of progressive tetraparesis, incoordination, and neck pain. Acute presentation usually occurs after minor trauma.

22. List problems with dorsal fixation of atlantoaxial luxations using a loop of orthopedic wire, nonabsorbable suture material, or autogenous graft (nuchal ligament).
- Failure of the suture or bone during initial fixation
- Tearing of the suture or wire through the dorsal arch of C1 or spinous process of C2
- Continued micromotion of C1-2 leading to fatigue and failure of the suture or orthopedic wire
- Spinal cord trauma as the fixation material is passed underneath the dorsal arch of C1
- Cannot relieve ventral spinal cord compression caused by an abnormally shaped odontoid process

23. List the advantages of ventral stabilization techniques for the surgical repair of atlantoaxial luxations.
- Accurate anatomic reduction of C1-2 for adequate decompression of the spinal cord.
  Pins placed in the most solid portion of C1-2.
  C1-2 can be arthrodesed through a ventral approach.
  Odontoidectomy can be performed through a ventral approach if necessary.

24. What is the most common complication after ventral cross-pinning for stabilization of atlantoaxial luxations?

Early pin migration in the postoperative period. Placing polymethyl methacrylate bone cement on the exposed surfaces of the pins can prevent pin migration.

25. Describe the proper pin placement for ventral cross-pinning of C1-2.

Two pins should be started close to the midline on the caudoventral surface of C2. Each pin should be directed medially toward the alar notch on the cranial edge of C1 with the point of the pin directed ventrally. Pins placed in this manner minimize the chances of penetrating and damaging the spinal cord.

26. Discuss special postoperative care for animals recovering from surgical stabilization of spinal fracture.

Caring for recumbent animals, especially large-breed dogs, can be challenging. Long-haired dogs should have the perineal area clipped to prevent urine scalding and fecal contamination. Animals should be encouraged to lie in a sternal position; if they are in lateral recumbency, they should be turned every 4 hours. Incontinent animals require frequent attention to prevent pressure sores and decubital ulcer formation. Water beds can also be used to decrease the chances of decubital ulcer formation. Urinary incontinence (urine retention) is ideally managed by manual expression of the bladder every 8 hours. If the animal cannot be expressed manually, an indwelling urinary catheter is sterilely inserted and connected to a close collection system. Animals should be constantly monitored for early signs of urinary tract infections. Walking slings and supports should be used with caution in the early postoperative period, especially in large-breed dogs in which repair techniques may be challenged by the forces associated with vertebral loading. Swimming and hydrotherapy are ideal for encouragement of motor function and hygiene. Passive physiotherapy should be instituted three times daily, taking each joint through a complete range of motion.

CONTROVERSY

27. Should a neck brace be used in the postoperative management of surgically stabilized atlantoaxial luxations?
     Some surgeons believe neck braces inadequately stabilize C1-2 and are impractical for use in veterinary medicine. Others report that regardless of whether a ventral or dorsal technique is used for the stabilization of C1-2, a neck brace should be placed on the animal. Because the goal is either obtaining a fibrous union of C1-2 (dorsal approach) or arthrodesis of C1-2 (ventral approach), rigid immobilization is important. Neck braces should be placed on the animal for a period of 4–6 weeks or until radiographic evidence of union has occurred. The neck brace should be checked weekly. Strict cage confinement should be part of the postoperative therapy.

BIBLIOGRAPHY

1. Carberry CA, Flanders JA: Nonsurgical management of thoracic and lumbar fractures/luxations in the dog and cat. J Am Anim Hosp Assoc 25:43–53, 1989.
2. Hawthorne J, Blevins WE: Cervical vertebral fractures in 56 dogs. J Am Anim Hosp Assoc 35:135–146, 1999.
3. McCarthy RJ, Lewis DD, Hosgood G: Atlantoaxial subluxation in dogs. Comp Cont Educ Pract Vet 17:215–220, 1995.
4. Selcer RR, Budd WJ, Walker TL: Management of vertebral column fractures in dogs and cats: 211 cases (1977–1985). J Am Vet Med Assoc 198:1965–1968, 1991.
5. Wheeler SJ, Sharp NJH: Small Animal Spinal Disorders, Diagnosis and Surgery. London, Mosby-Wolfe, 1994, pp 171–191.

91. NEOPLASMS OF THE SPINE

Otto I. Lanz, D.V.M., Dip. A.C.V.S.

1. What are the three basic tumor types that affect the spine?

PRIMARY NEURAL TUMORS	SECONDARY TUMORS	METASTATIC TUMORS
Spinal Cord	Bone	Mammary adenocarcinoma
Astrocytomas	Osteosarcoma	Lymphosarcoma
Ependymomas	Fibrosarcoma	Hemangiosarcoma
Medulloepithelioma	Chondrosarcoma	
Sarcoma	Meningioma tissue	
Spinal nerves	Meningioma	
Neurofibroma	Fibrosarcoma	
Neurofibrosarcoma		

2. What are the clinical signs in patients presented with spinal tumors?

LOCATION OF LESION	FORELIMBS	HIND LIMBS	OTHER
Cervical (C1-5)	UMN	UMN	Ataxia in all four limbs
Cervicothoracic (C6-T2)	LMN	UMN	Ataxia in all four limbs
Thoracolumbar (T3-L3)	Normal	UMN	Hind limb ataxia ± forelimb extensor rigidity
Lumbosacral (L4-S3)	Normal	LMN	LMN signs in perineal structures or tail

UMN = upper motor neuron, LMN = lower motor neuron.

3. Do tumors symmetrically involve the spinal cord and nerves?

No. Animals may present with asymmetric signs of spinal cord or nerve root involvement. Hemiparesis or hemiplegia may be seen with asymmetric cervical and cervicothoracic lesions. Monoparesis or monoplegia may be seen with tumors affecting only the brachial plexus on one side and in the hind limb with an asymmetric lumbosacral involvement. Neurofibromas of the nerve roots cause asymmetric signs early in the course of the disease. These animals may be exhibiting much discomfort (radicular pain) in only one limb. Animals with extradural or intradural extramedullary lesions are usually painful, whereas animals with intramedullary masses may not present with spinal hyperesthesia.

4. List the anatomic locations of spinal tumors.

- Intramedullary
- Intradural (extramedullary)
- Extradural

5. Describe the myelographic appearances of spinal cord tumors.

- **Extradural** tumors compress the spinal cord, causing the contrast column to deviate away from the mass, resulting in a widening of the epidural space.
- **Intradural, extramedullary tumors** act as a wedge displacing the dura mater abaxially and the spinal cord axially. As the contrast material surrounds the tumor, a **golf tee** configuration is formed.
- **Intramedullary tumors** cause compression of the spinal cord from within, resulting in a circumferential enlargement of the spinal cord. The swelling of the spinal cord results in diverging attenuation of the contrast material in all views.
- Multiple radiographic views (ventrodorsal, lateral, and oblique) are necessary to show the exact location of the mass. Further imaging modalities, such as CT or MRI scans, are helpful in localizing the tumor.

6. What are the most common intradural extramedullary tumors found in the dog?
Meningiomas and nerve sheath tumors.

7. What is the most common spinal tumor diagnosed in cats?
Lymphosarcoma.

8. What tumors have been shown to have a propensity for CNS metastasis?
- Mammary adenocarcinoma
- Melanoma
- Hemangiosarcoma
- Lymphosarcoma

9. Discuss abnormalities that are seen in CSF analyzed from animals with spinal tumors.
Sometimes, none. **Albuminocytologic dissociation** (increased protein in the absence of increased cells) has been described. Neoplastic cells are rarely seen. Tumor cells are seen when the tumor has invaded the subarachnoid space; an inflammatory response is more commonly observed

in CSF from animals with spinal tumors. Elevated CSF pressures have also been reported in animals with spinal tumors. Meningiomas have been associated with a neutrophilic pleocytosis.

10. Where is the best location, relative to the spinal mass, for a diagnostic spinal tap?
Caudad to the suspected tumor.

11. When is myelography contraindicated?
When CSF analysis indicates inflammation or infection. Myelography may potentiate clinical signs or spread of the infection within the CNS.

12. List characteristics of contrast agents to perform myelography.
Characteristics of an ideal myelographic contrast agent are:
• Nontoxic
• Miscible with CSF
• Water-soluble
• Radiopaque
• Absorbable
• Inexpensive

13. What myelographic contrast agents are specifically recommended?
• Iopamidol (Isovue)
• Iohexol (Omnipaque)

14. What are the radiographic findings of vertebral multiple myeloma?
Osteolysis in the spinous processes and pelvis.

15. Where does spinal cord compression secondary to spinal tumors occur, compared with disk-associated compression, when viewed on a myelogram?
Within the body of the vertebrae, whereas cord compression caused by intervertebral disk disease is dorsal to the intervertebral disk space.

16. Discuss the surgical approach recommended for the removal of spinal tumors.
The surgical approach is based on the location of the tumor and can be aided with enhanced diagnostic imaging (CT or MRI). Tumors with a ventral location in the thoracic or lumbar spine may be approached through a **hemilaminectomy.** Hemilaminectomies of the cervical spine have been reported in the veterinary literature; however, dorsal laminectomies are most often performed for tumors located in the cervical spine. **Dorsal laminectomies** may be used for tumors with a lateral location in the thoracic or lumbar spine. If exploration does not reveal evidence of a spinal tumor, a biopsy specimen of epidural fat should be obtained to rule out lymphosarcoma or myxosarcoma. A durotomy should also be performed to rule out an intradural extramedullary or intradural tumor. In this case, the dura should also be submitted for histopathology.

17. What adjunctive therapy can be combined with surgery for animals with spinal tumors?
   • **Chemotherapy** (steroids) has been used for animals with spinal lymphosarcoma.
   • **Radiation therapy** after surgical decompression and tumor removal increases surgical time in dogs with spinal tumors. Response to radiation therapy depends on tumor type, histologic grade, tumor extent, anatomic location, and metastasis.

BIBLIOGRAPHY

1. Levy MS, Kapatkin AS, Patnaik AK: Spinal tumors in 37 dogs: Clinical outcome and long-term surgical (1987–1994). J Am Anim Hosp Assoc 33:307–312, 1997.

2. Morrison WB: Cancer affecting the nervous system. In Morrison WB (ed): Cancer in Dogs and Cats. Philadelphia, Lippincott, 1999, pp 655–667.
3. Prata RG: Diagnosis of spinal cord tumors in the dog. Vet Clin North Am Small Anim Pract 7:165–185, 1997.
4. Siegel S, Kornegay J, Thrall DE: Postoperative irradiation of spinal cord tumors in 9 dogs. Vet Radiol Ultrasound 37:150–153, 1996.
5. Wheeler SJ, Sharp JH: Small Animal Spinal Disorders. London, Mosby-Wolfe, 1994, pp 156–168.

92. CERVICAL VERTEBRAL INSTABILITY

Thomas R. Fry, D.V.M., M.S., Dip. A.C.V.S.

1. What is cervical vertebral instability (CVI)?
A condition of large-breed dogs in which abnormalities of the cervical vertebrae and disks lead to spinal cord or nerve root compression resulting from mass effect, instability, or both. Chronic and progressive compression leads to demyelination and malacia.

2. What are synonyms for CVI?
- Cervical malformation-malarticulation syndrome
- Cervical spondylopathy
- Cervical spondylolisthesis
- Cervical spondylomyelopathy
- Wobbler

3. What is the signalment?
Great Danes and **Doberman pinschers** are predisposed, but other breeds are affected. Young Great Danes and Dobermans and middle-aged to older male Dobermans make up two distinct populations.

4. What is the pathogenesis of CVI?
1. **Congenital osseous malformation:**
Pedicles, arches, or facets become malformed. This syndrome occurs in young Great Danes and Doberman pinschers. Levels C3-7 are affected.
2. **Cervical vertebral instability with chronic degenerative disk disease:**
Chronic disk herniation leads to annular hypertrophy and static or dynamic spinal cord compression. This syndrome occurs in middle-aged male Dobermans. Levels C5-7 are predisposed.
3. **Vertebral tipping:**
Dorsal displacement of the cranial vertebral body into the spinal canal occurs, caused by or leading to disk degeneration. This type of abnormality is seen in middle-aged male Dobermans. C5-7 lesions are commonest.
4. **Ligamentum flavum disease or vertebral arch malformations:**
Instability leads to hypertrophy of the ligamentum flavum. Also, with vertebral arch or facet malformations, static or dynamic dorsal compression of the spinal cord may occur. Young Great Danes at dorsal C4-7 are predisposed. Malformations may be due to heritable tendencies, nutritional imbalances, trauma, or osteochondroses.
5. **Hourglass compression:**
Ligamentum flavum, dorsal annulus, and facet hypertrophy lead to simultaneous ventral, lateral, and dorsal spinal cord compression. This form also occurs in young Great Danes at all levels of the cervical spine.

5. What are typical clinical signs of CVI?
- Signs of radicular **involvement** include neck pain, root signature, or both.
- Signs of **myelopathy** include ataxia, rear limb weakness followed by forelimb weakness, and ambulatory tetraparesis progressing to nonambulatory tetraparesis. Dogs (as should the veterinarian) avoid dorsiflexion if a dynamic lesion is present.

6. How is CVI diagnosed?
- Survey radiographs do not allow for accurate diagnosis.
- Because of the potential dynamic nature of lesions, **myelography** is critical. Standard (lateral, ventrodorsal, oblique) and stress (linear traction, ventroflexed, and dorsiflexed) myelographic views are indicated.
- CT and CT myelography may be used but are not critical for diagnosis and surgical decision making.

7. Discuss elements of conservative treatment.
- **Rest:** Restrict activity to prevent neck trauma, and use chest harnesses instead of collars.
- **Nonsteroidal antiinflammatory drugs:** Relatively ineffective.
- **Corticosteroids:** Use judiciously. All patients on corticosteroids need to be closely monitored for gastrointestinal side effects, and steroid used should be discontinued if these occur.
  Dexamethasone: 0.1 mg/lb PO or IM once a day for 1 week, then taper.
  Prednisone or **prednisolone:** 0.25–0.5 mg/lb PO sid for 1 week then every other day.
  Methylprednisolone should be used only as a preoperative single dose at 60 mg/lb IV.

8. When should surgical intervention be recommended?
A static (3–4 weeks) or worsening neurologic status is an indication. Lack of response to medical management is common, so it is critical for the veterinarian to examine patients serially during conservative therapy.

9. Discuss surgical treatments for CVI.
Decompression includes dorsal laminectomy and ventral slot. Both approaches allow for spinal cord decompression, but they do not address dynamic lesions completely. Ventral slot may be combined with stabilization procedures indicated for dynamic compressive lesions. Ventral slot is used for single-level or two-level chronic disk herniation. It is ineffective for treatment of a dorsal component. Ventral slot may provide less than ideal decompression because of limited spinal canal access. Dorsal laminectomy may be used to treat all types of wobblers except chronic intervertebral disk herniation and vertebral tipping because there is a primary dorsal compressive component to the disease. Some surgeons treat greater than two-level herniations with dorsal laminectomy.

Stabilization procedures include use of cortical bone grafting of interspaces combined with polyvinylidine spinal plating, ventral Harrington rods, pins and methyl methacrylate, bone screw and washer, and an interbody polymethyl methacrylate plug. In these procedures, the spine is placed under traction to reduce compression from a dynamic lesion, and implants are used to stabilize the spine until osseous fusion occurs. With these techniques, most of the decompression is afforded indirectly via distraction of structures that are causing dynamic compression, versus the more direct decompression afforded by the slot of laminectomy procedures.

10. What factors affect the prognosis?
1. **Number of spinal levels involved:** Lesions involving more than two levels dramatically lower the prognosis.
2. **Anatomic abnormality:** Congenital osseous malformations do not have a favorable prognosis compared with chronic disks.
3. **Static versus dynamic lesions:** Static lesions may have a more favorable prognosis than dynamic lesions.

4. **Presenting neurologic status:** Pain alone or mild long tract signs carry a much more favorable prognosis than nonambulatory tetraparesis.

5. **Timing of surgical intervention is critical:** Success is more likely if surgery is performed before chronic changes (demyelination) have occurred.

11. What is the prognosis for CVI in general?

Animals that are moderately to severely tetraparetic, particularly with multiple spinal levels of involvement, have a guarded-to-poor prognosis. Dogs that present with single-level involvement in which surgical intervention is elected early have a good-to-excellent prognosis. Success rates approaching 80% are possible with early surgical intervention.

12. What postoperative care is necessary?
- Appropriate postoperative analgesic therapy is essential.
- Discontinue steroids and provide excellent nursing care to nonambulatory patients.
- Frequent turning, padding to avoid decubital ulcers, bathing, and prevention of urinary tract infection are critical.
- Pick appropriate surfaces for walking (rubber mats, carpet, lawn) and encourage daily exercise.
- Provide hydrotherapy and physical therapy (passive flexion and extension exercises) as necessary.
- Neck braces are required after Harrington rods and polyvinylidine plate surgeries for 6 weeks postoperatively.
- Vigorous activity should be avoided for 8 weeks postoperatively.

13. List the complications of surgery for wobbler's syndrome.

Intraoperative	Immediate postoperative	Long-term
• Hemorrhage	• Graft or implant failures	• Further instability (**domino** effect)
• Nerve trauma	• Worsening neurologic signs	
• Hypotension		• Urinary tract infection
• Cardiac dysrhythmia or arrest		• Pressure sores

14. How common are subsequent neurologic lesions after surgery?

Approximately 25% of dogs that undergo fusion develop disk herniations adjacent to the fused segment within 5 years of surgery.

BIBLIOGRAPHY

1. Dixon BC, Tomlinson JL: A modified distraction-stabilization technique using an interbody polymethylmethacrylate plug in dogs with CVI. J Am Vet Med Assoc 208:61–68, 1996.
2. Lyman R: Wobbler syndrome: Continuous dorsal laminectomy is the procedure of choice. Prog Vet Neurol 2:143–146, 1991.
3. McKee WM, Butterworth SJ: Management of cervical spondylopathy-associated disc protrusions using metal washers in 78 dogs. J Small Anim Pract 40:465–472, 1999.
4. Seim HB: Wobbler syndrome. In Fossum TW (ed): Small Animal Surgery. St. Louis, Mosby, 1997, pp 1071–1084.
5. Walker TL: Use of Harrington rods in caudal cervical spondylomyelopathy. In Bojrab MJ (ed): Current Techniques in Small Animal Surgery, 4th ed. Philadelphia, Lea & Febiger, 1998, pp 830–832.
6. Wheeler SJ, Sharp NJH: Small Animal Spinal Disorders Diagnosis and Surgery. London, Mosby-Wolfe, 1994, pp 135–155.

93. LUMBOSACRAL DISEASE

Lisa Klopp, D.V.M., M.S., Dip. A.C.V.I.M. (Neurology)

1. Outline the functional neuroanatomy of the lumbosacral spinal cord.

SPINAL CORD SEGMENTS AND NERVE ROOTS		MOTOR INNERVATION
L4-6	Femoral nerve	Quadriceps femoris m.
		Sartorius m.
		Iliopsoas m.
	Obturator nerve	Pectineus m.
		Adductor m.
		Gracilis m.
		External obturator m.
L6-S2	Cranial gluteal nerve (L6, L7, S1)	Middle and deep gluteal mm.
		Tensor fascia lata m.
	Sciatic nerve (L6, L7, S1, ±-S2)	Biceps femoris m.
	Branches of the sciatic nerve	
	Common peroneal n.	Cranial tibial m.
		Lateral digital extensor m.
		Long digital extensor m.
		Peroneus longus m.
	Tibial nerve	Deep and superficial digital flexor mm.
		Popliteus m.
		Gastrocnemius m.
		Semimembranosus m.
		Semitendinosus m.
	Caudal gluteal nerve (L7, S1, S2)	Middle and superficial gluteal mm.
S1–3	Pudendal nerve	External anal sphincter
		Urethralis m. (external urinary sphincter)
	Pelvic nerve (parasympathetic)	Detrusor m. (bladder muscle)

2. What is unique about the anatomy of the lumbosacral region?

A differential growth rate of the spinal cord and vertebral column results in **termination of the spinal cord at the L6 vertebra in the dog and L7 in the cat.** For this reason, lesions affecting the lumbosacral joint generally affect the cauda equina (CE) and not the spinal cord.

3. What is the difference between lumbosacral and CE syndromes?

- Lumbosacral syndrome encompasses spinal cord segments L4-S3.
- CE syndrome reflects the peripheral nerve roots in the caudal lumbar and sacral spinal canal. In essence, CE syndrome is a neuropathic disease rather than spinal cord disease.

4. What does the term lower motor neuron (LMN) mean?

LMNs that supply muscles of the pelvic limbs arise from L4-S2 spinal cord segments. Injury to this area of the spinal cord, peripheral nerves, or nerve roots may result in LMN signs in the pelvic limbs:

- Flaccid paresis or plegia
- Hyporeflexia to areflexia
- Neurogenic atrophy

5. What does the term upper motor neuron (UMN) mean?

UMNs arise from motor centers in the cerebrum (corticospinal tracts) and brain stem

(rubrospinal, medullary and pontine reticulospinal, vestibulospinal tracts). These neurons influence and modify LMNs. UMN signs involve:
- Normal tonicity to spastic paresis or plegia
- Normoreflexia to hyperreflexia
- Disuse atrophy if dysfunction is severe and prolonged

6. What is lumbosacral stenosis?
Narrowing of the L7 and sacral spinal canal secondary to congenital malformation or acquired degenerative changes.

7. What does the term lumbosacral disease encompass?
- Degenerative disk disease, type I or II.
- Congenital stenosis, malformation, or malarticulation.
- Degenerative changes and hypertrophy of:
    Ligamentum flavum
    Dorsal longitudinal ligament
    Articular facet joint capsule

8. What is spondylosis?
A common radiographic finding in asymptomatic middle-aged to older dogs characterized by ventral bone bridging between vertebrae. It rarely interferes with neural structures, unless severe lateral spondylosis causes nerve root impingement near the intervertebral foramen.

9. What is the signalment of dogs most commonly affected by lumbosacral disease?
Young to middle-aged, large-breed and working male dogs.

10. List the common signs of lumbosacral disease.
- Lumbosacral pain
- Intermittent or persistent hind limb lameness
- Mild paraparesis
- Proprioceptive deficits
- Tail paresis
- Incontinence

11. Why is it important to assess hock flexion specifically when performing the withdrawal reflex?
The tarsus can passively flex with flexion of the stifle and hip. Lumbosacral disease often affects the nerve roots that supply sciatic innervation to the distal musculature of the limb. Manual pressure in front of the stifle keeps it from flexing and allows evaluation of hock flexion specifically, which may be found to be depressed or absent with sciatic nerve dysfunction.

12. Why is the patellar reflex spared?
The sensory and motor components of the patellar reflex are supplied by the femoral nerve that arises from spinal cord and nerve roots L4–6. The last nerve root contributing to this reflex exits in the L6–7 intervertebral foramen.

13. List some methods to evaluate dogs for lumbosacral pain.
- Deep lumbosacral palpation
- Dorsal elevation of the tail base
- Pelvic limb wheelbarrow reaction

14. What condition is critical to rule out for dogs with lumbosacral disease?
Osteoarthritis of the hip joints.

15. What is pseudohyperreflexia?
A term used for an exaggerated patellar reflex secondary to loss of antagonistic muscles supplied by the sciatic nerve.

16. What is intermittent claudication?
From the Latin, *claudicato*—limping. A complex of symptoms characterized by absence of pain or discomfort in a limb at rest and the commencement of pain, tension, and weakness during exercise. Exercise increases metabolic demands for oxygen and nutrients by the spinal cord and cauda equina. The radicular arteries passing through the **stenotic intervertebral foramen** become compressed and cannot meet the metabolic demands of the nervous system. Nerve root ischemia results in radicular pain, which is referred to the back, perineum, and extremities.

17. What is paresthesia?
Abnormal sensation resulting from nerve root injury or compression. Signs of licking, chewing, and self-mutilation represent behavioral manifestations of paresthesia in animals.

18. What is dysesthesia?
An unpleasant, abnormal sensation with normal stimuli, such as touch or mild manipulation.

19. What is the source of pain in animals with lumbosacral disease?
Compression ischemia to a peripheral nerve produces dysfunction in large-caliber (heavily myelinated) nerve fibers first. Compression of sensory roots results in mechanical depolarization perceived by the central nervous system as radiating pain. Diskogenic pain also plays a role.

20. List common traumatic lesions of the lumbosacral area in dogs and cats.
- Lumbosacral fracture and luxations
- Pelvic fractures
- Sacroiliac luxation
- Sacrocaudal fracture and avulsion

21. List other diseases that affect the lumbosacral spine, peripheral nerves, and spinal cord and CE in dogs.
- Diskospondylitis
- Fibrocartilaginous emboli
- Spina bifida
- Neoplasia
- Neuropathies

22. List other diseases that affect the lumbosacral spine and spinal cord, peripheral nerves, and CE in cats.
- Aortic thromboembolism
- Diabetic neuropathy
- Metastatic neoplasia
- Sacrocaudal dysgenesis
- Traumatic ischemic myelopathy

23. What imaging procedures are used for lumbosacral disease?
- Survey radiography
- Myelography
- Epidurography
- Discography
- CT
- MRI

24. Which imaging procedures are best?
CT provides the best bone detail, whereas **MRI** is most accurate for soft tissue lesions.

25. What electrodiagnostic studies are helpful in the diagnosis of lumbosacral disease?
Needle electromyography is used to determine if there is normal muscle physiology and integrity of muscle membrane and physiology.

26. How is lumbosacral syndrome treated medically?

Most dogs with pain alone respond to antiinflammatory medications and short-term (4–6 weeks) exercise restriction. Slow return to more normal activity over a few months is recommended. Permanent lifestyle changes, including no jumping, climbing stairs, or excessive physical activity, are also helpful.

27. Discuss surgical options for lumbosacral disease.

Dorsal laminectomy or **hemilaminectomy** at L7-S1. Unilateral and bilateral facetectomy or foraminotomy may be used when pathology involves the lateral recesses or intervertebral foramen. Laminectomy allows access to the spinal canal for débridement of ruptured disk material, hypertrophied ligaments, and fibrous scar tissue. Diskectomy can be performed via this approach.

28. When is decompressive surgery indicated?

When animals are not responsive to medical (conservative) therapy or have multiple recurrences of clinical signs despite lifestyle changes. Animals with severe marked progressive neurologic dysfunction are surgical candidates. Adequate postoperative rest and convalescence is imperative for a positive outcome.

29. What are the complications of surgical treatment of lumbosacral disease?

- Injury to nerve roots and excessive hemorrhage.
- Dogs are often in pain and clinically worse for a few days (application of epidural anesthesia, e.g., morphine or morphine and metdetomidine, before surgical closure is beneficial in short-term postoperative pain control).

30. What is the recommended aftercare for surgical treatment of lumbosacral disease?

Strict rest with leash walks only for 6–8 weeks. Minimal controlled activity is warranted to provide physical therapy. Passive and active pelvic limb physical therapy is recommended for animals with neurologic dysfunction. After the initial 6–8 weeks of limited activity, it is best to retrain slowly and increase activity over 3–4 months. If it is not necessary for animals to work (jump, climb, hunt), permanent lifestyle restrictions are encouraged.

31. What determines the prognosis of animals with lumbosacral disease?

Nerve roots, which are ensheathed by meninges near the spinal cord and epineurium distally, are more resistant to injury than the spinal cord. Dogs with signs of back pain, mild neurologic dysfunction, or claudication have a good-to-fair prognosis. Animals with severe neurologic dysfunction or autonomic dysfunction warrant a more guarded-to-poor prognosis.

CONTROVERSY

32. Discuss controversial issues regarding surgical treatment of lumbosacral disease.

Dorsal fusion and fixation entails distraction of the dorsal aspect of the lumbosacral laminae, pin placement through the articular facets of L7 and S1, and bone graft over the dorsal laminae. Laminectomy is not performed. The aims are to enlarge the intervertebral foramen, relieve the compressive radiculopathy, and stabilize the lumbosacral articulations. This procedure has merit in congenital instability before secondary acquired stenosis. It does not address acquired stenosis secondary to disk extrusion and fibrous proliferation of soft tissues in the lumbosacral joint. Middle-aged to older animals that undergo surgery for acquired stenosis rarely have obvious gross instability evaluated intraoperatively. Performing dorsal fusion and fixation without entering the canal may not truly address the primary pathology. Complications with this procedure include fracture of articular facets, pin migration, and improper pin placement.

BIBLIOGRAPHY

1. Palmer RH, Chambers JN: Canine lumbosacral diseases: Part II. Definitive diagnosis, treatment, and prognosis. Comp Cont Educ Pract 13:213–221, 1991.

2. Prata RG: Cauda equina syndrome. In Slatter D (ed): Textbook of Small Animal Surgery, 2nd ed. Philadelphia, W.B. Saunders, 1993, pp 1094–1109.
3. Ramirez O, Thrall DE: A review of imaging techniques for cauda equina syndrome. Vet Radiol Ultrasound 39:283–296, 1998.
4. Slocum B, Devine T: L7-S1 fixation-fusion for treatment of cauda equina compression in the dog. J Am Vet Med Assoc 188:31–35, 1986.
5. Wheeler SJ: Lumbosacral disease. Vet Clin North Am 22:937–951, 1992.
6. Wheeler SJ, Sharp NJH: Lumbosacral disease. In Wheeler SJ, Sharp NJH (eds): Small Animal Spinal Disorders. London, Mosby-Wolfe, 1994, pp 122–134.

94. PERIPHERAL NERVE SURGERY

C. W. Dewey, D.V.M., M.S., D.A.C.V.S., D.A.C.V.I.M. (Neurology)

1. How frequently is peripheral nerve surgery performed in veterinary patients?
Not often.

2. What are indications for peripheral nerve surgery?
- The most common indication is a diagnostic procedure: nerve **biopsy** for suspected neuropathies.
- Less frequently, perineural **dissection** has been performed for patients with sciatic neuropathy resulting from fibrous tissue entrapment subsequent to trauma in the region of the proximal femur. In such cases, it is important to find normal, nonentrapped nerve, and establish a dissection plane between nerve and fibrous tissue. Microsurgical equipment and magnification head loupes are used for this type of delicate surgery.
- Uncommonly the brachial plexus area is explored if a nerve sheath tumor in the axillary region is suspected.
- Surgical procedures for reanastomosis (neurorrhaphy) of major nerve trunks are well described in the veterinary literature, but rarely performed.

3. How does one perform a nerve biopsy?
A readily accessible nerve, such as the ulnar or common peroneal, is selected for biopsy. A small (<30% diameter) longitudinal sample of nerve fascicles is removed for histologic examination. Stay sutures are placed at the proximal-distal aspects of the nerve biopsy ends, and the segment is cut using a No. 11 blade or fine iris scissors.

4. Discuss surgical procedures that are recommended for brachial plexus avulsions.
Typically, the procedure of choice in complete brachial plexus avulsions is **thoracic limb amputation.** Nonavulsion or cranial plexus (radial nerve spared) injuries are uncommon. The prognosis for salvaging a functional limb is poor in most brachial plexus injuries. Surgical reestablishment of innervation at the point of injury with nerve grafts, nerve transfers, or nerve root reimplantation into the spinal cord have been suggested. Even if this type of difficult surgery is successfully performed, the chance for functional recovery in a veterinary patient is quite low because the distance the axons must regrow to reach target muscles is considerable. Most likely, the target muscles will become fibrotic before the axons reach them. Also, recovery of a dog or cat's thoracic limb function is translated into weight bearing, and this degree of functional recovery is unrealistic, compared with the degree of recovery that is considered successful in human cases.

With suspected brachial plexus avulsion, it is appropriate to provide time (4–6 months) for axonal regeneration, in case the nerve roots are not physically torn from the spinal cord. If at any time during this period the patient excoriates or begins to self-mutilate the foot, amputation of the dysfunctional limb should be performed. Dogs and cats, with few exceptions, do well with three legs.

BIBLIOGRAPHY

1. Rodkey WG: Peripheral nerve surgery. In Slatter D (ed): Textbook of Small Animal Surgery, 2nd ed. Philadelphia, W.B. Saunders, 1993, pp 1135–1141.
2. Shores A: Peripheral nerve injury and repair. In Bojrab MJ, Ellison GW, Slocum B (eds): Current Techniques in Small Animal Surgery, 4th ed. Philadelphia, Williams & Wilkins, 1998, pp 73–82.

95. BRAIN INJURY

C. W. *Dewey*, D.V.M., M.S., D.A.C.V.S., D.A.C.V.I.M. (*Neurology*)

1. What are common causes of brain injury in dogs and cats?
Trauma from automobiles, projectiles, bites, and falls.

2. What is the difference between primary and secondary brain injury?
Primary brain injury pertains to events at the time of trauma:
• Direct brain parenchymal damage
• Acute bleeding
Secondary brain injury primarily deals with the cascade of biochemical events after the primary injury:
• Elevation of brain extracellular glutamate levels (neurotoxic)
• Oxygen free radical production
• Increased intracellular calcium levels
• Decreased intracellular ATP levels in neurons

3. How should one neurologically assess the acutely brain-injured patient?
One should not. As with any other traumatic situation, physiologic aberrations (hypotension and hypoxia) most likely to end the patient's life need to be addressed first:
• **Fluid support** of the hypotensive brain injury patient is of paramount importance.
• **Airway, breathing, and cardiovascular system** need to be evaluated and supported.

4. What about determining prognosis for the acutely brain-injured patient via the neurologic examination, before potentially expensive therapy is initiated?
Attaching clinical significance to the mental status of a hypotensive, brain-injured patient is an inaccurate endeavor.

5. What fluid therapy should be given to brain injury patients?
Any fluid given in adequate volume to correct hypotension and sustain normal blood pressure. **Hetastarch combined with crystalloids** for maintenance fluid support, once normovolemia is attained, is a good approach.

6. What about volume limiting the brain-injury patient to decrease intracranial pressure (ICP)?
Pressure autoregulation serves to keep ICP fairly constant through systemic blood pressure extremes between 50 and 150 mm Hg. The volume of blood in the brain can be varied mainly by vasodilation or vasoconstriction of cerebral capillaries and veins. Pressure autoregulation remains intact in most brain injury victims, but it may be partially lost in others, so that the lower limit to autoregulation is set to a higher value (e.g., 80 mm Hg, rather than 50 mm Hg). Combine the concept of pressure autoregulation with the following formula: **CPP = MAP − ICP.** CPP stands for **cerebral perfusion pressure** and represents the forward driving force at the brain arteriolar level.

Adequate CPP allows for oxygen and nutrients to reach the brain parenchyma. MAP refers to **mean arterial pressure.** If the patient with severe brain injury remains in a hypotensive state (low MAP), CPP falls. This is deleterious to the brain. The brain vasculature (mainly capillaries and veins) dilates in response to the drop in MAP, in an effort to preserve blood flow. ICP subsequently increases, further lowering CCP.

7. How should one administer supplemental oxygen to the brain-injured patient?

Most patients benefit from nasal oxygen administration. If cribriform fractures are present, inserting a nasal O_2 catheter too far can have disastrous consequences. With a nasal O_2 catheter, flow rates of 100–200 mL/kg/min should provide an oxygen environment of approximately 40%. Intubation and hyperventilation should be reserved for patients whose elevated ICP is likely to be due to hypercarbia. These are typically patients that are close to or have lost consciousness. Hyperventilation as a primary method of decreasing ICP may cause excessive brain arteriolar vasoconstriction in the nonhypercarbic animal; this may adversely affect CPP.

8. Should mannitol be administered once the patient is stabilized?

Yes. Mannitol decreases ICP. Theoretical contraindications to mannitol administration in veterinary brain injury patients (brain hemorrhage exacerbation) continue to be raised, despite the fact that they do not seem to occur clinically. Restricting mannitol administration to three doses in a 24-hour period prevents problems in most cases.

9. What about other therapies for brain-injured patients?

Despite exhaustive investigations into numerous potential drugs (e.g., DMSO) for brain injury, there are no compelling data to support their use in clinical patients. There is convincing evidence in human medicine that moderate hypothermia (a drop in body temperature of 4°C) improves outcome in brain injury. This is believed to work primarily via inhibiting the release of glutamate and inflammatory cytokines. This mode of therapy is available to veterinary patients and is worth considering.

10. If the patient is not responding well to medical therapy, should one obtain imaging studies, such as skull radiographs, CT, or MRI?

- Skull radiographs seldom reveal any clinically useful information. Fracture location (over the cranial vault versus frontal sinus) and extent of fragment displacement are typically difficult to appreciate on standard skull films.
- **CT** is the preferred imaging modality for the brain-injured patient. It is rapid, is relatively inexpensive (compared with **MRI**), and images bone and acute hemorrhage quite well.

11. Discuss surgical intervention for brain injury in dogs and cats.

The indications for surgical intervention are not well defined in veterinary medicine. Some clear indications would be depressed or open skull fractures or focal intracranial hemorrhage in the face of deteriorating neurologic status. Focal intracranial hemorrhage may occur frequently after severe brain injury in dogs and cats, similar to the situation in humans. Knowledge of these conditions requires CT scanning. The value of craniectomy solely as a decompressive maneuver (to decrease ICP) is controversial in human medicine. Its benefit for veterinary brain injury victims that are responding poorly to medical therapy is unknown. Because it has been shown that craniectomy-durotomy decreases ICP by approximately 85% in normal dogs and cats, surgical intervention should be considered a potentially useful treatment option in canine and feline brain injury.

12. Discuss the prognosis for brain-injured dogs and cats.

Quite variable based on the extent of trauma among patients. With severe brain injury, in which severe disturbances of consciousness occurs, the prognosis is often guarded to poor. The absence of brain stem reflexes (physiologic nystagmus, gag or swallow reflex, blink reflex) is a poor prognostic indicator. Too much emphasis is placed on pupillary light reflexes in these cases. This is especially true if the patient's other brain stem reflexes are intact. Massive sympathetic discharge after brain injury leads to pupillary dilation. A cheap penlight with a weak battery may not affect dilated, nonresponsive pupils. Alternatively, cerebral injury can result in impressive miosis of the pupils. This observation is an indication that there is cerebral injury but is not a prognostic indicator. A pupillary light reflex may not be apparent because the pupils cannot constrict any more. Dogs and cats can recover from severe cerebral damage if they are provided proper nursing care and time.

CONTROVERSY

13. Should glucocorticoid therapy be used in the brain-injured patient?
The lack of evidence to support glucocorticoid use in the brain-injured patient is voluminous. However, there is some experimental evidence that a **high-dose** methylprednisolone protocol may provide some benefit in brain injury. This large dose of methylprednisolone is believed to exert its beneficial effects as an oxygen free radical scavenger and not via activation of glucocorticoid receptors. Hyperglycemia has been associated with poor outcomes in brain-injured humans. This is believed to be due to the shift to anaerobic metabolism and subsequent lactic acid production that occurs in the damaged, hypoxic brain. Elevated glucose levels may lead to subsequent increases in brain-damaging lactic acid. If the patient is already hyperglycemic, think twice about administering a big dose of steroids. High doses of methylprednisolone may produce gastric hemorrhage in normal dog, so mucosal protectants and antacids are warranted.

BIBLIOGRAPHY

1. Bagley RS: Intracranial pressure in dogs and cats. Comp Cont Educ Pract Vet 18:605–621, 1996.
2. Dewey CW: Emergency management of the head trauma patient: Principles and practice. Vet Clin North Am Small Anim Pract 30:207–225, 2000.
3. Proulx J, Dhupa N: Severe brain injury: Parts I, II. Pathophysiology and therapy. Comp Cont Educ Prac Vet 20:897–905, 993–1006, 1998.
4. Rohrer CR, Hill RC: Gastric hemorrhage in dogs given high doses of methylprednisolone sodium succinate. Am J Vet Res 60:977–984, 1999.

96. BRAIN TUMORS

C. W. *Dewey*, D.V.M., M.S., D.A.C.V.S., D.A.C.V.I.M. (*Neurology*)

1. What types of brain tumors affect dogs and cats?
Primary brain tumors arise from brain parenchyma, cells that line the brain tissue, or vascular elements of the brain:
- Meningiomas
- Gliomas (astrocytoma, oligodendroglioma)
- Choroid plexus tumors
- Ependymomas

Secondary brain tumors arise from structures that are not intrinsic to the brain and are less common:
- Pituitary tumors
- Invasive nasal–frontal sinus tumors
- Calvarial tumors (e.g., multilobular osteochondrosarcoma)
- Metastatic neoplasia

2. Name the most common primary brain tumor encountered in dogs and cats.

Meningiomas. Cats are unlikely to develop brain tumors other than meningioma.

3. Are these patients typically older animals?

Yes. The median age for dogs with brain tumors is 9 years and >10 years for cats.

4. Describe clinical signs in dogs and cats with brain tumors?

Most brain tumors are in the front part of the brain (cerebrum, diencephalon), and clinical signs such as seizures, circling, head-pressing, visual disturbances, and behavioral changes are common. Palpable neck pain is also common with forebrain tumors.

Dogs and cats with more caudally located (midbrain through medulla) tumors tend to have severe disturbances of consciousness, gait, and cranial nerve deficits (other than visual or CN II dysfunction). Animals with cerebellar tumors display intention tremors and hypermetria.

5. What is hemineglect or hemi-inattention?

In dogs and cats with structural forebrain (cerebrum-diencephalon) masses, the animal ignores environmental cues from the side opposite the tumor. Such a patient tends to eat from one side of the food bowl and responds to sounds and localizes noxious stimuli (skin pinch) on one side.

6. How is a brain tumor diagnosed?

Advanced imaging (**CT, MRI**) is needed to make the diagnosis. Imaging also provides information pertaining to the surgical accessibility of the tumor. Cerebrospinal fluid examination, without imaging, is unlikely to provide valuable information because tumor cells are rarely shed in the cerebrospinal fluids and abnormal cell counts or an elevated protein level are variable. At some institutions, a stereotactic CT-guided biopsy device is used to obtain a sample of the neoplasm at the time of imaging.

7. How are brain tumors treated?

Supportive therapy for secondary effects (edema, seizures) of tumor:
- Prednisone
- Anticonvulsants (phenobarbital, potassium bromide)

Definitive therapy to destroy tumor cells:
- Chemotherapy (nitrosoureas for gliomas)
- Surgery with or without irradiation
- Cobalt-60 irradiation for deep-seated lesions
- None (metastatic lesions, invasive nasal–frontal sinus carcinomas)

8. Discuss the surgical approach used for brain tumor removal.

For rostral tumors (olfactory bulb), a **transfrontal craniectomy** and limited lateral craniectomy are performed. Often the orbital ligament is transected near its attachment to the zygomatic process of the frontal bone on one or both sides of the craniectomy to remove the medial wall of the orbit. The eyeball, in its protective orbital sheath, can be gently retracted laterally once this ligament is transected. With this approach, the dorsal sagittal sinus may become lacerated. If the bleeding does not stop with application of a hemostatic agent (Surgicel), the sinus can be ligated at this rostral location. This approach necessitates invasion of the frontal sinus. It is imperative to create a barrier between the brain and frontal sinus during any craniotomy-craniectomy. One option is to pack the sinus area with cephalothin-impregnated polymethyl methacrylate after removing the sinus lining. The dural defect is closed with temporalis fascia or synthetic dura. Failure to separate the brain from the frontal sinus area can lead to encephalitis or pneumocephalus.

A **caudal approach** is used to remove cerebellar masses. One of the transverse sinuses can be sacrificed (bone wax into these areas to occlude the vessel) to remove a tumor at the cerebellomedullary angle. Attempts to ligate this sinus lead to further hemorrhage. With a caudal approach, the confluens sinuum (where the two transverse sinuses converge) can be lacerated if the surgeon carries the craniectomy too far dorsally.

9. How does one get the tumor out?
- Gentle traction (feline meningioma)
- Microsurgical brain tumor instrumentation
- Suction and bipolar cautery
- Cavitron ultrasonic aspirator

10. List difficult aspects of the postoperative convalescence.
- Extensive hospital and home aftercare
- Pharyngeal dysfunction and aspiration pneumonia (1–2 days postoperatively)
- Pulmonary atelectasis (recumbency) and subsequent pneumonia
- Acute idiopathic anemia (feline patients, 1–3 days postoperatively)
- Overmedication (confusing dementia with pain)

11. What is the prognosis for the brain tumor patient?
With supportive therapy alone, most dogs and cats with brain tumors either die or are euthanized because of worsening neurologic dysfunction within 3 months of initial presentation. In cats with meningiomas, the prognosis appears good after surgical removal, with median survival times of about 1 year. The prognosis for canine brain tumor patients treated with various definitive therapies is considerably more vague. Radiation therapy alone, for gliomas and meningiomas, may provide median survival times of approximately 10 and 12 months. Carmustine therapy may be effective in treating canine gliomas. Several canine meningioma patients (Texas A&M University) treated with a combination of surgery and radiation therapy have lived well beyond a year. Although not well documented at this time, most accessible canine primary brain tumors should be irradiated after surgery, to maximize the chance of long-term patient survival.

BIBLIOGRAPHY

1. Brearley MJ, Jeffery ND, Phillips SM: Hypofractionated radiation therapy of brain masses in dogs: A retrospective analysis of survival of 83 cases (1991–1996). J Vet Intern Med 13:408–412, 1999.
2. Dewey CW, Coates JR, Bahr A: How I treat primary brain tumors in dogs and cats. Comp Cont Educ Pract Vet (in press).
3. Lecouteur RA: Current concepts in the diagnosis and treatment of brain tumors in dogs and cats. J Small Anim Pract 40:411–416, 1999.

V. Oncologic Surgery

97. PRINCIPLES OF ONCOLOGIC SURGERY

Nicole Ehrhart, V.M.D., M.S., Dip. A.C.V.S.

1. Is the "chance to cut, a chance to cure"?
Yes, especially in surgical oncology. Surgery, as a single modality, is responsible for curing more cancer than any other single treatment.

2. Why does the first surgery have the best chance for cure in cancer patients?
Once the surgeon intervenes, normal tissue planes are disrupted, tissues that serve as natural tumor barriers are removed, and seroma or hematoma fluids accumulate in the tumor bed. If any tumor cells are remaining in the patient, they disseminate along previously inaccessible tissue planes via normal movement of muscles and spread of seroma fluid. Conservative excision performed on known malignancy may enhance tumor spread. The first surgery should be performed with curative intent.

3. Besides removing the primary tumor, what are other roles of surgery in the management of cancer?
- Prevent cancer (neutering).
- Treat oncologic emergencies (hemorrhage, intestinal or airway obstruction).
- Alleviate pain and infection associated with cancer (removal of necrotic or ulcerated masses).

4. What are the three questions every clinician should ask before proceeding with treatment of an animal with cancer?
1. **What is it?** This question should be answered using cytologic or histologic examination (or both) before excision.
2. **Where is it?** This is the staging process using a set of tests, including blood work, thoracic radiography, abdominal ultrasonography, and examination of peripheral lymph nodes.
3. **How bad is it?** This question is answered by palpation of the lesion, preoperative biopsy, tumor grading (when possible), and special imaging such as computed tomography, magnetic resonance imaging, ultrasound, or scintigraphy.

5. What is the oncologic optimal treatment plan?
A protocol developed before surgery to provide optimal control of systemic tumor spread and local growth with minimal patient morbidity, including hospitalization. This plan varies for each patient and involves multimodality therapies. The most frequent compromise of the optimal treatment plan is removal of a malignant mass without first obtaining a fine-needle aspirate or biopsy specimen to ascertain the tumor type.

6. Define the term surgical dose.
The amount of surgery (or margin of normal tissue removed around the tumor) required to provide long-term local tumor control.

7. What is the tumor pseudocapsule?
An area of compressed stromal cells and tumor cells resembling a fibrous capsule that surrounds a neoplasm. A reactive zone surrounds the tumor pseudocapsule and is a region of normal tissue response that includes fibrosis and increased blood supply.

8. What is wrong with "peeling out" a tumor that seems encapsulated?
Peeling out a tumor leaves the pseudocapsule, reactive zone, and neoplastic cells behind. **Encapsulated** tumors are not benign.

9. Describe the four types of excision techniques (surgical doses) used in oncologic surgery.
  1. **Intracapsular excision**—piecemeal removal of a mass; dissection plane is intracapsular. If performed on a malignant tumor, intracapsular excision results in microscopic or macroscopic disease being left in the patient. **Indications:** cyst or abscess removal, débridement.
  2. **Marginal excision**—en bloc removal of mass and pseudocapsule; dissection is through the reactive zone surrounding the tumor (**peeling out**). If performed on a malignant tumor, marginal excision results in local recurrence if microscopic foci have separated from the primary tumor. **Indications:** benign lipoma, sebaceous adenoma.
  3. **Wide excision**—en bloc removal of mass, pseudocapsule, reactive zone, and 2-cm margin of normal tissue; dissection plane is in normal tissue. If performed on a malignant tumor, wide excision usually results in complete excision; however, skip metastases (bypass of draining lymph node) or metastases to draining lymph nodes are possible. **Indications:** well-localized or low-grade malignant tumors.
  4. **Radical excision**—regional removal of entire compartment containing the tumor (amputation, thoracic wall resection). Dissection plane is within normal tissue distant from the primary tumor and lymph nodes. If performed on a malignant tumor, radical excision usually results in complete excision. **Indications:** poorly localized or high-grade tumors.

10. When are preoperative fine-needle aspiration and cytologic interpretation indicated?
Nearly always. The only contraindication is abscessation within a body cavity.

11. When is preoperative biopsy indicated?
  • If the type (radiation versus surgery) or extent (marginal versus radical excision) of treatment would be altered by knowing the tumor type.
  • If the owner's willingness to treat would be altered by knowing the tumor type.
  • If the tumor is in a difficult place for reconstruction, and the method of reconstruction would be altered based on knowledge of the surgical dose needed to achieve long-term tumor control.
  • When cytologic interpretation is inconsistent with clinical findings or is nondiagnostic.
  • Any time that more knowledge about the type of tumor would aid in refining the optimal treatment plan.

12. Are there any contraindications to pretreatment biopsy?
  • When the biopsy procedure would be as difficult or dangerous as the definitive removal of the tumor (brain tumor)
  • When the surgical procedure would be the same regardless of the disease process present (testicular mass)

13. Do all masses need to be submitted for histologic evaluation once removed, even if one has a cytologic or histologic diagnosis before excision?
Yes, for several reasons:
  1. Although cytology provides excellent cellular detail, it does not allow interpretation of tissue architecture or invasiveness.
  2. For some tumor types, cytology cannot discern between the malignant and benign forms of a neoplastic process.
  3. Discernment between inflammation and neoplasia on cytologic samples may be difficult.

4. Even when tissue is acquired for analysis (as in the case of preoperative biopsy), tumors are not homogeneous.

5. Pathologists often change the diagnosis when they look at the entire specimen.

6. Submission of the excised specimen allows the pathologist to provide information about the completeness of surgical excision.

14. What basic surgical principles are common to all oncologic surgeries?
- Tumors should be removed in one piece with a layer of surrounding normal tissue.
- Manipulation of the tumor should be minimized to prevent rupture of the mass or embolic showers.
- Avoid excessive undermining of tissue planes.
- Minimize contamination of normal tissues by protective drapes, laparotomy sponges, and copious lavage.
- Ligate veins early in the procedure to prevent embolization of tumor cells into the bloodstream.
- Minimize hematoma or seroma formation by using meticulous hemostasis and closure of dead space.
- Once surgical excision of a tumor is performed, all instruments, gloves, and drapes are considered contaminated. Change gloves, and instruments between excisions of different masses or when performing new procedures.
- If you remove it, submit it.

15. Is placement of surgical drains to obliterate dead space a good idea in the oncology patient?
For the most part, surgical drains are contraindicated because they can seed tumor cells throughout the entire draining tract. If the margins are dirty, the field for reexcision or radiation therapy needs to incorporate the drain site, increasing the amount of normal tissue to be removed or irradiated to achieve local tumor control. If a drain is necessary, it should be an active rather than a passive drain, and the exit site should be close to the incision so that the drain tract can be excised easily or irradiated en bloc with the surgical wound.

16. What is a surgical margin?
A tissue plane on the outside boundary of a resected specimen, **the tissue beyond which is left in the patient.**

17. What if the surgical margin is dirty?
When the pathologist describes a **dirty** or incomplete excision, the surgeon should intercede immediately with reexcision, including 2–3 cm margins around the entire surgical scar, or perform radiation therapy of the site.

18. Is it necessary to remove the entire surgical scar with 2–3 cm margins if the margin was dirty only in one site?
Yes. Once the surgical instruments have passed through the tumor in any area, any tissue that the instruments touch is contaminated. Reexcision (or radiation) of the entire wound bed with 2–3 cm margins is required to ensure that all tumor cells have been removed.

19. List some methods to mark margins before submission that aid the pathologist in evaluating the completeness of excision.
- **Suture tags**—differing numbers or colors of sutures can be used to denote different sites.
- **Inks**—India ink or color inking systems can be used by the surgeon to **paint** the surgical margins.
- **Specimen sketch on the submission form**—indicates areas of concern.
- **Multiple tumor bed samples submission**—if samples contain tumor, the margin is dirty.

BIBLIOGRAPHY

1. Ehrhart N: Principles of tumor biopsy. Clin Tech Small Anim Pract 13:10–15, 1998.
2. Ehrhart N: Tumor biopsy principles and techniques. In Bojrab MJ (ed): Current Techniques in Small Animal Surgery. Baltimore, Williams & Wilkins, 1998, pp 13–71.
3. Withrow SJ: The science of surgical oncology: Past progress and future direction. Vet Clin North Am 25:225–227, 1995.

98. BONE TUMORS

Nicole Ehrhart, V.M.D., M.S., Dip. A.C.V.S.

1. List the types of tumors that arise in bone.

Osteosarcoma (most common)

Chondrosarcoma

Hemangiosarcoma

Fibrosarcoma

Multiple myeloma

Lymphoma

Metastatic bone neoplasia

Giant cell tumor of bone

Multilobular osteochondrosarcoma

Synovial cell sarcoma

2. If a primary bone tumor is suspected based on diagnostic imaging and clinical signs, what are the chances that it is osteosarcoma?

- In **dogs,** 85%
- In **cats,** 70%–80%

3. What are the typical locations for osteosarcoma in the dog?

"Away from the elbow and toward the knee."

- Distal radius
- Proximal humerus
- Distal femur
- Proximal tibia

4. What is the typical signalment of a dog with osteosarcoma?

Large to giant breed in middle or old age.

5. What is the incidence ratio of appendicular to axial skeletal occurrence of osteosarcoma?

4:1.

6. Describe the common radiographic changes of osteosarcoma.

Appendicular osteosarcoma is generally monostotic (single bone), is metaphyseal, and rarely crosses the joint. The overall radiographic appearance of the lesion can be highly variable, ranging from lytic to osteoproductive. Cortical lysis is a common feature, and soft tissue extension with soft tissue swelling may be present. Tumor bone (osteoid) forms in a palisading pattern radiating from the axis of the cortex in a **sunburst** pattern. More subtle radiographic changes include loss of the fine trabecular pattern in the metaphysis and punctate areas of lysis.

7. What is Codman's triangle?

A radiographic characteristic caused by periosteal elevation and rapid deposition of dense new bone (tumor bone) under the periosteum. This process produces a wedge or triangular structure along the periosteal surface at the periphery of the lesion. It is not pathognomonic for osteosarcoma, but it suggests an aggressive osteoblastic process.

8. How is metastatic bone neoplasia distinguished from osteosarcoma?

Metastatic bone neoplasia is more commonly located near the medullary artery, whereas **primary osteosarcoma** is located in a metaphyseal region. Bone tumors that occur in appendicular sites that are atypical of osteosarcoma (e.g., near the elbow) should be viewed as suspicious. A history of a previous tumor raises the index of suspicion for metastatic bone neoplasia. Definitive differentiation can be made only via **biopsy.**

9. Name some nonneoplastic diseases that have radiographic features that mimic primary bone neoplasia.

- Osteomyelitis (bacterial, fungal)
- Severe degenerative joint disease
- Bone cyst
- Bone infarct

10. In what clinical stage of disease do dogs with appendicular osteosarcoma typically present?

Stage IIB: The tumor is confined to the limb but has extramedullary extension.

11. What percentage of dogs have clinically evident metastasis at the time of osteosarcoma diagnosis?

<10%

12. What percentage of dogs have microscopic metastatic disease at the time of diagnosis?

90%. If amputation is performed, greater than 90% of dogs die of metastatic disease within the first year.

13. What organs are at risk for metastasis from osteosarcoma?

In order of frequency:
- Lungs
- Bone
- Liver
- Lymph node
- Other soft tissues and brain

14. What is the preferred method of bone biopsy?

- **Trephine biopsy** provides a large specimen for analysis, but it requires an open approach to the bone and leaves a large defect that may increase the risk of pathologic fracture.
- A **Jamshidi bone marrow** biopsy needle does not require an open approach, creates a small defect, and provides a small specimen. It is the preferred method for limb salvage candidates.
- **Open biopsy** and curettage is preferred in lytic lesions that cannot be examined by the aforementioned techniques.

15. Does a biopsy report describing reactive bone rule out osteosarcoma?

No. If signalment, history, physical examination, and radiographic signs are consistent with osteosarcoma, the periphery of the lesion and not representative tissue may have been obtained for biopsy. Osteosarcoma and other primary bone tumors tend to arise in the medullary canal, causing expansion and bone reaction at the periphery of the tumor. It would be best to obtain another biopsy specimen from the center of the lesion.

16. Discuss the treatment options for osteosarcoma in dogs.

- **Curative-intent therapy** involves surgical removal of the tumor followed by adjuvant chemotherapy to treat the micrometastatic disease present in 90% of patients. Surgical options for appendicular osteosarcoma involve either limb salvage or amputation. Chemotherapy protocols use platinum-containing agents (carboplatin or cisplatin), doxorubicin, or combinations.

- **Palliative therapy** is controlling pain and preventing pathologic fracture. No aggressive attempt is made to prolong survival; disease progression is expected. Palliative therapy usually involves radiation therapy (with or without chemotherapy) and nonsteroidal anti-inflammatory drugs, opioids, or bisphosphonates.

17. What is limb salvage surgery?

En bloc resection of bone, replacement with a fresh-frozen cortical allograft, stabilization, and arthrodesis with a bone plate.

18. What anatomic site is most amenable to limb salvage surgery in the dog?

Distal radius and ulna. Dogs with tumors located in the ulna, proximal humerus, scapula, or portions of the pelvis may also be candidates for limb salvage.

19. What constitutes candidacy for a limb salvage procedure?

- Tumor confined to a single site amenable to limb salvage.
- Tumor involves less than 50% of the bone length and no evidence of metastatic disease.
- Otherwise healthy dog expected to live at least 1 year.
- Absence of a pathologic fracture.

20. Do large dogs function well after limb amputation?

Yes; regardless of forelimb or hind limb surgery or arthritis in other joints.

21. List the contraindications for amputation in dogs with osteosarcoma.

- Previous amputation of another limb
- Progressive or severe neurologic disorders
- Metastasis to bone

22. How is amputation performed?

Complete (including scapula) forelimb or hind limb (coxofemoral disarticulation) resection.

23. What is the prognosis for osteosarcoma if amputation is performed as the sole treatment?

The average dog survives osteosarcoma 3–4 months.

24. What is the prognosis for osteosarcoma if amputation is followed by adjuvant chemotherapy?

Median survival time, 10–14 months.

25. Are there any survival differences between dogs that receive limb salvage surgery versus those that receive amputation?

No. Limb salvage followed by chemotherapy has a similar prognosis to amputation followed by chemotherapy.

26. List the most common complications associated with limb salvage surgery.

- **Cortical allograft infection** (most common, occurs in 44%)
- Local recurrence of tumor (does not negatively affect survival if neoplastic tissue is removed in a **respare** procedure)
- Implant loosening
- Fracture of the allograft

27. Which procedure, amputation or limb salvage, has a higher incidence of complications?

Limb salvage (also more expensive).

28. What is the prognosis for canine appendicular osteosarcoma compared with axial osteosarcoma?

Osteosarcoma of the axial skeleton has a poorer prognosis (median survival, 5 months) than appendicular skeleton when curative intent treatment is performed. Lesions in the axial skeleton are more difficult to resect completely. The exception is osteosarcoma of the mandible, which has been associated with longer survival than other axial sites.

29. What is the biologic behavior and prognosis of canine versus feline osteosarcoma?

Prognosis for feline osteosarcoma is better because the tumor is less aggressive, and the rate of metastasis is lower. Complete excision can result in cure; remissions greater than 2 years are reported in the literature.

30. Should cats with osteosarcoma routinely receive cisplatin chemotherapy?

No. **"Cisplat splats cats!"** It causes rapid, fatal pulmonary edema. In contrast, carboplatin can be administered safely.

BIBLIOGRAPHY

1. Bergman PJ, MacEwan EG, Kurzman ID: Amputation and carboplatin for treatment of dogs with osteosarcoma: 48 cases (1991–1993). J Vet Intern Med 10:76–81, 1996.
2. Bitetto WV, Patnaik AK, Schrader SC: Osteosarcoma in cats: 22 cases (1974–1984). J Am Vet Med Assoc 190:91–93, 1987.
3. Cooley DM, Waters DJ: Skeletal neoplasms of small dogs: A retrospective study and literature review. J Am Anim Hosp Assoc 33:11–23, 1997.
4. O'Brien MG, Withrow SJ, Straw RC: Recent advances in the treatment of canine appendicular osteosarcoma. Comp Cont Educ Pract Vet 15:939–945, 1993.
5. Straw RC: Tumors of the skeletal system. In Withrow SJ, MacEwan EC (eds): Small Animal Clinical Oncology. Philadelphia, W.B. Saunders, 1996, pp 287–315.

99. SOFT TISSUE SARCOMAS

Nicole Ehrhart, V.M.D., M.S., Dip. A.C.V.S.

1. What are soft tissue sarcomas?

Common, malignant tumors arising from the nonbone connective (mesenchymal) tissues, including a variety of tumor types that differ morphologically but share similar biologic behavior.

2. What tumor types are included in the soft tissue sarcoma category?

SOFT TISSUE SARCOMA	CELL OF ORIGIN
Fibrosarcoma	Fibrocytes
Hemangiopericytoma	Pericytes of blood vessels
Liposarcoma	Lipocytes
Rhabdomyosarcoma	Skeletal muscle cells
Malignant fibrous histiocytoma	Fibrous tissue and histiocyte
Myxosarcoma	Myxomatous tissue
Malignant nerve sheath tumors	Nerve sheath
Neurofibrosarcoma	
Schwannoma	
Undifferentiated sarcoma	Primitive mesenchymal cell
Mesenchymoma	
Spindle cell tumor	

3. List the biologic features common to soft tissue sarcoma tumors.
- Can arise from any anatomic site
- Are pseudoencapsulated tumors with poorly defined histologic margins
- Can infiltrate through fascial planes
- Metastasis (through hematogenous routes) occurs late in the course of disease
- Common local recurrence after conservative excision
- Poor response to chemotherapy and radiation therapy when gross tumor is present

4. Can all tumors with a sarcoma suffix be considered soft tissue sarcomas if they arise in soft tissue?

No. Examples include osteosarcoma, synovial cell sarcoma, lymphangiosarcoma, hemangiosarcoma, and chondrosarcoma. These tumors (with the exception of chondrosarcoma) have a higher metastatic rate than the classic soft tissue sarcomas.

5. What organs are at risk for metastasis with soft tissue sarcomas?

Any organ in the body; the **lungs** are most commonly affected.

6. List diagnostic tests that should be included in staging for soft tissue sarcomas.
- Fine-needle aspiration cytology to support diagnosis (rule out mast cell tumor)
- Palpation of the tumor to determine the degree of extension
- Palpation of the draining lymph nodes
- Thoracic radiography (three views)
- Complete blood count and chemistry panel
- Abdominal ultrasonography
- Radiography of the primary tumor site if the tumor is fixed to bone
- A pretreatment biopsy when the tumor is difficult to resect with large margins

7. When is advanced imaging, such as computed tomography and magnetic resonance imaging, helpful?

To determine the extent of underlying tissue involvement before resection. Reconstructive options can be planned using the CT or MR image as a guide, and the surgeon can gain an idea for successful (wide) excision with clean margins by evaluating nearby structures.

8. What is the primary treatment for soft tissue sarcomas?

Aggressive wide excision should always be performed as the first surgery. Conservative excision leaves microscopic disease in the patient and results in local recurrence. The surgeon should remove the tumor en bloc with a 2–3 cm cuff of normal tissue in all planes (including deep) surrounding the tumor. The tumor should be submitted for histologic evaluation to assess completeness of margins and histologic grade of the tumor.

9. Discuss the factors associated with prognosis.

Size, location, histologic grade, previous treatment attempts, and completeness of surgical margins influence prognosis. **Size** has a negative effect on local tumor control when surgery is used alone. When adjuvant radiation therapy is used before or after surgery, size does not influence prognosis. Tumors **located** in areas where wide margins are difficult to obtain are not easily resected with histologically clean borders. **Previous conservative excision** and subsequent regrowth have a negative influence on prognosis because normal anatomic barriers are disrupted, exposing previously uninvolved tissue planes to remaining tumor cells; the field size of remaining microscopic disease to be removed or irradiated is increased; and the most aggressive subpopulation of cells at the tumor edge is left behind.

10. What is histologic grade?

Histologic criteria based on necrosis, mitotic index, differentiation, and invasion. Tumor grade is predictive of biologic behavior and characterized as **low (I), medium (II),** or **high (III).**

11. How does histologic grade influence prognosis in soft tissue sarcomas?

High-grade tumors are five times more likely to metastasize than low-grade tumors. A low histologic grade (grade I) indicates a better prognosis.

12. When should adjuvant chemotherapy be used?

In animals that have high-grade tumors or when the tumor has already metastasized. Chemotherapy agents with efficacy against soft tissue sarcomas include doxorubicin, carboplatin, mitoxantrone, and cisplatin. Chemotherapy as the sole form of therapy is rarely effective for soft tissue sarcomas. Chemotherapy for adjuvant treatment, when microscopic disease is present after surgery, has not been thoroughly evaluated.

13. When should adjuvant radiation therapy be used?

When incomplete excision has been performed and the remaining disease is microscopic. Radiation therapy should be initiated as soon as inadequate margins are confirmed. As long as there is no tension on the surgical closure and the skin is healthy, radiation can be safely started before suture removal. The use of megavoltage radiation therapy after incomplete excision results in a favorable 70%–80% control rate at 1 year. Radiation therapy can also be used before surgery to sterilize the tumor margin, allowing less aggressive excision. Radiation therapy used preoperatively may not shrink the tumor because of the large stromal content in the mass.

14. What are the treatment options when the tumor has been excised and margins are dirty?

Reexcision or **radiation therapy.** The entire surgical wound is considered contaminated with tumor cells, and reexcision of the wound must be performed with wide margins (2–3 cm) around the **entire** surgical bed; likewise, the radiation field must incorporate the entire surgical wound bed.

15. What is the prognosis associated with completely excised soft tissue sarcomas?

- Local recurrence rates are 13%–32% for all soft tissue sarcomas treated with wide margin excision.
- Strict attention to oncologic surgical principles results in an 80% control rate with a high potential for cure.
- A higher rate of metastasis is associated with poorly differentiated (grade III) tumors, and the prognosis is poorer.

CONTROVERSY

16. Are feline injection-site sarcomas included in the soft tissue sarcoma category?

No. Cats can develop the typical soft tissue sarcomas (usually fibrosarcomas). These tumors behave in a similar manner to canine soft tissue sarcomas and usually occur in older cats on the extremities. The sarcomas that arise in cats at vaccination or injection sites are high grade, and local regional recurrence is extremely high despite aggressive surgical attempts at removal. The median age for cats with injection-site sarcomas is significantly younger than the typical sarcoma. Injection site sarcomas can be of any histologic type in the mesenchymal category. Fibrosarcoma and fibrous histiocytomas are commonly diagnosed, but osteosarcoma, rhabdomyosarcoma, and chondrosarcoma have all been reported. Conservative surgery may enhance tumor regrowth. It is likely that multimodality therapy is needed to improve local tumor control. Most veterinary cancer treatment centers use a combination of radiation therapy and aggressive surgery to prevent local tumor recurrence, but further study is needed to develop the optimal treatment regimen for these tumors. Reported rates of metastasis are 11%–27%.

BIBLIOGRAPHY

1. Dernell WS, Withrow SJ, Kuntz CA: Principles of treatment for soft tissue sarcomas. Clin Tech Small Anim Pract 13:59–63, 1998.

2. Kuntz C, Dernell WS, Powers BE: Prognostic factors for treatment of soft tissue sarcomas in dogs: 75 cases (1986–1996). J Am Vet Med Assoc 211:1147–1150, 1997.
3. Ogilvie GK, Moore AS: Tumors of the skin and surrounding structures. In Ogilvie GK, Moore AS (eds): Managing the Cancer Patient, A Practice Manual. Trenton, NJ, Veterinary Learning Systems, 1995, pp 473–518.
4. Powers BE, Hoopes PJ, Ehrhart EJ: Tumor diagnosis, grading and staging. Semin Vet Med Surg 10:158–163, 1995.
5. Withrow SJ, MacEwen EC: Soft tissue sarcomas. In Withrow SJ, MacEwen EC (eds): Small Animal Clinical Oncology. Philadelphia, W.B. Saunders, 1996, pp 211–226.

100. ORAL TUMORS

Bernard Seguin, D.V.M., M.S., Dip. A.C.V.S.

1. List the four commonest cancers of the mouth in dogs.
1. Malignant melanoma
2. Squamous cell carcinoma
3. Fibrosarcoma
4. Osteosarcoma

2. List the two commonest oral cancers in cats.
1. Squamous cell carcinoma
2. Fibrosarcoma

3. What other tumor arises from the periodontal ligament and is commonly found in dogs but rarely in cats?
Epulides. There are three different types: (1) acanthomatous, (2) ossifying, and (3) fibromatous.

4. Which of the four previously mentioned tumors in the dog has the highest metastatic rate?
Malignant melanoma.

5. Which of the four previously mentioned tumors in the dog has the highest local recurrence rate?
Fibrosarcoma.

6. Are there any concerns if a biopsy specimen from a mass in the mouth of a dog comes back fibroma?
Yes. You may be dealing with a **histologically low-grade yet biologically high-grade** fibrosarcoma. If the tumor is rapidly growing, recurrent, or invading bone, aggressive therapy is indicated despite the histologic diagnosis.

7. What is the treatment for the four commonest oral neoplasms of the dog when they are located on the gingiva?
Small lesions (<2 cm in diameter) that are fixed or minimally invasive into bone can be treated with **cryosurgery.** Larger or more extensive lesions require **mandibulectomy** or **maxillectomy.** A minimum 2-cm margin is advised to provide the best local control. **Radiation therapy** can be used as an adjuvant after incomplete tumor removal. When used as the sole mode of treatment, megavoltage irradiation has provided good median progression-free intervals for oral cancers (8 months for malignant melanoma, 26 months for fibrosarcoma, and 36 months for squamous cell carcinoma). Because of the high metastatic rate of malignant melanomas, **adjuvant chemotherapy** is indicated. Currently, platinum drugs appear to be the best option.

8. What is the most serious complication of a maxillectomy?
Wound dehiscence because it can lead to an oronasal fistula. It occurs in 7%–33% of cases.

9. List two factors that are known to promote wound dehiscence after maxillectomy?
1. Excessive tension on the suture line (caudad maxillectomies)
2. Use of electrocoagulation during the surgery

10. What are the positive prognostic factors specific for malignant melanoma in the dog?
- Lesions smaller than 2 cm
- Lesions treated with clean margins with the first attempt
- No evidence of metastasis

11. When performing a maxillectomy or mandibulectomy, does the prognosis depend on tumor site?
Yes. Tumors in a rostral location have a better prognosis.

12. Do mandibular and appendicular osteosarcomas have a similar prognosis?
No.
- Dogs treated with surgery alone for appendicular osteosarcoma have a 10% 1-year survival.
- Dogs with mandibular osteosarcoma treated with surgery alone have a 71% 1-year survival.

13. What is the age of dogs with papillary squamous cell carcinoma?
Young dogs, 2 months to 2 years old.

14. What is the treatment for papillary squamous cell carcinoma?
Surgical debulking and curettage followed by radiation. If the lesion is amenable to complete resection, maxillectomy or mandibulectomy should be curative. No metastasis has been reported, and long-term control is achieved.

15. List treatments for acanthomatous epulides.
- Mandibulectomy
- Maxillectomy
- Radiation therapy

16. What is the prognosis after treatment for acanthomatous epulides?
Recurrence rate after surgery is less than 5%. Control rate greater than 90% is achieved with irradiation. Malignant cancer developing in the irradiated site can occur in 20% of the cases, especially when orthovoltage is used. It can take several years for these malignancies to develop.

17. What is the treatment for fibromatous or ossifying epulides?
Conservative blade excision. The base can be treated with electrocautery or cryosurgery if it invades bone or if the lesion has recurred.

18. What is the commonest primary neoplasm of the tonsils in dogs?
Squamous cell carcinoma.

19. What is the treatment for tonsillar squamous cell carcinoma?
- Tonsillectomy is rarely curative because greater than 90% of cases develop metastases after tonsillectomy. Only 10% of animals survive for more than 1 year. Tonsillectomy remains a palliative treatment in most cases and should be performed bilaterally because of the high percentage of bilateral disease.

- Radiation can control local disease in greater than 75% of cases, but systemic disease remains the problem.
- Chemotherapy provides limited success.

20. What are the commonest lingual tumors in dogs?
Squamous cell carcinoma, followed by granular cell myoblastoma, melanoma, mast cell, and fibrosarcoma.

21. Is squamous cell carcinoma of the tongue more likely to metastasize than gingival squamous cell carcinoma?
Yes.

22. What percentage of the tongue can be removed for rostrally located tumors?
40%–60%.

23. What is the treatment and prognosis for lingual granular myoblastoma?
The treatment is **surgical resection,** and the prognosis is good. The surgery requires only conservative, close margins and is often curative (in >80% of cases). Local recurrence can be treated by surgical resection again.

24. What is the treatment for viral papillomatosis?
None in the majority of patients. Most patients undergo spontaneous regression of the disease within 4–8 weeks.

25. What is the treatment for oral squamous cell carcinoma in cats?
There is no effective treatment at this time. Surgical excision followed by radiation therapy may offer the best option. Local control of this disease remains challenging because the tumor is locally invasive. One-year survival rarely exceeds 10% in the cat.

BIBLIOGRAPHY

1. Berg J: Principles of oncologic orofacial surgery. Clin Tech Small Anim Pract 13:38–41, 1998.
2. Carpenter LG, Withrow SJ, Powers BE, et al: Squamous cell carcinoma of the tongue in 10 dogs. J Am Anim Hosp Assoc 29:17–24, 1993.
3. Morrison WB: Cancers of the head and neck. In Morrison WB (ed): Cancer in Dogs and Cats. Baltimore, Williams & Wilkins, 1998, pp 511–519.
4. Salisbury SK: Aggressive cancer surgery and aftercare. In Morrison WB (ed): Cancer in Dogs and Cats. Baltimore, Williams & Wilkins, 1998, pp 265–321.
5. Withrow SJ: Tumors of the gastrointestinal system: A. Cancer of the oral cavity. In Withrow SJ, MacEwen EG (eds): Small Animal Clinical Oncology, 2nd ed. Philadelphia, WB Saunders, 1996, pp 227–240.

101. CUTANEOUS AND SUBCUTANEOUS TUMORS

Bernard Seguin, D.V.M., M.S., Dip. A.C.V.S.

1. List the three classes of cutaneous and subcutaneous tumors.
   1. Epithelial
   2. Mesenchymal
   3. Round cell

2. What is the basis for this classification?

The tissue of origin as well as certain cytologic features.

3. Should a fine-needle aspirate be performed on cutaneous and subcutaneous masses?

Always. Although a fine-needle aspirate may not be able to identify an epithelial or mesenchymal tumor, it can usually identify round cell tumors.

4. What are the round cell tumors?

- Lymphoma
- Plasma cell tumor
- Histiocytoma
- Mast cell tumor
- Transmissible venereal tumor
- Melanoma

5. What if the fine-needle aspirate is nondiagnostic?

Biopsy is the next procedure. The biopsy can be excisional or incisional. The decision to perform one over the other depends on whether the results of the biopsy would change the therapeutic plan.

6. What else should be performed in the diagnostic evaluation before definitive treatment?

If the tumor is known or suspected to be malignant, the patient needs to be evaluated for metastases (**radiography or ultrasound**) and overall health (**hematology and chemistry profiles**).

7. List the tumors of epithelial origin.

- Basal cell tumor
- Sweat gland tumors
- Trichoepithelioma
- Pilomatricoma
- Squamous cell carcinoma
- Papillomas
- Sebaceous gland tumor
- Perianal gland tumor
- Anal sac adenocarcinoma

8. What are the tumors of mesenchymal origin?

- Soft tissue sarcomas
- Lipomas
- Hemangiomas/hemangiosarcomas

9. As a general rule, what is the treatment of choice for cutaneous and subcutaneous tumors?

Surgical excision.

10. Define actinic keratosis.

A condition induced by solar radiation that occurs frequently in poorly haired, pale-skin areas, such as the nose and the pinnas. It is **not** a neoplastic disease **but** can progress to become squamous cell carcinoma. It is not possible to tell the two conditions apart grossly; a biopsy is required. Because the potential exists for actinic keratosis lesions to progress into squamous cell carcinoma, surgical excision or cryosurgery is recommended.

11. What is squamous cell carcinoma *in situ?*

A superficial cluster of neoplastic keratinocytes confined to the epidermis, hair follicles, or both. It may invade the basement membrane and dermis to become **invasive squamous cell carcinoma** with the potential for local invasion and distant metastasis.

12. What are hepatoid tumors?

Tumors arising from the perianal glands, which are modified sebaceous glands. Most tumors are located in the perineum, but 10% are at other locations, such as the base of the tail or abdomen. Most are adenomas, but adenocarcinomas are possible.

13. Discuss the treatment for perianal adenomas.

Because most dogs affected by these tumors are intact males, **castration** is the treatment of choice. Estrogen therapy is also effective, but the risk of myelosuppression prohibits its use. Ninety-five percent of adenomas regress after castration.

If the tumor is large or in female dogs, **surgical excision** is necessary. Adenocarcinomas of perianal glands do not regress after castration and need to be surgically excised.

The role of radiation therapy and chemotherapy when margins are dirty after surgical excision or when metastases are present remains questionable.

14. Describe anal sac tumors.

Anal sac adenocarcinoma is the commonest tumor of anal sac, the other one being **adenoma.** Adenocarcinomas arise from apocrine glands in the anal sac. Some studies have reported female dogs as being more prevalent, and others have failed to show a gender predilection.

15. What is the commonest paraneoplastic syndrome associated with anal sac adenocarcinoma?

Hypercalcemia. The pathogenesis involves the tumor producing parathyroid hormone–related protein.

16. Describe the biologic behavior of cutaneous melanomas in dogs.

Cutaneous melanomas can be benign or malignant (over 85% are benign). This distinction may be hard to make because some crossover occurs in biologic behavior. Mitotic index seems to be a good predictor of biologic behavior. Malignant melanomas can metastasize in greater than 50% of patients, preferentially to the regional lymph nodes and lungs.

17. What are the tumors of the digits in dogs?
- The commonest is **squamous cell carcinoma.** It is locally invasive and can metastasize.
- The second commonest is malignant melanoma. It is less likely to have local bony lysis on radiographs than squamous cell carcinoma, but more likely to metastasize.
- The third commonest is mast cell tumor.

18. What is the treatment for tumors of the digits?

Amputation is the treatment of choice for all three. Adjuvant chemotherapy is indicated for malignant melanoma, but its benefit is questionable. Adjuvant chemotherapy for mast cell tumor is indicated depending on the grade and stage of the disease.

19. Describe the biologic behavior of histiocytomas.

Histiocytomas generally occur in young dogs 1 to 2 years of age. It is a benign tumor arising from the monocyte-macrophage cell line. Most spontaneously regress within weeks to 4 months.

20. How are histiocytomas treated?

If histiocytomas are not causing any problems, **no treatment** is the best approach at first. If they become ulcerated or self-trauma occurs, they are surgically removed. Topical and systemic corticosteroids have been reported to cause regression of multiple lesions.

CONTROVERSY

21. How are mast cell tumors staged, and what is the significance of the staging scheme?

Mast cell tumors preferentially metastasize to the regional lymph nodes, the spleen, the liver, and the bone marrow. They rarely metastasize to the lungs. Staging involves looking for disease in these areas by aspirating regional lymph nodes, performing ultrasound of the abdomen, aspirating the spleen and liver, and performing a bone marrow aspirate. A buffy coat examination can also be performed, but most agree that the bone marrow aspirate is more sensitive. Controversy arises when mast cells are seen in the spleen or liver or when mastocytemia is present. Normal dogs can have mast cells in the spleen or liver, and a report has shown that dogs with mastocytemia are more likely to have a disease other than mast cell tumor. In an animal that presents with a mast cell tumor on the skin, does finding mastocytemia or mast cells in the spleen or liver mean that the tumor has metastasized?

22. What are the four deadliest words in the American language referring to a lump on a patient?
    "Let's just watch it" (*S. J. Withrow*)

BIBLIOGRAPHY

 1. Thomas RC, Fox LE: Tumors of the skin and subcutis aggressive cancer surgery and aftercare. In Morrison WB (ed): Cancer in Dogs and Cats. Baltimore, Williams & Wilkins, 1998, pp 489–510.
 2. Vail DM, Withrow SJ: Tumors of the skin and subcutaneous tissues. In Withrow SJ, MacEwen EG (eds): Small Animal Clinical Oncology, 2nd ed. Philadelphia, W.B. Saunders, 1996, pp 167–191.

VI. Dental Surgery

102. EXODONTIA

Sandra Manfra Marretta, D.V.M., Dip. A.C.V.S., Dip. A.V.D.C.

1. What is exodontia?
Portion of dentistry that deals with the extraction of teeth.

2. What is the commonest indication for exodontia in dogs and cats?
- In **dogs**—advanced periodontal disease.
- In **cats**—odontoclastic resorptive lesions.

3. List other indications for exodontia in dogs and cats.
- Overly retained deciduous teeth
- Supernumerary teeth
- Dental crowding
- Fractured teeth with pulpal exposure (not candidates for endodontic therapy)
- Teeth with fractured roots
- Teeth with severe dental caries
- Maloccluded teeth causing tissue trauma in which owners decline alternative therapy

4. Name three extraction techniques commonly used in dogs and cats.
1. Simply (small, single-rooted teeth affected by periodontal disease).
2. Multirooted (tooth sectioned into single-rooted segments).
3. Complicated or surgical extraction (canine, mandibular first molar, maxillary fourth premolar).

5. List important steps of a surgical extraction.
1. Creation of a mucoperiosteal flap
2. Location of the furcation and sectioning of a multirooted tooth
3. Removal of buccal alveolar bone as needed
4. Elevation and extraction of segments
5. Performance of an alveoloplasty
6. Curettage and flushing of the alveolus and flap
7. Repositioning and closure of the mucoperiosteal flap

6. How can tension on a mucoperiosteal flap be relieved before closure?
Tension on a mucoperiosteal flap when closing a surgical extraction site or an oronasal fistula repair can be released by incising the innermost layer of the flap, the inelastic periosteum, at the apical portion of the flap.

7. When performing a mucoperiosteal flap for the surgical extraction of the maxillary fourth premolar, what structures should be carefully avoided?
- When making the mesial (rostral) portion of the incision, the **infraorbital artery, vein,** and **nerve** should be avoided as they exit the infraorbital canal immediately rostral to the periapical bone of the mesiobuccal root of the maxillary fourth premolar.
- When making the distal (caudad) part of the incision, the **parotid** and **zygomatic salivary duct papillae** should be visualized and avoided.

8. What factors may lead to failures in extraction?
- Ankylosis
- Supernumerary roots
- Abnormal direction of the roots
- Hypercementosis with bulbous swelling on the apical portion of the root

In addition, if the operator is elevating against the bone or the tooth itself, no progress can be made.

9. How can extraction failures be avoided?
- Dental radiography
- Conversion to a surgical extraction

10. How should a case be treated when ankylosis is documented radiographically (absence of periodontal ligament space)?
- Call the client and raise your estimate.
- Find a comfortable chair to complete the extraction using a surgical extraction technique, and cancel the next two to eight appointments, depending on how many teeth that are ankylosed require extraction.
- Have your associate complete the extraction and go out for a long lunch.

11. Discuss two approaches for surgical extraction of mandibular canine teeth.

The **labial** approach uses a mucoperiosteal flap located on the labial aspect of the tooth, whereas a **lingual** approach uses a lingually located flap. Equal amounts of alveolar bone are present buccally and labially so that there is no advantage of one technique over the other with regard to bone removal. The mental artery, vein, and nerve exit through the mental foramen located near the labial aspect of the apex of this tooth. A lingual approach avoids potential damage to these structures.

12. What factors aid in the localization of broken-off root tips during exodontia?
- Adequate lighting
- Magnification
- Dental radiographs

13. What distinguishing characteristics can be used to differentiate fractured root tips from surrounding alveolar bone?
- **Color:** The root tip is white and the bone is off-white.
- **Blood:** The hard tissue of the tooth does not bleed, whereas the bone does.
- **Tissue density:** The root tip is hard and cannot be penetrated with the tip of a dental explorer; the bone is softer and can be penetrated with an explorer tip.

14. Once a fractured root tip is localized, how can it be removed?

Once the root is visualized and the periodontal space is located around the root, the dental elevator is inserted into this space and advanced apically around the retained fractured root tip. If necessary, the root can be retrieved using a surgical extraction technique.

15. What ophthalmic complications may be associated with dental extractions?
- Penetration of the retrobulbar space with the potential for bacterial inoculation
- Laceration of periorbital vessels
- Perforation of the globe, including laceration of the retina or lens
- Postoperative corneal ulcers (may occur if the eyes are not adequately lubricated intraoperatively or the cornea is inadvertently abraded during the dental procedure)

16. How can ophthalmic complications be prevented?

Use of a short finger stop (index finger positioned near the elevator tip), especially when extracting the maxillary fourth premolars and the first and second molars

17. What factors predispose to ophthalmic complications?
- Periodontal or endodontic disease of the maxillary fourth premolars and the first and second molars may increase the risk of ophthalmic complications because the periapical bone may be compromised in these patients
- Brachycephalic breed dogs and cats have a shallow orbit, which is in close approximation to the maxillary fourth premolars and molars, increasing the risk of ophthalmic complications in these animals.

BIBLIOGRAPHY

1. Manfra Marretta S: Oropharynx. In Birchard S, Sherding R (eds): Saunders Manual of Small Animal Practice. Philadelphia, W.B. Saunders, 1994, pp 607–629.
2. Smith MM: Lingual approach for surgical extraction of the mandibular canine tooth in dogs and cats. J Am Anim Hosp Assoc 32:359–364, 1996.
3. Ramsey DT, Manfra Marretta S, Hamor RE, et al: Ophthalmic manifestations and complications of dental disease in dogs and cats. J Am Anim Hosp Assoc 32:215–224, 1996.

103. PALATAL DEFECTS

Sandra Manfra Marretta, D.V.M., Dip. A.C.V.S., Dip. A.V.D.C.

1. Name the two basic categories of congenital palatal defects.
- **Primary:** incisive bone or hare lip
- **Secondary:** hard and soft palates

2. Where, in the hard palate, are congenital defects located?
On the midline and usually associated with midline soft palatal defects.

3. What relationship exists between hard and soft palatal defects?
Although soft palatal defects may occur when hard palatal defects are absent, they are more frequently identified when hard palatal defects are present.

4. What are the causes of congenital palatal defects?
- The two palatine shelves fail to fuse during fetal development.
- Incomplete closure of either the primary or secondary palate is attributed to:
    Inherited (recessive or irregular dominant, polygenic traits) factors
    Nutritional factors
    Hormonal factors (steroids)
    Mechanical factors (*in utero* trauma)
    Toxic (including viral) factors

5. What are the two basic techniques used for the repair of congenital hard palatal defects?
1. The epithelial margins of the defect are removed with apposition of the edges of the defect after the creation of bilateral releasing incisions along the upper dental arcade.

2. Overlapping-flap technique: A large mucoperiosteal flap is created unilaterally along the dental arcade and hinged at the edge of the palatal defect. It is placed beneath the other edge of

the defect through a mucoperiosteal flap raised from the edge of the defect and held in place with vest-over-pants sutures.

6. **List three reasons why the overlapping-flap technique is preferred.**
   1. Less tension on the suture line
   2. Suture line not located directly over the defect
   3. Larger area of opposing connective tissue resulting in a stronger scar

7. **Briefly describe the technique for closing midline soft palatal defects.**
   Incisions are made along the medial margin on each side of the palatal cleft. The palatal tissue is divided into dorsal and ventral components. The two dorsal flaps are apposed and the two ventral flaps are apposed until the soft palate edge reaches the midpoint or caudad end of the tonsils and touches the tip of the epiglottis.

8. **List the causes of acquired palatal defects.**
   - Dental disease
   - Blunt head trauma
   - Bite wounds
   - Electric shock
   - Gunshot wounds
   - Foreign body penetration
   - Pressure necrosis
   - Iatrogenic (post–axillectomy procedures, post–radiation therapy)

9. **Where are acquired palatal defects located?**
   Defects secondary to dental disease are located in the region of the dental arcade, whereas defects secondary to other causative agents may be located anywhere in the hard palate. Rarely, acquired palatal defects may be located in the soft palate.

10. **What clinical signs are associated with palatal defects?**
    - Sneezing
    - Chronic unilateral or bilateral mucopurulent nasal discharge

11. **When should traumatically acquired palatal defects be repaired?**
    Acquired palatal defects are not life-threatening lesions. The acute inflammatory reaction and the overall clinical status of the patient with acute trauma should be managed before surgical intervention of palatal defects.

12. **What are the guidelines for successful palatal reconstruction?**
    - Treat only symptomatic animals.
    - Choose the appropriate procedure based on location of the defect.
    - Make flaps as large as possible.
    - Suture cut edges together, not intact epithelial edges.
    - Use two-layer closure when possible.
    - Do not locate a suture incision over defect if possible.
    - Maintain blood supply to the flap.
    - Control hemorrhage with firm pressure, and avoid use of electrocautery.
    - Avoid creating tissue closure that is under tension.

13. **List the various surgical techniques that can be used to repair acquired palatal defects.**
    - Buccal flaps
    - Rotation flaps
    - Advancement flaps
    - Tongue flaps
    - Split palatal U-flaps

14. What are the indications for use of buccal flaps?
Closure of:
- Oronasal and oroantral fistulas
- Maxillectomy and mandibulectomy procedures
- Peripherally located palatal defects

15. What inelastic structure located in the mucoperiosteal flap, if not incised, may result in tension across the incision line and dehiscence of the flap?
Periosteal layer of the mucoperiosteal flap.

16. What are the indications for use of rotation flaps?
Closure of small circular defects (especially defects located lateral to the midline).

17. What are the indications for advancement flaps?
Closure of wide defects of the caudad hard palate.

18. When are split palatal U-flaps recommended?
To repair acquired hard palatal defects located in the caudad hard palate. The edges of the palatal defect are debrided and a large U-shaped flap is created rostral to the defect. The major palatine arteries are preserved during the creation of the U-flap. The U-flap is divided on the midline. One side of the U-flap is rotated 90° into the defect and sutured in place. The second side of the U-flap is rotated 90° and sutured to the previously rotated flap.

19. What occurs postoperatively at the site on the palate from which the mucoperiosteal flap is harvested?
The harvest site appears as denuded palatal bone. Within 2 to 3 weeks, this site is filled with granulation tissue, which is covered with epithelium in 4 to 8 weeks.

20. The ventral approach to the nasal cavity or nasopharynx involves the creation of a midline palatal incision and, possibly, removal of midline palatal bone. What are the indications for this infrequently used surgical approach?
- Removal of nonendoscopically retrievable, ventral nasal foreign bodies
- Biopsy and removal of ventral nasal tumors (previous nondiagnostic biopsy techniques)
- Surgery for nasopharyngeal stenosis in cats
- Surgery for choanal atresia

CONTROVERSIES

21. Discuss the most appropriate treatment for hypoplasia or congenital absence of the soft palate.
Various recommendations have been made ranging from surgical correction to euthanasia. Surgical correction of this condition involves bilateral overlapping buccal mucosal flaps based at the palatoglossal arches with the mucosal surface of flaps forming the caudad nasopharynx and oropharynx. Surgical intervention, however, does not resolve the clinical signs associated with this condition. Persistent clinical signs include sneezing, mucopurulent nasal discharge, and chronic rhinitis. These clinical signs persist because the newly created soft palate lacks appropriate neurologic function. Euthanasia has been recommended as the treatment of choice for this condition because of the poor prognosis even with surgical correction. This condition has been successfully managed long-term by the author with conservative medical management. Conservative treatment includes feeding from an elevated platform, drinking from a water bottle, and treatment of intermittent rhinitis with antibiotics.

22. What is the clinical indication for the use of tongue flaps, and how successful is this procedure?
Treatment of large rostral palatal defects. This technique has a high incidence of dehiscence, and alternative techniques to tongue flaps are recommended whenever possible.

BIBLIOGRAPHY

1. Harvey CE, Emily PP: Oral surgery. In Harvey CE, Emily PP (eds): Small Animal Dentistry. St. Louis, Mosby, 1993, pp 312–377.
2. Hedlund CS: Congenital and acquired oronasal fistulas. In Fossum TW (ed): Small Animal Surgery. St. Louis, Mosby, 1997, pp 211–222.
3. Manfra Marretta S: Maxillofacial surgery. Vet Clin North Am Small Anim Pract 28:1285–1296, 1998.
4. Nefen S, Sager S: Use of buccal mucosal flaps for the correction of congenital soft palate defects in three dogs. Vet Surg 27:358–363, 1998.
5. Nelson AW: Upper respiratory system. In: Slatter D (ed): Textbook of Small Animal Surgery, 2nd ed. Philadelphia, W.B. Saunders, 1993, pp 733–776.

VII. Veterinary Surgery as a Specialty

104. ACADEMIC VERSUS PRIVATE PRACTICE

Joseph Harari, M.S., D.V.M., Dip. A.C.V.S.

1. What is one of the major trends of the past 5 years in the development of small animal surgery as a specialty field?

Increasing influx of residency applications into academic training programs and concomitant efflux of trained residents and faculty into private specialty practices.

2. Why is this trend occurring?

Perceived and real financial rewards in the private sector along with professional and personal independence. Academia lacks respect and understanding of clinical specialists compared with researchers. In the real world, the reverse situation exists; surgeons choose the path of least resistance.

3. Is this a bad situation?

No. Positive market forces reward surgeons (specialists) for their training and competence. Society, including animals, benefits from an ample supply of sophisticated veterinary surgical care. Academic surgeons (as well as other specialists) will be recruited and retained at a higher value than before as university administrators receive the wake-up call of competition.

4. What are the benefits of a surgical position in academia?
- Intellectual stimulation and prestige of a university environment
- Reduced influence of finances on salary, case management, and work schedule
- Off-clinic time devoted to personal development, research, and teaching
- Guaranteed salary, health and retirement benefits
- Academic rewards for teaching students and training young surgeons
- Ability to focus on and refine a narrow field of interest
- Ability to rise administratively and effect positive changes based on clinical experiences
- Intraoperative assistance from students and trainees
- Access to a university library system and multimedia offices

5. List the disadvantages of a surgical position in academia.
- Inefficient, nonclinical, bureaucratic system
- Reduced salaries compared with the private sector
- Unpredictable rewards system
- Burdensome team approach for case management, negatively affected, at times, by academic specialists with little practical experience and large egos

6. List some advantages of a private practice position.
- Increased, direct and controllable financial rewards
- Professional and personal freedoms not encumbered by university policies
- Increased efficiency, quality, and quantity of case management
- Desirable geographic locations

7. List some disadvantages of a private surgical practice.
- Lack of time for personal and professional development
- Persistent financial pressure to complete cases

- Variable technical assistance
- Inconsistent interaction with other specialists for intellectual stimulation
- Reduced access to a university library system and multimedia centers

8. Is there a middle ground between academic and private surgical practices in terms of advantages and disadvantages?

Yes. Established and well-known clinical centers, such as Angell Memorial in Boston and the Animal Medical Center in New York City. These centers provide high-case exposure in a frenetic, quasiintellectual environment contained in a unique (nonacademic) bureaucratic system.

9. Why should young surgeons seek training in a university setting?

ADVANTAGES	DISADVANTAGES
Intellectual environment	Inefficient bureaucracy
Faculty diversity for training	Faculty with little practice or stagnant university experiences
Introduction to writing, research, and teaching	Low salary for long work schedule, including emergencies
Financial support for continuing education programs	Unyielding hierarchical structure
Time off for personal development	Academic (classes, laboratoriess) conflicts with clinical interests
University prestige	
Access to library and multimedia centers	

10. Why should young surgeons seek training in a private referral setting?

ADVANTAGES	DISADVANTAGES
Efficient case management	Lack of faculty diversity
High surgical caseload	Mediocre ancillary training in anesthesia, medicine, and pathology
Future job security (regionally)	Reduced time off for professional development

11. What types of academic positions are available for surgeons?

- Instructorships following a residency
- Clinical (nontenure), renewable faculty positions
- Tenure tract (assistant, associate, and full professors) positions
- Temporary or visiting (nontenure tract, assistant, associate, and full professors) faculty positions

12. What type of positions are available in private practice?

Owner or employee (with an option to buy-in) in:
- Solo venture
- Small or large group containing other specialists
- General practice

13. What type of private practice has become popular nationwide during the past 5 years?

A mobile practice delivering surgical care to individual general practices or emergency centers.

14. What is the future of small animal surgery as a specialty field?

Brighter than ever; diverse employment opportunities are available around the world with increasing salaries in referral practice, academia, and industry.

105. SURGEONS IN INDUSTRY

Lynetta J. Freeman, D.V.M., M.S., Dip. A.C.V.S.

1. How many veterinary surgeons are employed in industrial positions?

2% of the 752 diplomates of the American College of Veterinary Surgeons (about 15 total).

2. Why consider a position in industry?

1. Veterinary surgeons may be interested in industry if they want to apply their surgical skills to help people.

2. Some areas of industrial research benefit veterinary and human patients.

3. Having the ability to focus on a specific research area and to be on the cutting edge of new developments are also attractive options.

3. How does one find out about positions in industry?

Usually the position is advertised in a professional journal, and applicants submit their resume for consideration. Sometimes, professional employment recruiters are used to help companies identify potential applicants. Companies also post employment opportunities on their Internet sites.

4. Why do firms hire veterinary surgeons?

Most positions in industry are with companies that manufacture medical devices. Such devices must be evaluated in animals to meet U.S. Food Drug Administration regulatory requirements and ensure the devices are safe and effective before they are used in human surgery. Veterinary surgeons participate in designing the preclinical (animal) test protocols, conducting the studies, and reporting the results. In doing so, they ensure that alternatives to animal testing are considered, minimal number of animals are used for evaluation, and the highest standards of animal care are provided, as specified by the Animal Welfare Act. Veterinary surgeons use their surgical skills to perform the procedure using a medical device on an animal, as it would be performed in a human operating room.

5. In addition to surgical skills, what other credentials are required?

- Research experience
- Managerial experience
- Analytical, communication, and interpersonal skills

6. What factors influence job satisfaction for veterinary surgeons in industry?

- Job duties
- Independence
- Salary
- Benefits
- A feeling of making a difference in the health and welfare of humans
- Satisfaction gained from development of special projects and publications that demonstrate the feasibility and benefits of performing surgery in animals

7. Discuss the duties and responsibilities of veterinary surgeons in industry.

Typical duties may include **designing, conducting,** and **reporting surgical studies** to support developing new products. Veterinary surgeons collaborate with physician specialists to perform research studies, develop surgical models, and perform product evaluations.

Veterinarians provide care of animals in compliance with company policy and government regulations. Veterinarians perform a literature search to ensure that no alternatives to animal testing are available and that the model selected provides the best representation for human anatomy. The search ensures that the study does not repeat work that may have been performed earlier at another institution. The veterinarian submits a study proposal to the Animal Care and Use Committee. The study proposal details the procedures to be performed, the numbers of animals used and the statistical methods used to arrive at that number, and the provisions for postoperative care and pain management for the animals in the study. Before surgery can begin, the protocol is reviewed, modified as needed, and approved by the committee.

Veterinarians commonly provide training for technical personnel and sales representatives to acquaint them with new products and their application. Because of the veterinarian's intimate knowledge of the product features and use, they may participate in training clinical investigators before the product is used in human surgery.

Because veterinarians have an intimate knowledge of medicine and surgery, they are able to provide input to product development teams working on devices for use in human surgery. Often the veterinary surgeon needs to develop a special expertise in an area beyond what he or she learned in the residency program. In some companies, veterinary surgeons are assigned an area of specialty (general surgery, breast care, cardiovascular, urology, and oncology) and given the responsibility to develop a research program to support the needs of that particular business unit.

8. How is performance determined and measured?

- Corporations allow veterinarians to set their own performance objectives to meet the corporate vision and mission.
- With input and guidance from the supervisor, associates develop a list of personal objectives, consistent with the goals of the corporation.
- Employees work with their supervisor to define what level of performance is expected, above expected, and outstanding for each stated objective.
- Achievement awards may be given for outstanding accomplishments beyond the scope of job duties.
- Special awards are often given to recognize inventors of patents and to teams that deliver their products ahead of schedule or go beyond what is expected.

9. How much job autonomy is allowed in a corporate environment?

Autonomy is allowed as long as performance expectations are met and resources are available. Independence is gained by level of job responsibility, a long record of excellent productivity, expert knowledge, and skills.

10. How do salary and benefits in industry compare with those in private practice and academia?

Salaries for Veterinarians

	MEAN STARTING SALARY FOR NEW GRADUATE VETERINARIANS IN 1998	MEAN PROFESSIONAL INCOME (1997)
Private practice	$36,724	$65,844
Academic position	$17,500	$75,984
Government and military	$43,533	$68,153
Industry	Insufficient data*	$109,941

Note. According to the 1997 Compensation Survey by the American Association of Industrial Veterinarians, the mean salary (including bonuses) was $105,664. This salary was associated with a management position (for at least 5 years), in industry for at least 10 years with at least 5 years in the present job. Post-DVM training or Board certification, the geographic area, and the nature of the employer (e.g., whether a human pharmaceutical or device company or an animal health company) may influence salaries.
*There were insufficient data on starting salaries entering industry and commercial positions because there were only three respondents (this may be an indication that new college graduates may have difficulty finding industry positions).

11. Do salaries increase with time in grade and increased responsibility?

Yes. Corporate salary growth may be determined by a corporate compensation committee that determines the average overall merit increase based on the company's overall productivity. Extra compensation is available for promotions and increased job responsibility.

12. What benefits are offered?

1. Most companies offer paid vacation time and may pay for professional liability, health, and disability insurance.

2. Individuals may participate in retirement programs, with the company matching individual contributions up to a certain level.

3. Some firms furnish a company car.

4. Firms provide educational assistance by paying for attendance at professional meetings, professional dues and subscriptions, and tuition for continuing education.

5. Industry positions may allow veterinarians to participate in new product royalties, profit sharing, or company stock purchase programs.

13. Discuss potentially negative aspects of working in industry.

Company policy and administration may be outside of an individual's control. In the competitive market, frequent changes in company direction may be needed to reach the objectives identified by the corporation. Successful people are flexible and able to negotiate and lead others through changes as they occur. As with any position, an unpleasant relationship with one's supervisor, colleagues, or subordinates can lead to job dissatisfaction.

14. Is industry considered a collegial environment?

Yes; however, the environment is different from that of an academic position. In the university setting, one interacts with various specialists—radiologists, surgeons, internists, large animal practitioners, small animal practitioners, and emergency department veterinarians—to make a diagnosis and provide the best care for the animal, consistent with the owner's wishes. In industry, a veterinarian's peers may not be other veterinarians. Instead, they may be a physician, a bench chemist, an electrical engineer, a regulatory specialist, or a marketing manager.

15. Are work days (evenings and weekends) shorter in industry compared with practice or academia?

Although some veterinarians may be attracted to an industry career because there is little emergency or after-hours duty, people may, in fact, spend more hours at work, not less, because they enjoy it so much.

16. How much travel is involved?

Travel is a form of reward. To be asked to travel is one means of being recognized as a corporate expert. As a company representative, one is entrusted with additional responsibility for overseeing the outcome of a project. The amount of travel varies greatly, depending on the specific project assignment.

17. What are potential career paths for veterinary surgeons in industry?

Technical positions offer scientists the opportunity to develop their technical knowledge and skills, to contribute innovative ideas for products that become commercialized, and to devote a portion of their time to pursue personal research interests. Senior technical staff are expected to serve as role models and mentors for young scientists. A typical technical career path might be as follows: assistant scientist, scientist, senior scientist, principal scientist, research fellow, senior research fellow, and distinguished research fellow.

Managerial positions include team leaders, managers, directors, and vice-presidents. The team leader is responsible for a group of 10 to 12 people directed toward a specific goal (e.g., developing a product for market introduction in 12 months.) Managers oversee a department that may include diverse work areas. Directors usually oversee four to five team leaders or managers. Vice-presidents oversee a group of directors. A distinguished research fellow on the technical career ladder can be equivalent to a vice-president on the managerial career ladder in terms of salary, budgetary authority, recognition, and responsibility.

18. How is leadership developed?

Whether on the technical or the managerial path, developing leadership skills is critical. Leadership is developed at all levels in the organization. Classes and training are offered to help develop leaders. A 360-degree performance feedback program gives individuals input from managers, peers, and subordinates to help associates strengthen leadership skills. Veterinary surgeons are well suited for the task of bringing together the right group of people, asking the right questions, and guiding others to understanding and potential solutions: This is leadership.

19. What are future roles for veterinary surgeons in industry?

Because of the broad training offered in the professional curriculum and the skills developed on the job or before entering industry, veterinarians are well suited to assume increasing levels of responsibility. There are **excellent opportunities** for veterinarians to fill other roles in the company beyond preclinical product evaluation:

1. A veterinary surgeon may serve as a team leader for innovation teams, ensuring a steady supply of innovative medical devices to enhance the quality of life for human surgical patients.

2. Veterinarians may provide technical input necessary to assess new business opportunities.

3. Veterinary surgeons are entering areas of research in gene therapy; in tissue engineering; and in screening, detection, diagnosis, and therapy for cancer.

BIBLIOGRAPHY

1. AVMA Centers for Information Management: Employment, starting salaries, and educational indebtedness of 1998 graduates of U.S. veterinary medical colleges. J Am Vet Med Assoc 214:488–490, 1999.
2. AVMA Centers for Information Management: 1997 income of U.S. veterinarians. J Am Vet Med Assoc 214:1489–1491, 1999.
3. Brown JP, Silverman JD: The current and future market for veterinarians and veterinary medical services in the United States. Executive Summary, May 1999. J Am Vet Med Assoc 215:161–183, 1999.
4. Gehrke BC, et al, AVMA Center for Information Management: Veterinary human capital—knowledge, skills, and abilities that enhance employment opportunities outside private practice. J Am Vet Med Assoc 214:1781–1784, 1998.

INDEX

Page numbers in **boldface type** indicate complete chapters.

Dehiscence (*cont.*)
    of mucoperiosteal flaps, 349
    tracheal, as subcutaneous emphysema cause, 91
Dehydration, fluid requirements for correction of, 42
Delayed-onset muscle soreness (DOMS), 293
Denervation, as muscle injury mechanism, 290
Dental occlusion, restoration of, by jaw fracture repair, 209
Dermatologic disorders, acupuncture therapy for, 26
Deroofing, 153, 154
Detrusor areflexia, 308–309
Developmental diseases, of bone, **251–255**
Devita pin method, for coxofemoral luxation stabilization, 268
Dexamethasone, as cervical vertebral instability therapy, 318
Diabetes, effect on wound healing, 3
Diaphragm
    pelvic, anatomy of, 155
    tears of. *See* Hernia, diaphragmatic
Diaphragmatic advancement, 100
Diazepam, hepatotoxicity of, 33
Dietary factors, in osteochondrosis, 258
Dietary management. *See also* Nutritional support, perioperative
    of chylothorax, 96
Digits, tumors of, 343
Disinfection, differentiated from antisepsis, 7
Disk disease. *See* Intervertebral disk disease
Diskospondylitis, 322
Disseminated intravascular coagulation (DIC)
    gastric dilatation-volvulus-related, 131
    pyometra-related, 185
Distraction index (DI), 263–264, 265
Diuretics, as chylothorax therapy, 96
DNA (deoxyribonucleic acid) synthesis, enhanced, 3
Doberman pinschers
    cervical vertebral instability in, 317
    nontraumatic carpal laxity syndrome in, 222
Dogs. *See also* specific breeds
    brachycephalic breeds, 78, 79
    chondrodysplastic breeds, 253
    functional skills rehabilitation in, 32
    giant-breed
        gastric dilatation-volvulus in, 130
        pericardial effusion in, 115
    show dogs, ulnar ostectomy in, 245
    small breeds, mitral valve insufficiency in, 106
Doppler flow probe, use in skin flap dissection, 68
Dorsal fusion and fixation, as lumbosacral disease treatment, 323
Double bubble sign, of gastric dilatation-volvulus, 131
Doxorubicin, as bladder cancer therapy, 181
Drains/drainage
    omentum pedicle, of chylothorax, 97, 98
    use in oncologic surgery, 332
    open peritoneal, **144–148**
    pleural, as idiopathic chylothorax therapy, 96

Drains/drainage (*cont.*)
    postablation placement in ear canal, 75
    postural, 30, 31–32
    sump-Penrose, 146
Dressings, **36–40**. *See also* Bandages
    adherent, 36
    functions of, 36
    nonadherent, 2, 36–38
Ductus arteriosus
    anatomy of, 100–102
    patient. *See* Patent ductus arteriosus
Ductus deferens, ureter mistakenly identified as, 199
Ductus venosus, as single intrahepatic portosystemic shunt, 124
Durotomy, 308
Dysesthesia, 322
Dysphoria, opioids-related, 20, 21
Dysplasia
    definition of, 251
    of the elbow. *See* Elbow, dysplasia of
    hepatic microvascular, 125
    of the hip. *See* Hip, dysplasia of
    tricuspid valve, 111
Dyspnea, chylothorax-related, 95

Ear canal
    ablation of, 73, 74–75
    resection of, 73
    tumors of, 73–75
Echocardiography
    of patent ductus arteriosus, 103–104
    of pericardial effusions, 115
    of pulmonic stenosis, 108
Ectopia, patellar, 271
Edema, pulmonary
    patent ductus arteriosus-related, 104
    reexpansion, 121
Effleurage, 31
Effusions
    biliary, bile peritonitis-related, 129
    chylous, 95
    pleural, 43
        as pericardiectomy complication, 117
Ehmer, Anton Emerson, 39
Elbow
    arthrodesis in, 293, 296
        contraindication to, 295
    arthroscopic examination of, 47, 48, 261
    dysplasia of, 253, **259–262**
    incongruity of, 246, 261
    luxation of, 270–271
        congenital, 254, 259
    osteochondrosis of, 257
Electrical burns, 69
Electrical stimulation, use in physical therapy, 29, 30, 31
Electroacupuncture, 27, 28
Electrocardiography, 41
    for pericardial effusion evaluation, 115
Electrocautery
    differentiated from laser therapy, 55
    use during flap dissection, 59

364 Index

Electromyography
for laryngeal paralysis diagnosis, 83
needle, for lumbosacral disease diagnosis, 322
Electroscapel dissection, in subtotal prostatectomy, 196
Electrosurgery, use in minimally-invasive surgery, 44
Elephant's foot callus, 242
Emboli, fibrocartilaginous, 322
Embolization, transcatheter coil, 104, 106
Embryonal carcinoma, 199
Emphysema
bullous, 94
subcutaneous, 87, 91
Empty abdomen syndrome, 122–123
Endocardiosis, 106
Endoscopy, use in removal of gastrointestinal foreign bodies, 138
English bulldogs
as chondrodysplastic breed, 253
gastric outflow obstruction in, 134
laryngeal paralysis in, 82
pulmonic stenosis in, 108
uroliths in, 178
English springer spaniels, patent ductus arteriosus in, 103
Enteral nutrition, 33–34, 35
Enteropexy, after intestinal reduction or resection, 142
Enterotomy, for intestinal foreign body removal, 139
Enthesophyte (periosteal bone) formation, on radial styloid process, 222
Ependymoma, 314, 327
Epicondyle, ununited medial, 257, 261
Epidermal cell cancer, tracheal, 89
Epidermal growth factor, 2
Epididymitis, 199–200
Epidural anesthesia/analgesia, 21
Epidural space, as drug administration site, 21
Epinephrine, contraindication as acepromazine antidote, 15
Episioplasty, 188–189
Episiotomy, 187–188
Epithelial tumors, 341, 342
Epulides, 339, 340
Escherichia coli infections
as cholecystitis cause, 128
as osteomyelitis cause, 297
prostatic, 195
of surgical wounds, 9
Escherichia coli infections, uterine, 185
Esophagostomy tube feeding, 35
of burn patients, 71
Esophagraphy, use in persistent right aortic arch evaluation, 113
Esophagus
entrapment in persistent right aortic arch, 112, 113
foreign bodies in, **118–120**
holding layer of, 119
Estrogen
in pyometra, 185
secretion by neoplastic testicles, 200

Estrogen receptors, in mammary gland tumors, 189
Estrus cycle, effect on coxofemoral joint laxity, 264
Ethylene oxide, as sterilant, 10
Etodolac, as osteoarthritis therapy, 302
Euthanasia, for hypoplasia, 349
Eventration, 3, 4
Evisceration, 3, 4
Excision techniques, in oncologic surgery, 331, 332
Exercise
active, 32
by osteoarthritis patients, 301
passive, 32
Exodontia, **345–347**
Exostoses, multiple cartilagenous, 252
External fixation
complications of, 243
of tibial fractures, 232, 233, 234
transarticular, for tarsal shearing injury repair, 236
External fixation splint, KE (Kirschner-Ehmer), 206
External fixators
acrylic, 206, 207, 236
circular, 203, 207, 208
in femoral fracture repair, 229
skeletal, effect on physeal growth, 241

Facial nerve, ear canal ablation-related injury to, 74
FCP (fragmented medial coronoid process of the ulna), 260–261
Feminization, testicular tumor-related, 199, 200
Femoral head, arthroplasty of, as hip dysplasia treatment, 265, 266
Femoral neck
anteversion and retroversion of, 272
arthroplasty of, as hip dysplasia treatment, 265, 266
fractures of, 227–228
lengthening procedure for, 265
Femoral nerve
as lumbosacral spine innervation, 320
pelvic fracture-related injury to, 224
Femur
distal
fractures of, 229, 230
growth deformities of, 272
fractures of, 201, **227–231**
as quadriceps muscle contracture cause, 292
severely comminuted, bone grafts for, 250
total hip replacement-related, 265
tension band surface of, 205
Fentanyl
epidural administration of, 21
as supplemental intraoperative analgesia, 19
Fentanyl patch, 19, 21
Ferrets
adrenal tumors in, 159, 160
insulin-secreting islet cell tumors in, 164
Fibroblast growth factors, 2
Fibromyoma, 194
Fibrosarcoma
of bone, 333
lingual, 341
oral, 339

Physes (*cont.*)
  premature closure of, 244, 245, 246
  radial, distal, premature closure of, 245, 246
  ulnar
    distal, premature closure of, 245
    retained ulnar cartilage cores of, 253
Physical therapy, **29–33**
  initiation after muscle repair, 290
Pillar sign, of gastric dilatation-volvulus, 131
Pin-and-plate combination, for femoral fracture repair, 228
Pins. *See also* Intramedullary pins (IM)
  anatomic landmarks for placement of, in vertebral bodies, 312–313
  for cervical vertebral ventral cross-pinning, 313
  complications of, 243
  use in coxofemoral luxation stabilization, 269
  positive-profile, end-threaded, 207
  predrilling for insertion of, 207
  transfixation, 207
  use in spinal fracture-luxation stabilization, 312
Pituitary tumors, 327
Plasmalyte-A, 13
Platelet-derived growth factor, 2
Plate-rod construct, for fracture fixation, 206
Plates. *See also* Bone plates
  clamp-on, 233
  complications of, 243
  effect on physeal growth, 241
  spinous process, 312
Pleural effusion, 43
  as pericardiectomy complication, 117
Pleurodesis, 97
Pleuroperitoneal diaphragmatic hernia, 120
Pneumonia
  aspiration
    in persistent right aortic arch patients, 113, 114
    in tracheal resection patients, 90
  chronic, pulmonary abscess associated with, 93–94
Pneumothorax, spontaneous, bullous emphysema associated with, 94
Polydioxanone sutures, 180
Polyethylene mesh, use in thoracic wall reconstruction, 100–101
Polyglactin 910 sutures, 180
Polyglycolic acid sutures, 180
Polymethyl methacrylate mesh, use in spinal fracture-luxation stabilization, 312
Polypropylene mesh
  use in superficial digital flexor tendon stabilization, 288
  use in thoracic wall reconstruction, 100–101
Polyps
  acquired pyloric, 134
  of ear canal, 73, 75
Polysulfated glycosaminoglycans
  as hip dysplasia therapy, 266
  as osteoarthritis therapy, 303
Pomeranians
  cryptorchidism in, 197
  patent ductus arteriosus in, 103

Poodles
  cryptorchidism in, 197
  miniature, mucoceles in, 77
Portal vein, ligation of, 124
Posteroperative period, patient monitoring during, **40–43**
Postoperative care
  for brain tumor patients, 329
  for cervical vertebral instability patients, 319
  for diaphragmatic hernia patients, 122
  for intussusception patients, 142
  for necrotizing pancreatitis patients, 162
  rehabilitation in, 31–32
Postresuscitation injury, 143
Potassium, in burn wounds, 70, 71
Pouch skin flap, 68
Prednisolone, as cervical vertebral instability therapy, 318
Prednisolone sodium, as spinal injury therapy, 310
Pressure autoregulation, 325–326
Pringle maneuver, 123
Private practice, comparison with academic practice, **351–352**
Progesterone
  in pyometra, 185, 186
  secretion by neoplastic testicles, 200
Progesterone receptors, in mammary gland tumors, 189
Progestin, as benign prostatic hyperplasia therapy, 193
Propofol
  effect on cardiopulmonary function, 16
  use in cats, 17
  as postoperative wound infection risk factor, 8
Prostate cancer, 193, 194
Prostatectomy
  subtotal, 57, 196
  total, 196
Prostate gland
  abscess of, 144, 195, 196
  in cats, 199
Prostatic diseases, **193–196**
Prostatitis, 195–196
Protein restriction, as portosystemic shunt therapy, 126
Proteoglycans, osteoarthritis-related loss of, 299
Proteus infections
  as osteomyelitis cause, 297
  prostatic, 195
Prothrombin time (PT), 42
Proximal intertarsal joint, 236
Proximate linear cutters, 53
Proximate linear staplers, 53
PR (prothrombin time), 42
Pseudoarthrosis, 242
Pseudocapsule, of tumors, 330–331
Pseudocyst, pancreatic, 163
Pseudohermaphroditism, 185
Pseudohyperreflexia, 322
Pseudomonas infections
  as osteomyelitis cause, 297
  prostatic, 195
  of surgical wounds, 9

Small breeds, mitral valve insufficiency in, 106
Small intestine
    foreign bodies in, 138
    wound healing in, 3
Sneezing, palatal defect-associated, 348
Sodium, in burn wounds, 70–71
Soft-tissue reconstruction techniques, for patellar
        stabilization, 274
Soft-tissue sarcoma, **336–339**
Sonipuncture, 27
Spaying. *See* Ovariohysterectomy
Spermatocele, 199–200
Sphincter hypertonus, 308–309
Spica bandages, 217
Spica splints, 39
Spinal cord
    compression of, 316
    tumors of, 314–317
Spinal nerves, tumors of, 314, 315
Spinal tap, location for, 316
Spindle cell tumors, 336
Spine
    fractures of, **310–314**
    tumors of, **314–317**
    vertebral fracture-associated injury to, 310
Spleen
    functions of , 165
    mast cells in, 343–344
    most common diseases of, 165
    vascular ligation of, 166
Splenectomy, **165–168**
    complications of, 167
    indications for, 132
Splenic arteries, ligation of, 166, 167
Splenic cancer, 167
Splenomegaly, 166
    law of two-thirds for, 167–168
Splints, 39
    complications of, 243
    controindication as premature physeal closure-
        related curvature treatment, 245
    Schroeder-Thomas, 230
Split palatal U-flaps, 349
Split ring technique, of tracheal anastomosis, 89
Spondylolithesis, cervical, 317
Spondylosis, 321
Sprains, ligamentous, classification of, 221
Squamous cell carcinoma
    of the digits, 343
    of ear canal, 74
    in situ, 342
    lingual, 341
    nasal, 57
    oral, 339
        in cats, 341
        papillary, 340
    prostatic, 193
    renal, 171
    tonsillar, 340–341
    tracheal, 89
Stack pinning, of fractures, 204
Stainless steel external fixators, 206

Stainless steel plates, for scapular fracture repair,
        213
Staphylectomy, 80
Staphylococcus infections
    as osteomyelitis cause, 297
    of surgical wounds, 9, 50
Stapling
    advantages and disadvantages of, 53
    in hepatic lobectomy, 124
    in intestinal anastomosis, 141
    in partial splenectomy, 167
    in pulmonary lobectomy, 92–93
Starvation, in critically-ill patients, 33
Stenosis
    aortic, 109–111
    of the ear canal, 73
    lumbosacral, 321
    pelvic, 226
    pulmonic, 108–109
    pyloric, 134, 137
    tracheal, 86
    vestibulovaginal, 188
    vulvar, 187
Sterilization
    differentiated from asepsis, 7
    of instruments and packs, 10
    of tissue, laser-based, 57
Sternotomy, median, 92, 116
Steroids. *See also* Corticosteroids
    as chylothorax therapy, 96
Stifle joint
    arthrodesis in, 293
        contraindication to, 295
    arthroscopic examination of, 46, 47
    fibrous ankylosis of, 292
    hyperextension of, as cranial cruciate ligament
        rupture cause, 275
    laxity of, as cranial cruciate ligament tear cause,
        276
    osteochondrosis of, 257
    "terrible triad injury" to, 282
    traumatic derangement of, 282
Stoma, for cholecystenterotomy, 129
Stomach
    foreign bodies in, 138–139
    vascular ligation of, 166
Stomach cancer, 134–135, 137
Stomatitis, feline, 57
Stool softeners, as perianal fistulae therapy, 154
Strain, as fracture cause, 202
Strains, muscular, 290–291
Streptococcus infections
    as osteomyelitis cause, 297
    prostatic, 195
    of surgical wounds, 9
Strictures
    perianal urethrostomy-related, 184
    rectal, 149
    tracheal, postsurgical, 90, 91
Struvite urinary calculi, 172, 176, 179
    urinary tract infections associated with, 178
Subclavian artery, aberrant, 112, 113